Pediatrics

NOTICE

Medicine is an ever-changing science. As new research and clinical experience broaden our knowledge, changes in treatment and drug therapy are required. The editors and the publisher of this work have made every effort to ensure that the drug dosage schedules herein are accurate and in accord with the standards accepted at the time of publication. Readers are advised, however, to check the product information sheet included in the package of each drug they plan to administer to be certain that changes have not been made in the recommended dose or in the contraindications for administration. This recommendation is of particular importance in regard to new or infrequently used drugs.

Pediatrics:
PreTest® Self-Assessment and Review

Second Edition

Edited by
Richard P. Lipman M.D., F.A.A.P.
Associate Clinical Professor of Pediatrics
Tufts University School of Medicine
Boston, Massachusetts

Chief of Medicine
North Shore Children's Hospital
Salem, Massachusetts

McGraw-Hill Book Company
Health Professions Division
PreTest Series

New York   St. Louis   San Francisco
Auckland   Bogotá   Guatemala   Hamburg
Johannesburg   Lisbon   London   Madrid
Mexico   Montreal   New Delhi   Panama
Paris   São Paulo   Singapore   Sydney
Tokyo   Toronto

Library of Congress Cataloging in Publication Data
Main entry under title:

Pediatrics: PreTest self-assessment and review.

    Bibliography: p.
    1. Pediatrics—Examinations, questions, etc.
I. Lipman, Richard P. [DNLM: 1. Pediatrics—
Examination questions. WS 18 P371]
RJ48.2.P42   1982   618.92′00076   80-39951

ISBN 0-07-050973-5

Editor: *Jane Edwards*
Project Editor: *Ellen Murray*
Editorial Assistant: *Donna Altieri*
Production: *Rosemary J. Pascale, Judith M. Raccio*
Designer: *Robert Tutsky*
Printer: *Hull Printing Company*
Cover Illustration: *"The Doctor" by Joseph Tomanek
(after Sir Luke Fildes, R.A.) courtesy of
Wyeth Laboratories, Philadelphia, Pa.*

Copyright © 1982 1978 by McGraw-Hill, Inc. All rights reserved. Printed in the United States of America. Except as permitted under the Copyright Act of 1976, no part of this publication may be reproduced or distributed in any form or by any means, or stored in a data base or retrieval system, without the prior written permission of the publisher.

3 4 5 6 7 8 9 HUHU 8 7 6 5 4 3 2

Contents

List of Contributors	vii
Introduction	ix
Preface	xi
General Pediatrics	
Questions	1
Answers, Explanations, and References	13
The Newborn Infant	
Questions	30
Answers, Explanations, and References	45
The Cardiovascular System	
Questions	59
Answers, Explanations, and References	71
The Gastrointestinal Tract	
Questions	84
Answers, Explanations, and References	95
The Urinary Tract	
Questions	108
Answers, Explanations, and References	119
The Neuromuscular System	
Questions	130
Answers, Explanations, and References	141
Infectious Diseases and Immunology	
Questions	155
Answers, Explanations, and References	169
Hematologic and Neoplastic Diseases	
Questions	188
Answers, Explanations, and References	201
Endocrine, Metabolic, and Genetic Disorders	
Questions	220
Answers, Explanations, and References	230
Bibliography	243

List of Contributors

Harvey L. Chernoff, M.D.
Associate Professor of Pediatrics
Tufts University School of Medicine
Pediatric Cardiologist
New England Medical Center Hospital
  (Boston Floating Hospital for Infants and Children)
Lecturer in Pediatrics
Boston University School of Medicine
Boston, Massachusetts

Jerome S. Haller, M.D.
Associate Professor of Pediatrics
  (Neurology)
Tufts University School of Medicine
Boston, Massachusetts

Julie R. Ingelfinger, M.D.
Assistant Professor of Pediatrics
Harvard Medical School
Associate in Medicine
The Children's Hospital Medical Center
Boston, Massachusetts

Richard P. Lipman, M.D., F.A.A.P.
Associate Clinical Professor of Pediatrics
Tufts University School of Medicine
Attending Pediatrician in Infectious Diseases
New England Medical Center Hospital
  (Boston Floating Hospital for Infants and Children)
Boston, Massachusetts
Chief of Pediatrics
North Shore Children's Hospital
Salem, Massachusetts

Marcellina Mian, M.D.C.M.
Department of Paediatrics
The Hospital for Sick Children
Toronto, Ontario
Assistant Professor of Paediatrics
Faculty of Medicine
University of Toronto
Toronto, Ontario

Uma S. Rai, M.D., F.A.A.P. (deceased)
Assistant Professor of Pediatrics
  (Hematology)
Tufts University School of Medicine
Boston, Massachusetts
Pediatric Hematologist
St. Elizabeth's Hospital
Brighton, Massachusetts

William F. Rowley, Jr., M.D.
Medical Director
North Shore Children's Hospital
Salem, Massachusetts
Assistant Professor of Pediatrics
Tufts University School of Medicine
Boston, Massachusetts

Abdollah Sadeghi-Nejad, M.S., M.D., F.A.A.P.
Associate Professor of Pediatrics
Tufts University School of Medicine
Pediatric Endocrinologist
New England Medical Center Hospital
  (Boston Floating Hospital for Infants and Children)
Boston, Massachusetts

John B. Watkins, M.D.
Director, Division of Gastroenterology
  and Nutrition
Children's Hospital of Philadelphia
Associate Professor of Pediatrics
University of Pennsylvania School of
  Medicine
Philadelphia, Pennsylvania

Introduction

Pediatrics: PreTest Self-Assessment and Review, 2nd Ed., has been designed to provide medical students, as well as physicians, with a comprehensive and convenient instrument for self-assessment and review within the field of pediatrics. The 500 questions provided have been designed to parallel the format and degree of difficulty of the questions contained in Part II of the National Board of Medical Examiners examinations, the Federation Licensing Examination (FLEX), the Visa Qualifying Examination, and the ECFMG examination.

Each question in the book is accompanied by an answer, a paragraph explanation, and a specific page reference to either a current journal article, a textbook, or both. An eight page bibliography, listing all the sources used in the book, follows the last chapter.

Perhaps the most effective way to use this book is to allow yourself one minute to answer each question in a given chapter; as you proceed, indicate your answer beside each question. By following this suggestion, you will be approximating the time limits imposed by the board examinations previously mentioned.

When you finish answering the questions in a chapter, you should then spend as much time as you need verifying your answers and carefully reading the explanations. Although you should pay special attention to the explanations for the questions you answered incorrectly, you should read **every** explanation. The authors of this book have designed the explanations to reinforce and supplement the information tested by the questions. If, after reading the explanations for a given chapter, you feel you need still more information about the material covered, you should consult and study the references indicated.

This book meets the criteria for up to 22 credit hours in Category 5(d) for the Physician's Recognition Award of the American Medical Association. It should provide an experience that is instructive as well as evaluative; we also hope that you enjoy it. We would be very happy to receive your comments.

Preface

It is gratifying to have the opportunity to prepare the second edition of this book. Along with extensive revisions to incorporate new information and references, we have attempted to retain characteristics which would inform and teach rather than merely test the reader's factual knowledge. Thus, many brief clinical cases are presented, often as focal points for a discussion of large topics in pediatrics. Furthermore, the discussions intentionally deal not only with the correct but with many of the incorrect answers. We hope, therefore, that the reader will find this book interesting and thought-provoking as well as useful.

The tragedy of Dr. Uma Rai's death has greatly saddened all who knew him. Stricken suddenly in the prime of his life, his legacy as a teacher and physician will always remain in his many patients and students.

We are grateful to Jay Erdman, M.D. and to Jane Edwards for their editorial assistance, and to Donald Darling, M.D. for the x-ray which depicts acute osteomyelitis. To my former professor, Dr. Louis Weinstein, goes my humble thanks for his example to a medical student and house officer many years ago as the epitome of clinician-teacher.

Richard P. Lipman, M.D.

General Pediatrics

William F. Rowley, Jr.

DIRECTIONS: Each question below contains five suggested answers. Choose the one best response to each question.

1. Although the exact cause of sudden infant death syndrome is unknown, all of the following statements concerning this syndrome are true EXCEPT that

(A) it affects female and male infants equally
(B) it typically involves infants two to four months of age
(C) it is more common among siblings of affected infants
(D) it has a higher incidence among illegitimate infants
(E) it has a higher incidence among infants of lower socioeconomic status

2. To induce vomiting at home in a child who has ingested a poison, the recommended agent of choice would be

(A) copper sulfate
(B) mustard in warm water
(C) apomorphine
(D) fluid extract of ipecac
(E) syrup of ipecac

3. The causative agent of molluscum contagiosum, which chiefly affects preschool children and adolescents, is

(A) rickettsial
(B) mycobacterial
(C) viral
(D) fungal
(E) unknown

4. A nine-year-old boy who injured his groin while sledding is brought to the emergency room complaining of pain in the left scrotum, nausea, and vomiting. Elevation of his left testis, which is swollen and painful, does not relieve the pain. Which of the following statements about the boy's disorder is true?

(A) It probably is epididymitis
(B) It probably is orchitis
(C) It probably is testicular torsion
(D) Surgery is rarely required
(E) Bed rest and sitz baths constitute proper therapy

5. The child pictured below has the most common type of generalized skeletal dysplasia. This disorder is

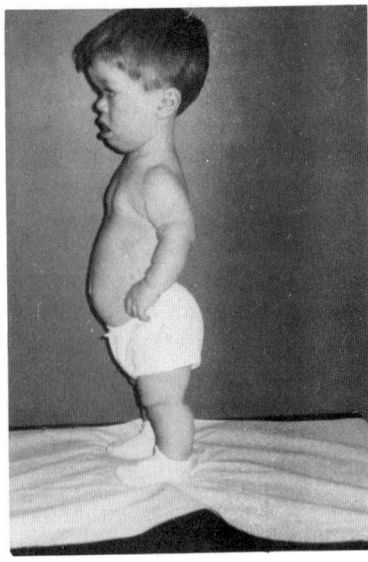

(A) achondrogenesis
(B) achondroplasia
(C) metatropic dwarfism
(D) thanatophoric dwarfism
(E) chondroectodermal dysplasia

6. Idiopathic scoliosis most frequently affects

(A) newborn infants
(B) preschool girls
(C) preschool boys
(D) adolescent girls
(E) adolescent boys

Questions 7-8

An eight-month-old girl is admitted to a hospital because of poor weight gain despite a voracious appetite. The presence of steatorrhea and a right upper lobe pneumonia points to cystic fibrosis.

7. If cystic fibrosis is the correct diagnosis, results of her sweat test would be expected to show

(A) low sodium and chloride concentrations
(B) low sodium concentration and a high chloride concentration
(C) normal sodium and chloride concentrations
(D) a high sodium concentration and a normal chloride concentration
(E) high sodium and chloride concentrations

8. The parents of the girl described above want to know whether future offspring also will be born with cystic fibrosis. They should be advised that the chance that their next child will have the disease is approximately

(A) 0 percent
(B) 25 percent
(C) 33 percent
(D) 50 percent
(E) 100 percent

9. Iridocyclitis (anterior uveitis), which is depicted in the photograph below, is most likely to be associated with which of the following disorders?

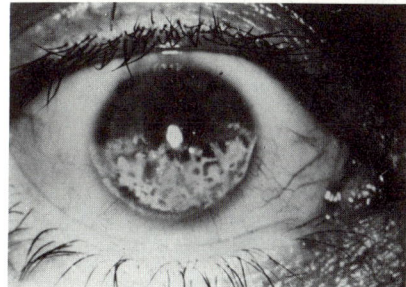

(A) Juvenile rheumatoid arthritis
(B) Slipped femoral epiphysis
(C) Schönlein-Henoch purpura
(D) Legg-Calvé-Perthes disease
(E) Osgood-Schlatter disease

10. All of the following are manifestations of chronic hypervitaminosis A EXCEPT for

(A) hepatomegaly
(B) alopecia
(C) desquamation of palms and soles
(D) tender swelling of bones
(E) subcutaneous calcifications

11. A ten-month-old infant is brought to a physician's office because of irritability and resistance to movement. The child prefers to assume a pithed-frog position with some flexion of the thighs and legs and outward rotation of the hips. The most likely diagnosis of this child's condition is

(A) rickets
(B) syphilis
(C) poliomyelitis
(D) scurvy
(E) trauma

12. Salicylate poisoning, the most common type of accidental poisoning in preschool children, is most likely to be associated with which of the following conditions?

(A) Respiratory acidosis followed by metabolic alkalosis
(B) Respiratory alkalosis followed by metabolic alkalosis
(C) Respiratory alkalosis followed by metabolic acidosis
(D) Metabolic acidosis superimposed upon respiratory alkalosis
(E) Metabolic acidosis superimposed upon respiratory acidosis

13. Osgood-Schlatter disease, one of several disorders classified as osteochondrosis, involves the

(A) tarsal navicular
(B) metatarsal head
(C) capital femoral epiphysis
(D) tibial tuberosity
(E) body of the sternum

14. Treatment of a child who has acute lead encephalopathy should include prompt administration of

(A) edetate calcium disodium (Ca EDTA)
(B) edetate calcium disodium and dimercaprol (British anti-lewisite)
(C) D-penicillamine
(D) D-penicillamine and dimercaprol
(E) D-penicillamine, edetate calcium disodium, and dimercaprol

15. The developmental assessment of children is an integral part of pediatric care. At which of the following age intervals should a child be able to run and turn without losing balance, lace shoes (without tying them), and count to four?

(A) One to two years of age
(B) Two to three years of age
(C) Three to four years of age
(D) Four to five years of age
(E) Five to six years of age

16. In children, the most commonly recognized form of familial hyperlipidemia is

(A) hypertriglyceridemia
(B) hypercholesterolemia
(C) hyperchylomicronemia
(D) combined hyperlipidemia
(E) type V hyperlipoproteinemia

17. The only immunoglobulin that can be transported across the placenta to a fetus is

(A) IgA
(B) IgD
(C) IgE
(D) IgG
(E) IgM

18. Atopic dermatitis, which often begins in infancy with the development of weepy erythematous patches on the cheeks, usually becomes quiescent when affected children reach

(A) two years of age
(B) five years of age
(C) eight years of age
(D) eleven years of age
(E) fifteen years of age

19. A six-year-old asthmatic child is brought to the emergency room because of severe coughing and wheezing during the prior 24 hours. The child had been taking ephedrine and theophylline as prescribed without relief and had vomited four times in the last hour. Physical examination reveals a child who is anxious, has intercostal and suprasternal retractions, expiratory wheezing throughout all lung fields, and a respiratory rate of 60 per minute. Initial treatment should include the administration of

(A) intravenous aminophylline
(B) parenteral phenobarbital
(C) subcutaneous epinephrine (Adrenalin)
(D) subcutaneous crystalline epinephrine suspension (Sus-Phrine)
(E) isoproterenol by intermittent positive-pressure breathing

20. Of the types of lice that are obligate parasites of man, the vector of typhus, trench fever, and relapsing fever is

(A) *Pediculus humanis capitis*
(B) *Pediculus humanis pedis*
(C) *Pediculus humanis corporis*
(D) *Phthirus pubis*
(E) *Dermacentor andersoni*

21. The child shown below has been brought to the emergency room because of an inability to urinate. The most likely diagnosis is

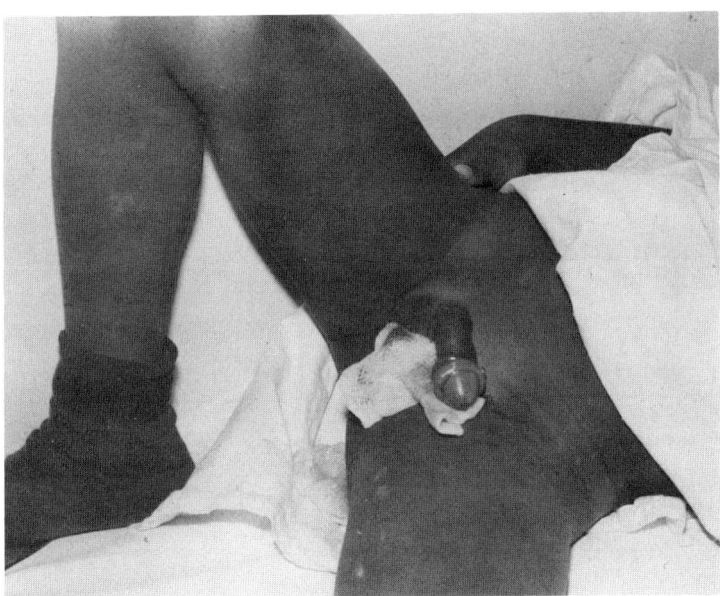

(A) priapism
(B) balanitis
(C) balanoposthitis
(D) phimosis
(E) paraphimosis

22. Accurate estimation of the surface area of a burn requires knowledge of how the body's total surface area is apportioned among the various parts. The chief difference between infants and adults relative to surface area is that infants have a proportionally

(A) smaller surface area for the trunk
(B) smaller surface area for the genitals
(C) smaller surface area for the hands and feet
(D) larger surface area for the head and neck
(E) larger surface area for the buttocks

23. The prognosis for near-drowning victims routinely can be determined on the basis of

(A) their state of consciousness upon recovery
(B) the presence or absence of apnea upon recovery
(C) radiographic examination
(D) whether the incident occurred in freshwater or saltwater
(E) none of the above

24. A buccal smear is performed on a child to determine the presence and number of Barr bodies; the nucleus of a buccal cell is shown below. The sex-chromosome pattern of this child is

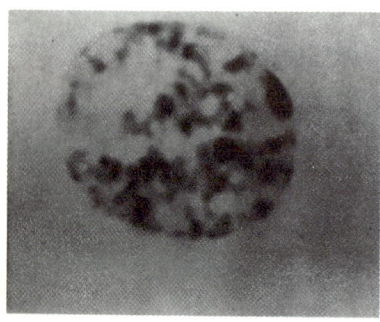

(A) XO
(B) XY
(C) XX
(D) XXX
(E) XXXX

DIRECTIONS: Each question below contains four suggested answers of which **one** or **more** is correct. Choose the answer:

A	if	**1, 2, and 3**	are correct
B	if	**1 and 3**	are correct
C	if	**2 and 4**	are correct
D	if	**4**	is correct
E	if	**1, 2, 3, and 4**	are correct

25. Mucocutaneous lymph node syndrome (Kawasaki disease), originally reported from Japan, is now seen in the United States. The diagnosis is based on a constellation of signs that includes

(1) stomatitis
(2) erythema multiforme-like rash
(3) conjuctivitis
(4) uveitis

26. In addition to characteristic skin lesions, Schönlein-Henoch purpura (anaphylactoid purpura) also is associated with which of the following conditions?

(1) Arthritis
(2) Abdominal pain
(3) Nephritis
(4) Paresis

27. At 28 weeks of age a normal baby should be able to

(1) sit with support
(2) roll over
(3) utter repetitive vowel sounds
(4) reach for and grasp large objects

28. Children who have ankylosing spondylitis may present with peripheral joint involvement. In the differentiation of this disorder from juvenile rheumatoid arthritis, it is helpful to know that ankylosing spondylitis

(1) occurs predominantly in males
(2) characteristically involves the dorsal spine
(3) frequently involves the heel
(4) has a significant familial incidence

29. Plumbism (lead intoxication) can be associated with which of the following hematologic findings?

(1) Decreased activity of delta-aminolevulinic acid dehydratase
(2) Decreased level of erythrocyte protoporphyrin
(3) Increased urinary excretion of delta-aminolevulinic acid
(4) Increased uptake and utilization of iron

30. Excessive weight gain in a pregnant woman can indicate the presence of which of the following congenital disorders in the fetus?

(1) Anencephaly
(2) Trisomy 18
(3) Duodenal atresia
(4) Renal agenesis

Pediatrics

SUMMARY OF DIRECTIONS				
A	B	C	D	E
1, 2, 3 only	1, 3 only	2, 4 only	4 only	All are correct

31. Because of its availability in many nonprescription drug preparations, iron (ferrous salts) often causes poisoning in children. Clinical effects of iron poisoning include

(1) gastrointestinal irritation
(2) hepatic damage
(3) shock
(4) alkalosis

32. A foreign body lodged in a child's trachea can cause hoarseness, cough, and dyspnea. Other physical findings are likely to include

(1) an audible expiratory slap
(2) a palpable expiratory thud
(3) asthmatoid wheezing
(4) cyanosis

33. Organisms recovered from the tracheobronchial tree of children who have cystic fibrosis are likely to include

(1) *Pseudomonas aeruginosa*
(2) *Streptococcus viridans*
(3) *Staphylococcus aureus*
(4) *Streptococcus (Diplococcus) pneumoniae*

34. Down's syndrome can be associated with which of the following chromosomal patterns?

(1) t(15q21q) centric fusion
(2) 46,XX
(3) Trisomy 21
(4) D/G translocation

35. The child pictured below has Down's syndrome. Her surgical scar and purpuric lesions are likely to be associated with

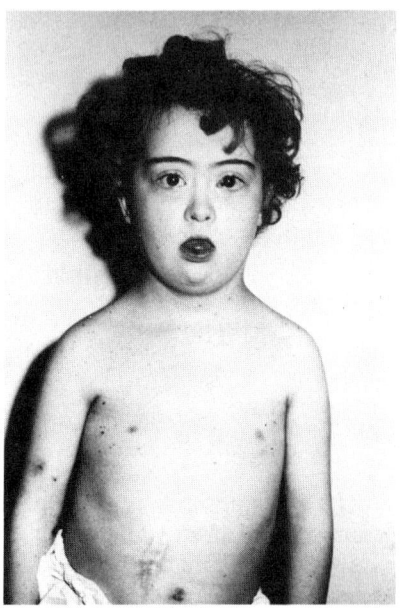

(1) leukemia
(2) thrombotic thrombocytopenic purpura
(3) congenital duodenal atresia
(4) intussusception

36. The rash that characteristically occurs in a high percentage of children who have the systemic form of juvenile rheumatoid arthritis is typically

(1) fleeting
(2) recurrent
(3) macular
(4) red-pink in color

37. Children who are moderately retarded (i.e., have an IQ between 35 and 50) generally have the potential for
   (1) economic independence
   (2) social adjustment within a neighborhood
   (3) basic literacy
   (4) attention to basic physical needs

38. Parents of an eight-month-old infant are concerned about their child's strabismus. They can be informed that
   (1) it is most likely due to a refractive error
   (2) early identification and treatment improve the outcome
   (3) children generally outgrow strabismus
   (4) a small degree of strabismus may lead to amblyopia ex anopsia

39. Children who have been abused in their home can develop which of the following psychological reactions?
   (1) Inability to sustain loving relationships
   (2) Tendency to resort to provocation when dealing with loss
   (3) Decreased threshold for impulsive behavior
   (4) Tendency to seek affectionate attention from sexual contacts

40. Anorexia nervosa, which is increasing in frequency, is associated with which of the following symptoms?
   (1) Decreased pulse rate
   (2) Hyperactivity
   (3) Diminished leukocyte count
   (4) Increased body temperature

41. The vitamins that must be provided in the diet to maintain good health include
   (1) thiamine
   (2) nicotinic acid
   (3) folic acid
   (4) biotin

42. The increasing use of organophosphate insecticides has led to a rise in the number of organophosphate poisonings. Physical findings associated with organophosphate intoxication can include
   (1) tachycardia
   (2) muscle fasciculations
   (3) hypotension
   (4) wheezing

43. Scabies has a worldwide distribution and affects children of all ages. However, the clinical picture in infants differs from that in older children and adolescents in that
   (1) burrows are frequently absent
   (2) face and scalp are frequently involved
   (3) bullae and pustules are common
   (4) there is often a superimposed eczematous dermatitis

44. Teenage pregnancies and their complications are an increasing problem that calls for a comprehensive approach. In teenage pregnancy there is an increased incidence of
   (1) preeclampsia and eclampsia
   (2) premature delivery
   (3) mental retardation in offspring
   (4) nutritional disorders

Pediatrics

SUMMARY OF DIRECTIONS

A	B	C	D	E
1, 2, 3 only	1, 3 only	2, 4 only	4 only	All are correct

45. Subdural hematoma is the most common cause of death in abused children. Children with this type of injury almost always have

(1) skull fracture
(2) bruising of scalp
(3) swelling of scalp
(4) retinal hemorrhage

46. Which of the following clinical signs can help differentiate acute otitis externa from acute otitis media?

(1) Pain heightened by movement of the tragus
(2) A red tympanic membrane
(3) Preauricular adenitis
(4) A foul-smelling discharge

General Pediatrics

DIRECTIONS: The groups of questions below consist of lettered choices followed by several numbered items. For each numbered item select the **one** lettered choice with which it is **most** closely associated. Each lettered choice may be used once, more than once, or not at all.

Questions 47-52

Drug and alcohol abuse is a problem that endangers a significant percentage of the adolescent population in the United States. For each of the specific drugs listed below that are currently abused, select the class to which it most likely belongs.

(A) Opiates
(B) Hallucinogens
(C) Cannabis
(D) Stimulants
(E) Hypnotic sedatives

47. Marihuana
48. Phencyclidine
49. Alcohol
50. Cocaine
51. Heroin
52. Mescaline

Questions 53-56

For each of the following syndromes that can cause childhood deafness, select the clinical finding with which it is most likely to be associated.

(A) Pulmonary stenosis
(B) White forelock
(C) Goiter
(D) Retinitis pigmentosa
(E) Polydactyly

53. Waardenburg's syndrome
54. Pendred's syndrome
55. Usher's syndrome
56. Leopard syndrome

Questions 57-61

For each disorder that follows, select the dietary deficiency that is most likely to be responsible.

(A) Caloric deficiency
(B) Thiamine deficiency
(C) Niacin deficiency
(D) Vitamin D deficiency
(E) None of the above

57. Marasmus
58. Kwashiorkor
59. Pellagra
60. Beriberi
61. Rickets

Questions 62-65

For each disorder listed below, select the age and sex distribution with which it is most likely to be associated.

(A) Males 4 to 10 years of age
(B) Males 13 to 18 years of age
(C) Females 4 to 10 years of age
(D) Females 10 to 16 years of age
(E) None of the above

62. Legg-Calvé-Perthes disease
63. Slipped capital femoral epiphysis
64. Idiopathic scoliosis
65. Subluxation of the head of the radius

Questions 66-70

Some of the numerous forms of dwarfism recognizable at birth or within the newborn period have distinguishing features that are useful in differential diagnosis. For each distinguishing feature listed below, select the disorder with which it is most likely to be associated.

(A) Achondrogenesis
(B) Diastrophic dwarfism
(C) Thanatophoric dwarfism
(D) Chondrodystrophia calcificans congenita
(E) Chondroectodermal dysplasia

66. Marked micromelia
67. Congenital heart disease
68. Flattened vertebral bodies
69. Natal teeth
70. Swollen ears

General Pediatrics

Answers

1. **The answer is A.** *(Kelly, Pediatrics 63:355-360, 1979. Vaughan, ed 11. pp 1980-1981.)* The sudden infant death syndrome (crib death, SIDS) typically affects infants two to four months of age and rarely occurs after six months of age. Male infants are affected more frequently than female infants and premature infants more frequently than full-term infants. This syndrome has a higher than normal incidence among infants who are illegitimate or who come from socioeconomically deprived families. Crib deaths tend to recur within families; siblings of affected infants are four to seven times more likely to experience crib death than infants in the general population. However, no distinct genetic pattern has yet been established. The occurrence of periodic breathing (repeated apneic spells) during sleep in infants with near-miss SIDS suggests a causative relationship in some cases.

2. **The answer is E.** *(Rudoph, ed 16. pp 783-785.)* Except where emesis is contraindicated, such as in the ingestion of kerosene, syrup of ipecac is the usual treatment of choice in the management of children who have ingested poisons. It is highly effective and, in an oral dose of 15 to 30 ml, usually induces vomiting within 10 to 30 minutes. (It is important not to confuse syrup of ipecac with fluid extract of ipecac, which is highly toxic and should not be kept in the home.) Apomorphine, which must be given by injection, is generally not available in the home, and copper sulfate and tartar emetics are not recommended because of their toxicity. Mustard and warm water is an ineffective emetic preparation. In contrast to induction of emesis, gastric lavage is less effective in removing ingested tablets; moreover, it carries a risk of perforation. Gastric lavage is necessary, however, for treatment of comatose patients. Other important methods for removing ingested poisons include the administration of a cathartic and an adsorbant, activated charcoal.

3. **The answer is C.** *(Vaughan, ed 11. pp 1925-1926.)* The skin disease molluscum contagiosum is caused by a DNA virus that infects the cytoplasm of epithelial cells. The characteristic lesions are waxy papules that range in size from 1 to 5 mm; these lesions, which have a central umbilication, can occur on any skin surface except the palms and soles. The shelling out of lesions is effective treat-

ment for individuals who have molluscum contagiosum. The disease is acquired by contact with an infected person or contaminated objects. The incubation period is thought to be between two and eight weeks, and the lesions are spread by autoinoculation.

4. **The answer is C.** *(Vaughan, ed 11. pp 1572-1573.)* Trauma to or excessive rotation of an especially mobile testis can lead to torsion. Presenting symptoms include pain and tenderness of a swollen testis, followed by development of fever, nausea, and vomiting. Elevation of an affected testis does not reduce the pain of torsion (a negative Prehn's sign); on the other hand, epididymitis and orchitis, which occur rarely during childhood, are associated with a positive Prehn's sign. Surgical correction of the torsion and fixation of the testis to scrotal tissues are essential. If affected boys are untreated during the first 24 hours after injury, infarction and necrosis almost invariably ensue. If, during surgery, the contralateral testis also is discovered to be abnormally mobile, it too should be affixed to scrotal tissue.

5. **The answer is B.** *(Rudolph, ed 16. pp 2004-2008.)* Achondroplasia is the most common form of skeletal dysplasia, occurring with an incidence of approximately 1 in every 9000 deliveries. Affected individuals bear a striking resemblance to one another and are identified by their extremely short extremities, prominent foreheads, short, stubby fingers, and a marked lumbar lordosis. Although they go through normal puberty, affected females must have children by cesarean section because of an associated pelvic deformity.

6. **The answer is D.** *(Vaughan, ed 11. pp 1822-1823.)* Scoliosis, or lateral curvature of the spine, can be divided into two major subgroups. In **functional** scoliosis, the most common type, spinal curvature may result from trauma that produces muscle spasm or, more often, from the presence of a short leg; bending toward the convex aspect of the curve or, for a short leg, placing a lift under the affected leg can correct the disorder. Functional scoliosis does not progress to **structural** scoliosis, the second subgroup. Structural scoliosis, which is a fixed scoliosis that cannot be corrected by bending, may develop due to hemivertebra, paralysis of muscles, fusion of the ribs, neurofibromatosis, infectious or neoplastic disease that destroys vertebrae, or other causes. Most often, however, structural scoliosis is idiopathic, affecting adolescent girls more frequently than other groups. Treatment, which involves mechanical correction and use of appliances such as the Milwaukee brace, has improved significantly the prognosis of children who have idiopathic scoliosis. Screening for idiopathic scoliosis is an important part of the examination of schoolchildren.

General Pediatrics

7. **The answer is E.** *(Vaughan, ed 11. p 1995.)* The sweat test remains the most reliable test for cystic fibrosis. In children, chloride levels in sweat that are greater than 60 mEq/L are diagnostic of cystic fibrosis; sodium concentrations are approximately 10 mEq/L higher. (Results of sweat tests in adults are harder to interpret, because sweat electrolyte concentrations normally are higher in adults than in children.) The mechanism governing this alteration of sweat electrolyte levels is unknown. Glycogen storage disease, vasopressin-resistant diabetes insipidus, untreated adrenal insufficiency, and a type of ectodermal dysplasia are among the small number of disorders that also may be associated with elevation of sweat electrolyte concentrations; none of these conditions, however, is likely to be confused clinically with cystic fibrosis.

8. **The answer is B.** *(Vaughan, ed 11. pp 1988-1989.)* It is believed that cystic fibrosis is inherited as an autosomal recessive trait, and statistical evidence exists to support this contention. As a result, each child born to parents who have had one child with cystic fibrosis has a 25 percent chance of being affected, a 50 percent chance of being a carrier, and a 25 percent chance of not carrying the gene (or genes) at all. Heterozygotes (carriers) for cystic fibrosis are clinically asymptomatic.

9. **The answer is A.** *(Rudolph, ed 16, p 374.)* Up to 25 percent of children who have the monoarticular or pauciarticular form of juvenile rheumatoid arthritis have iridocyclitis as their only significant systemic manifestation. Because this eye disorder may develop without signs or symptoms, it is recommended that all children with this form of arthritis have a slit-lamp eye examination every three months. Iridocyclitis cannot be discovered by regular ophthalmoscopic examination.

10. **The answer is E.** *(Vaughan, ed 11. pp 219-220.)* Chronic hypervitaminosis A develops due to excessive intake of vitamin A over a period of a month or more. Initial symptoms are nonspecific and include anorexia, pruritus, failure to gain weight, irritability, and tender swelling of bones associated with cortical hyperostosis. Among other manifestations of chronic hypervitaminosis A are hepatomegaly, alopecia, craniotabes, desquamation of palms and soles, seborrheic cutaneous lesions, and signs of increased intracranial pressure, including papilledema and bulging of the fontanelles. Daily intake of vitamin A should be at least 1500 IU for infants and 2000 to 5000 IU for older children.

11. The answer is D. *(Rudolph, ed 16. pp 230-232, 240-241.)* The clinical picture presented in this question, particularly the infant's characteristic pithed-frog position, is highly suggestive of scurvy, which usually affects children older than four months of age. Pain in the extremities is not characteristic of rickets. Trauma alone seldom produces the symmetric distribution of symptoms that is associated with scurvy. A child who has scorbutic pseudoparalysis of the lower extremities may be misdiagnosed as having poliomyelitis. However, tenderness in the legs is usually much more marked in children who have scurvy, and proper testing will demonstrate that these children do not have actual paralysis. Although some of the features of osteochondritis associated with congenital syphilis may suggest scurvy, syphilitic osteochondritis occurs almost exclusively in infants younger than those typically affected with scurvy.

12. The answer is D. *(Vaughan, ed 11. pp 2013-2014.)* The initial symptoms of salicylate poisoning are caused by vagal stimulation of the respiratory center. Minute volume consequently increases, and protraction of the expiratory phase causes the P_{CO_2} to decrease. The respiratory alkalosis thus produced is soon followed by renal compensation, which increases urinary excretion of bicarbonate and decreases loss of chloride, which then cause plasma chloride levels to rise and serum base levels to fall. In addition to these effects, salicylates also interfere with carbohydrate metabolism, and a persistent ketosis develops. Because the ketoacidosis further induces depletion of base through renal excretion, a true metabolic acidosis becomes superimposed upon the respiratory alkalosis. The ingested salicylates account directly for only a small portion of the acidosis; it is their interference with the Krebs cycle that causes accumulation of lactic acid, a more significant factor in the resultant metabolic acidosis. The effect on the Krebs cycle is due to an uncoupling of oxidative phosphorylation. This is also the cause of hyperpyrexia, another manifestation of salicylism, to which unknowing parents often respond with additional salicylates.

13. The answer is D. *(Vaughan, ed 11. pp 1819-1820.)* Osgood-Schlatter disease, a juvenile osteochondrosis, is most probably due to repeated trauma to the tibial tuberosity caused by excessive use of the quadriceps muscle. The disease causes pain and swelling over the tibial tubercle and tenderness on palpation. Irregular mineralization of the tibial tubercle is usually visible on x-ray. Avoidance of strenuous activity for one to two months is usually sufficient treatment. If this does not control symptoms, a cast may be required.

14. The answer is B. *(Rudolph, ed 16. pp 797-806.)* The three chelating agents used in the United States to treat individuals who have plumbism are edetate calcium disodium (Ca EDTA), dimercaprol (British anti-lewisite), and D-penicillamine. In children having the highest soft-tissue lead content (i.e., those who have acute encephalopathy), chelating agents must be administered in molar amounts in excess of those of the ingested lead; otherwise, the lead may once again disseminate within tissues of the body and cause further toxicity. Both edetate calcium disodium and dimercaprol should be given promptly in the treatment of a child affected with acute lead encephalopathy; D-penicillamine may be administered later during therapy. Careful restriction of parenteral fluids should be maintained so that further increase in cerebral edema does not occur.

15. The answer is D. *(Rudolph, ed 16. pp 35-36.)* Children between four and five years of age should be able to run and turn without losing their balance. A three-year-old child may begin to button and unbutton clothing but, unlike a five-year-old child, normally cannot lace up shoes. The concept of numbers shows a similar increase in understanding; children between four and five years of age generally can count to four, while children one year older are able to count at least to ten.

16. The answer is B. *(Rudolph, ed 16. pp 734-740, 742, 744.)* Familial hypercholesterolemia (classic type II hyperlipoproteinemia) is the most common form of familial hyperlipidemia occurring in childhood. The incidence of affected heterozygotes has been estimated at between 0.2 and 0.5 percent. The disorder is characterized by elevation of total cholesterol as well as low-density lipoprotein cholesterol levels in the plasma. Manifestations of familial hypercholesterolemia include the presence of tendon xanthomas, an increased likelihood of premature ischemic heart disease, and development during childhood of corneal arcus. Although a heterozygous child may be asymptomatic up to the age of ten, homozygous children may have physical signs, particularly planar xanthomas, from birth.

17. The answer is D. *(Vaughan, ed 11. pp 471-472, 583-585.)* Because immunoglobulin G (IgG) is the only immunoglobulin able to pass through the placenta to a fetus, newborn infants have serum levels of IgG approaching those of adults. Other immunoglobulins are present in considerably lower concentrations. Immunoglobulin M (IgM) antibodies are the first to be developed by the fetus; thus, increased cord blood levels of IgM can be considered an indication of intrauterine infection; however, it should be borne in mind that false positive results are common when IgM cord blood or early neonatal sera levels are used as screening tests for such infections.

18. The answer is B. *(Vaughan, ed 11. pp 636-637.)* Children affected as infants with atopic dermatitis often begin to show improvement at three years of age; in most children the disease becomes quiescent by five years of age. Some children, however, will continue to have eczema on scattered locations, such as the face, wrists, and especially the antecubital and popliteal fossae. A common complication of atopic dermatitis in infants and children is secondary bacterial infection, usually with staphylococci or β-hemolytic streptococci. Secondary infection in a patient with atopic dermatitis as a result of smallpox vaccination or contact with a vaccinated individual is no longer a problem since routine smallpox vaccination has been discontinued in the United States. However, herpes simplex can cause a severe secondary infection (Kaposi's varicelliform eruption); thus children with eczema should be kept away from people with herpetic infections.

19. The answer is C. *(Vaughan, ed 11. pp 632-633.)* Children in acute and obvious distress because of an episode of asthma usually respond to treatment with subcutaneous epinephrine (Adrenalin). Two or three injections may be required before symptoms are relieved. Once their asthmatic episodes have abated, affected children may be given a long-acting form of epinephrine, such as crystalline epinephrine suspension (Sus-Phrine), before going home. For children who do not respond to epinephrine, isoproterenol given by intermittent positive-pressure inhalation therapy may prove efficacious. If neither epinephrine nor isoproterenol is effective and respiratory distress persists, the patient should be considered to be in status asthmaticus and hospitalized immediately. Management then includes measurement of arterial blood gases and pH, intravenous administration of aminophylline and corticosteroids, and inhalation therapy with humidified oxygen and bronchodilators. Intravenous hydration and correction of acidosis are essential, and in some children previously unresponsive to epinephrine, may make subsequent injections of epinephrine more effective. Theophylline toxicity should be suspected in children who develop vomiting, irritability, or seizures, and xanthine administration should cease until accurate blood measurements can be obtained. Sedatives, which may cause respiratory depression, are contraindicated in the treatment of children with respiratory distress.

20. The answer is C. *(Vaughan, ed 11. p 1929.)* Of the three types of lice that are obligate parasites of man, *Pediculus humanis capitis, Phthirus pubis,* and *Pediculus humanis corporis,* only the body louse, *Pediculus humanis corporis,* is a vector for typhus, trench fever, and relapsing fever. Pediculosis capitis may cause intense pruritus, and secondary infection is common; although the lice may not be seen, the nits may be found attached firmly to hairs, particularly in the occipital region and above the ears. While pediculosis pubis is usually encountered among adolescents, young children may occasionally acquire the disease through close contact. Pediculosis corporis is usually associated with poor hygiene since the lice are most often transmitted via infested clothing or bedding, the nits and lice collecting in the seams of the cloth. Gamma benzene hydrochloride, in lotion or shampoo form, is effective for all three types of lice. Clothing and bedding should be carefully laundered.

21. The answer is E. *(Rudolph, ed 16. p 1335.)* Paraphimosis occurs when a retracted prepuce remains behind the glans; edema develops, preventing reduction of the paraphimosis. If untreated, the disorder can lead to gangrene of the glans. Reduction of the paraphimosis usually necessitates sedation; occasionally, slitting of the constricted ring may be required. All affected children should be circumcised once the inflammation has disappeared. Phimosis is characterized by an inability to retract the foreskin of the penis due to a narrowing of the preputial opening. Balanitis and balanoposthitis are inflammatory disorders affecting the glans penis and, in the case of balanoposthitis, the prepuce; these disorders develop when persistent adhesions between the foreskin and glans penis cause retention of smegma mixed with urine and lead to infection or chemical irritation.

22. The answer is D. *(Rudolph, ed 16. pp 771-772.)* The percentage of total surface area taken up by the head and neck of a one-year-old child is almost twice that for the same region in a ten-year-old child and nearly three times that in an adult. The percentage of surface area of the hands, feet, trunk, and genitals remains fairly constant despite the overall increase in total surface area. The surface area of the buttocks is proportionally less in an infant than in an adult.

23. The answer is E. *(Rudolph, ed 16. pp 766-770.)* Prognosis for near-drowning victims is affected by several factors, including the length of time of submersion and the volume of fluid aspirated. The prognosis cannot be predicted by the initial clinical state of the near-drowning victim. Hospitalization and monitoring, preferably in an intensive-care facility and for at least 24 hours following submersion, are indicated for all affected individuals. A lack of demonstrable pulmonary radiographic findings does not rule out the possibility of significant pathology; generally, however, the severity of radiographic abnormalities correlates with the severity of clinical problems. Although the clinical course may differ depending on whether the near-drowning incident occurred in freshwater or saltwater, this distinction will not help to determine the prognosis.

20   Pediatrics

24. The answer is C. *(Rudolph, ed 16. p 285.)* In human somatic cells, only one X chromosome is physiologically active in replication. All additional X chromosomes become inactivated and condensed; these are visible within the nuclei of interphase cells as sex-chromatin bodies (Barr bodies). Thus, the number of sex-chromatin bodies in a cell is one less than the total number of X chromosomes (the Lyon hypothesis). Microscopic examination of a buccal smear from a normal female (XX) would show one Barr body in every cell nucleus, as shown below:

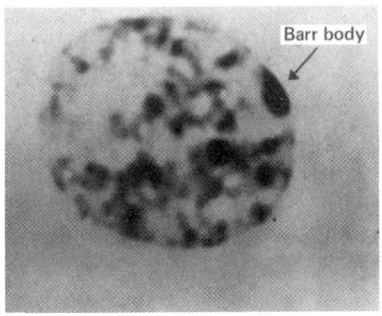

A similar preparation from a normal male (XY) shows no Barr bodies.

25. The answer is A (1, 2, 3). *(Vaughan, ed 11. pp 673-674.)* Over 12,000 cases of mucocutaneous lymph node syndrome (Kawasaki disease) have been documented in Japan since 1962. Clinical manifestations include prolonged high fever, lymphadenopathy, conjunctivitis, palmar and plantar erythema, and erythema multiforme-like rashes. Approximately 2 percent of the children with this disease die from coronary vasculitis, and it is estimated that as many as 40 percent of the affected children have some inflammation of the coronary arteries. Other complications that may occur during the course of the disease are pyuria or proteinuria, aseptic meningitis, arthralgia or arthritis, pneumonitis, and a mild form of hepatitis.

26. The answer is E (all). *(Vaughan, ed 11. pp 670-672.)* The clinical manifestations of Schönlein-Henoch purpura are due to vasculitis. Acute inflammation in the skin causes characteristic lesions that begin as urticarial wheals or red maculopapules and progress to purpura, usually on the buttocks and legs. An exudate containing lymphocytes, polymorphonuclear leukocytes, eosinophils, and red blood cells tends to accumulate around the small blood vessels of the corium. Inflammation and hemorrhage also may occur at other sites, notably joints, kidneys, the gastrointestinal tract, and the central nervous system. The arthritis associated with Schönlein-Henoch purpura usually involves the larger joints, particularly the knees and ankles. Nephritis can develop and lead to chronic renal disease, and gastrointestinal symptoms, although usually limited to colicky abdominal pain and bleeding, rarely can result in intussusception. Central nervous system involvement is infrequent, but when it does occur corticosteroid therapy is indicated.

27. The answer is E (all). *(Vaughan, ed 11. pp 42, 57.)* A 28-week-old infant should be able to sit briefly with pelvic support, roll over, reach for and hold large objects, and utter vowel sounds. At 40 weeks of age, an infant should creep or crawl, sit up without support, and make consonant sounds in a repetitive fashion ("dada," "mama"). At about one year, infants generally are able to walk with assistance. Evaluation of a child's development can be affected by a variety of circumstances, such as hunger, fatigue, or illness, which can impede a child's performance. Serial examinations are therefore much more reliable in assessing accurately a child's development.

28. The answer is E (all). *(Vaughan, ed 11. pp 663-665.)* Although ankylosing spondylitis generally is considered to be a disease of young and middle-aged adult males, it can occur in children as young as six years of age. The disorder is associated with a significant familial incidence. Radiographic evidence of destruction of the sacroiliac joint usually is evident within three to four years of onset; spinal involvement then progresses upward to the lumbar, then the dorsal, and finally the cervical spines. In contrast, children who have juvenile rheumatoid arthritis commonly have involvement of the cervical spine but not of the dorsal or lumbar spines. Heel pain, common in children who have ankylosing spondylitis, is unusual in children with juvenile rheumatoid arthritis. It is important to differentiate between these two disorders, because drug therapies may differ.

29. The answer is B (1, 3). *(Rudolph, ed 16. p 799.)* Lead disrupts the production of hemoglobin by inhibiting several steps in the manufacture of heme. In addition to decreased activity of delta-aminolevulinic acid dehydratase and increased excretion of delta-aminolevulinic acid in the urine, lead poisoning leads to increased erythrocyte protoporphyrin levels and decreased uptake and utilization of iron. Lead also interferes with the synthesis of globin in maturing erythrocytes. As a result of these impairments, a hypochromic, microcytic anemia ensues and basophilic stippling of red blood cells occurs. Red blood cell survival time is shortened and a very mild hemolytic anemia may result.

30. The answer is A (1, 2, 3). *(Vaughan, ed 11. pp 386-387.)* It is generally presumed that duodenal atresia leads to hydramnios (polyhydramnios) by interference with reabsorption of swallowed amniotic fluid. Abnormal production or release of antidiuretic hormone by fetuses who have anomalies of the central nervous system is considered to be responsible for hydramnios during their gestations. Hydramnios also is associated with approximately 80 percent of infants who have trisomy 18. Oligohydramnios occurs in association with congenital abnormalities of the fetal kidneys, such as renal agenesis, that inhibit formation of fetal urine.

31. **The answer is A (1, 2, 3).** *(Vaughan, ed 11. pp 2019-2020.)* Iron toxicity can produce life-threatening hemodynamic changes that are brought on by the action of vasodepressor agents (notably ferritin) and that lead to shock and depression of the central nervous system. Early in its course, iron poisoning causes vomiting and bloody diarrhea due to severe irritation or necrosis of gastrointestinal mucosa; iron also can cause direct damage to the liver. Pallor, lethargy, and, eventually, coma develop. Accumulation of lactic acid and citric acid results in acidosis. Administration of deferoxamine has proven to be of value in the treatment of children who have acute iron poisoning.

32. **The answer is E (all).** *(Vaughan, ed 11. p 1198.)* On expiration, the transient impaction below the glottis of a tracheal foreign body may cause both a palpable "thud" and an audible "slap." An asthmatoid wheeze and cyanosis also may be present in a child who has a foreign body lodged in the trachea. These findings, though significant and highly suggestive of a tracheal foreign body, are not necessarily diagnostic; bronchoscopy usually is required for definitive diagnosis.

33. **The answer is B (1, 3).** *(Vaughan, ed 11. pp 1992-1993.)* Chronic pulmonary disease afflicts almost all cystic fibrosis patients. Of the organisms that may be recovered from the respiratory tract of these persons, *Staphylococcus aureus* and *Pseudomonas aeruginosa* are the most common. *Pseudomonas* has been increasingly found in patients with cystic fibrosis who have received intensive antibiotic therapy. The *Pseudomonas* is of the mucoid type in over 60 percent of these patients, in contrast to 2 percent of other patients. Patients with cystic fibrosis usually tolerate chronic *Pseudomonas* infections well. These infections can be suppressed but not cured.

34. **The answer is E (all).** *(Rudolph, ed 16. pp 1777-1779.)* Children who have Down's syndrome most commonly have trisomy 21; translocations, especially between D-group and G-group chromosomes—t(15q21q) centric fusion is the most common of these abnormalities—account for a small percentage of cases. Children who have trisomy 21, which is caused by nondisjunction, have 47 chromosomes; karyotypes of children with a translocation reveal a normal chromosome count of 46. The chromosomal defect causing translocation Down's syndrome can be carried by asymptomatic individuals, if the translocation is balanced (i.e., if the **amount** of chromosomal material is normal, regardless of

structural changes in the chromosomes). Therefore, chromosome analysis should be performed on members of an affected child's family, because the chance that future siblings will have Down's syndrome is significantly greater if translocation rather than nondisjunction is the etiology.

35. The answer is B (1, 3). *(Vaughan, ed 11. p 355.)* Down's syndrome is a major cause of clinically identifiable mental retardation. Affected children show moderate to severe retardation and have a variety of morphologic abnormalities. A small, flattened skull, an upward cast to the eyes, the presence of epicanthic folds, and a protruding tongue contribute to their characteristic facies. These children have a high incidence of duodenal atresia, which must be corrected surgically during the newborn period to relieve intestinal obstruction. Children who have Down's syndrome also have a higher incidence of congenital heart disease. First signs of leukemia, which is 10 to 20 times more likely to occur in Down's syndrome children than in the general population, may be petechiae and bruises, which occur because the uncontrolled proliferation of leukocytes in the bone marrow suppresses platelet production.

36. The answer is E (all). *(Vaughan, ed 11. pp 658-659.)* The systemic form of juvenile rheumatoid arthritis (JRA) can be distinguished from the polyarticular and pauciarticular forms by the prevalence of extra-articular manifestations in affected children. The most prominent of these manifestations are fever, rash, and hepatosplenomegaly or lymphadenopathy, all of which occur in more than 75 percent of cases. Because these symptoms are often the presenting complaints, a diagnosis of arthritis may not be considered in affected children. Joint manifestations usually develop within a few months. The characteristic rash, which is fleeting and recurrent, usually occurs during febrile periods; it also may appear due to skin trauma (isomorphic response). The rash consists of individual, red-pink macules that arise most often on the trunk and proximal extremities.

37. The answer is C (2, 4). *(Vaughan, ed 11. p 160.)* Children whose intelligence quotients (IQ) are between 35 and 50 (moderate retardation) are considered to be trainable but not educable. These children account for 5 to 10 percent of retarded children, and their mental disabilities generally are evident during the preschool period. They usually can be taught to care for their basic physical needs and to attain some economic productivity either at home or in a well-supervised work environment. Although these children are capable of adjusting adequately within certain social contexts, such as their home and neighborhood, they are not capable of an independent existence.

38. The answer is C (2, 4). *(Rudolph, ed 16. pp 1967-1968.)* Up until the age of about four months, transient strabismus in an infant need not be a cause for concern; however, transient strabismus in older infants or persistent strabismus in any individual warrants detailed ophthalmologic evaluation. Although the majority of cases of strabismus are due to faulty innervation of the rectus muscles, refractive errors and a number of intraocular diseases such as retinoblastoma and toxocariasis must be excluded. As an affected child becomes older, strabismus may appear to improve due to a decrease in convergence; children do not outgrow strabismus, however, and the risk of failure to develop binocular vision persists, even in cases of slight deviation. In children who have double vision, progressive loss of vision in the weaker eye (amblyopia ex anopsia) can occur. One of the leading causes of blindness, amblyopia ex anopsia is almost always avoidable and may be reversed if strabismus is recognized and treated before six years of age. Treatment consists of forcing children to use their weak eye (e.g., by patching or medicational mydriasis of the stronger eye) and of restoring binocular vision by surgical or optical corrections.

39. The answer is E (all). *(Rudolph, ed 16. pp 73-74.)* Battered children may be more permanently wounded psychologically than physically. Children who have been abused suffer multiple losses and, as a result, are fearful of personal closeness. These children are unable to forge lasting relationships and later look to their sexual contacts for affection. Tendencies toward provocative and impulsive behavior also are common, and abused children may subsequently abuse their own children. It is imperative that physicians recognize that these factors may contribute to additional physical and psychological injuries and that the provoking child may urgently need psychological assessment and therapy.

40. The answer is A (1, 2, 3). *(Rudolph, ed 16. pp 89-90.)* Anorexia nervosa, a sometimes life-threatening disorder that primarily affects preadolescent and adolescent girls, is characterized by profound weight loss (25 to 30 percent or more of body weight). Despite vigorous investigation, no organic basis for anorectic weight loss has been found. Affected individuals have a distorted body image and are preoccupied with food. Body temperature may be as low as 35.6°C (96°F); pulse rate, blood pressure, and leukocyte count also are decreased. Anorectic individuals are hyperactive and expend a tremendous amount of energy. Therapy is difficult; skillful psychotherapeutic management is fundamental.

41. The answer is B (1, 3). *(Rudolph, ed 16. p 194.)* Vitamins can be divided into three groups: **obligatory** vitamins (vitamin A, thiamine, riboflavin, pyridoxine, folic acid, vitamin B_{12}, vitamin C, and vitamin D), which must be provided in the diet in order to maintain good health; **conditional** vitamins (nicotinic acid, choline, and vitamin K), which are required only if certain other nutrients are deficient; and **questionable** vitamins (including inositol, biotin, pantothenic acid, and vitamin E), which have not yet been proven to be essential dietary components.

42. The answer is C (2, 4). *(Rudolph, ed 16. pp 793-795.)* When the clinical signs of constricted pupils, bradycardia, and muscle fasciculations are associated with the sudden onset of neurological symptoms, progressive respiratory distress, diaphoresis, diarrhea, and overabundant salivation, a diagnosis of organophosphate poisoning should be suspected. Intake of organophosphate agents can occur by ingestion, inhalation, or absorption through skin or mucosa. Organophosphates inhibit carboxylic esterase enzymes, including acetylcholinesterase and pseudocholinesterase; toxicity depends primarily on the inactivation or inhibition of acetylcholinesterase.

Treatment consists of gastric lavage, if the poison has been ingested, or decontamination of the skin, if exposure has been through contact; maintenance of adequate ventilation and fluid and electrolyte balance also is indicated. All symptomatic children should receive atropine and, if severely affected, cholinesterase reactivating oximes as well. Cholinesterase reactivating oximes quickly restore consciousness by inhibiting the muscarinic and nicotiniclike synaptic actions of acetylcholine. Two cholinesterase reactivating oximes are pralidoxime iodide (PAM) and pralidoxime chloride (Protopam).

43. The answer is A (1, 2, 3). *(Vaughan, ed 11. pp 1927-1929.)* Preferred sites for scabies in older children are the interdigital spaces, wrist, groin, and genitalia, while areas near or on the head and neck are usually not involved; in infants lesions are often found on the face and scalp. In older children and adults the typical lesions consist of papules and vesicles, often with superimposed eczematous dermatitis. Bullae and pustules are common in infants, and consequently other more unusual bullous disorders of infants are often considered in the differential diagnosis. The correct diagnosis may be further obscured because the threadlike burrows typical of the mite bite are not seen in infants. Because gamma benzene hexacholoride may be readily absorbed percutaneously in infants, alternative therapy such as sulfur ointment should be prescribed to avoid potential neurotoxicity.

44. The answer is E (all). *(Vaughan, ed 11. pp 1711-1712.)* The main obstetric complications of teenage pregnancy are preeclampsia and eclampsia, which are thought to be due to inadequate prenatal care and nutrition. The rate of prematurity is high, and this in turn is thought to account for the increased incidence of mental retardation among children of teenage mothers. The incidence of repeat pregnancy is high, and too few communities make provisions for the mother to continue her education. A combination of medical, social, psychological, and educational resources must be made available to permit optimum health and development of the teenage mother and her child.

45. The answer is D (4). *(Vaughan, ed 11. p 123.)* Unfortunately, more than 50 percent of children with inflicted subdural hematoma have no skull fracture and no external evidence of trauma such as bruising or swelling of the scalp. It is thought that violent shaking of the child tears the bridging cerebral veins with subsequent bleeding into the subdural space. An eye examination is extremely important as retinal hemorrhages are almost always present and make the correct diagnosis more likely.

46. The answer is B (1, 3). *(Vaughan, ed 11. pp 1182-1183.)* The pain of otitis externa but not of otitis media is increased by movement of the tragus. In addition, the presence of preauricular, postauricular, or cervical adenitis, a feature of outer-ear but not middle-ear disease, aids in making the proper diagnosis. The tympanic membrane, if visualized in otitis externa, may appear normal or red; a red tympanic membrane also characterizes acute suppurative otitis media. The presence of a foul-smelling discharge may occur in association with either otitis externa or otitis media, following rupture of a tympanic membrane.

47-52. The answers are: 47-C, 48-B, 49-E, 50-D, 51-A, 52-B. *(Vaughan, ed 11. pp 127-131.)* In 1972, the National Commission on Marihuana and Drug Abuse reported that 7 percent of American youths were regular users of marihuana. Users of this drug may exhibit a variety of behavioral changes from simple euphoria to hallucinations. Users' response time and coordination may be impaired. A 1976 survey revealed that there seemed to be no increase in usage of marihuana in adolescents but that alcohol was assuming greater importance as an addictive substance.

Phencyclidine (PCP, angel dust) is one of the more common hallucinogens available on the "street." Because PCP may cause confusion and a wide variety of hallucinations, it is of especially high risk to individuals prone to psychiatric problems, in whom prolonged psychosis may be produced. Lysergic acid diethylamide (LSD) and PCP are often the active ingredients in substances sold as mescaline or psilocybin because they are relatively easy to produce.

Alcohol, while regarded by many as simply a beverage, is a depressant which, among other problems, accounts for an increasing number of automobile accidents. It has been reported that as many as 28 percent of adolescents in the United States are problem drinkers.

Cocaine is another stimulant that is increasingly available. Formerly, cocaine was used in combination with heroin, but it is now often used as a primary drug, even though it is very expensive. Dealing in drugs may be the easiest way for an adolescent to meet the cost of drug use.

Heroin, along with methadone and morphine, is an opiate. It is usually injected but occasionally is taken intranasally. Infections at the injection site, hepatitis, endocarditis, and tetanus are among the medical problems encountered in opiate users.

Mescaline, another hallucinogen, is more likely to be LSD or PCP. Prolonged use of hallucinogens may result in disturbed interpersonal relations, poor time and place orientation, and regressive behavior. With abstinence, hallucinogenic flashbacks may recur for months.

53-56. The answers are: 53-B, 54-C, 55-D, 56-A. *(Rudolph, ed 16. pp 967-968.)* Waardenburg's syndrome is the most common of several syndromes that are characterized by both deafness and pigmentary changes. Features of this syndrome, which is inherited as an autosomal dominant disorder, include a distinctive white forelock, heterochromia, unilateral or bilateral congenital deafness, and lateral displacement of the inner canthi.

Individuals who have Pendred's syndrome, inherited as an autosomal recessive trait, typically have a marked hearing loss and thyroid dysfunction. Goiter, which usually develops before affected children reach the age of ten years, may arise because their thyroid glands are unable to convert inorganic iodine into organic iodine. The benign goiter responds to thyroid replacement therapy.

Congenital deafness is also a symptom of the autosomal-recessive Usher's syndrome. Pigmentary changes in the retina (retinitis pigmentosa) can be detected in affected infants, and these degenerative changes continue throughout life. Early visual impairments include loss of night vision and development of tunnel vision. Functional blindness can arise in affected adolescents and adults.

Leopard syndrome is characterized by the presence of multiple l*en*tigines, *o*cular hypertelorism, p*ulmonary* stenosis, *abnormal* genitalia, *r*et*ardation* of growth, and profound *deafness*. The syndrome is inherited as an autosomal dominant disorder with variable penetrance.

57-61. The answers are: 57-A, 58-E, 59-C, 60-B, 61-D. *(Vaughan, ed 11. pp 212-214, 220-221, 222-223, 228-234.)* Marasmus (infantile atrophy) is due to inadequate caloric intake that may be linked with such factors as insufficient food resources, poor feeding techniques, metabolic disorders, and congenital anomalies. Symptoms of marasmus include progressive weight loss, constipation, muscular atrophy, loss of skin turgor, hypothermia, and edema. In advanced disease, affected infants are lethargic and suffer from starvation diarrhea, which is characterized by the presence of small, mucus-containing stools.

Kwashiorkor, which is caused by a severe deficiency of protein, is the most common—and most serious—type of malnutrition in the world. Caloric intake in affected children may be adequate. Children who have protein deficiency become more susceptible to infection; vomiting, diarrhea, muscle wasting, dermatitis, hepatosplenomegaly, edema, dyspigmentation of the skin and hair, and changes in mental status are among the many manifestations of this disease. The most important laboratory finding is a decrease in serum albumin level. Pellagra, which literally means "rough skin," is due to a deficiency of niacin. Niacin is an essential component of two enzymes—nicotinamide adenine dinucleotide (NAD) and nicotinamide adenine dinucleotide phosphate (NADP) needed for electron transfer and glycolysis. Pellagra is most prevalent in areas that rely on corn as a basic foodstuff (corn contains little tryptophan, which can be converted into niacin). The classic ("3-D") triad of clinical symptoms of pellagra consists of dermatitis, diarrhea, and dementia.

Beriberi results from a deficiency of thiamine, which is essential for the synthesis of acetylcholine and for the operation of certain enzyme systems in carbohydrate metabolism. Thiamine is present in fair amounts in cereals, fruits, vegetables, and eggs; meat and legumes also are good sources. Thiamine is destroyed by heat, and polishing of grains reduces their thiamine content by removing the coverings that contain most of the vitamin. Clinical disturbances stemming from thiamine deficiency are congestive heart failure, peripheral neuritis, and psychic disturbances.

Rickets is a disorder of bone characterized by defective mineralization—despite normal formation—of collagen, matrix, and osteoid. The type of rickets that responds to administration of normal doses of vitamin D is termed vitamin D-deficient rickets; children who have vitamin D-resistant rickets or rickets due to chronic renal disease are not helped by vitamin D therapy. Deficiency of vitamin D can lead to osseous changes, such as enlargement of the costochondral junctions ("rachitic rosary") and crainotabes, within a few months; advanced rickets may cause scoliosis, pelvic and leg deformities, "pigeon breast," rachitic dwarfism, and other disorders.

62-65. The answers are: 62-A, 63-B, 64-D, 65-E. *(Rudolph, ed 16. pp 1995-2031. Vaughan, ed 11. pp 1818, 1819, 1822-1823, 1827-1828.)* Legg-Calvé-Perthes disease (coxa plana) is aseptic necrosis and flattening of the capital femoral epiphysis; the cause of this disorder is unknown. Boys between the ages of four and ten years are most frequently affected. Presenting symptoms include a limp, pain in the knee or hip, or limitation of weight bearing.

Slipped capital femoral epiphysis occurs typically in adolescents; the disorder is slightly more common among boys than girls. The etiology is unknown. Onset of this disorder, which is more common in childhood, is gradual; pain referred to the knee is characteristic and may mask the hip pathology. Treatment aims at arresting the slippage by immobilization of the hip through cast or surgical fixation.

Idiopathic scoliosis occurs most frequently in adolescent girls and requires prompt evaluation. Treatment by bracing, spinal fusion, or both is sometimes necessary. Unrecognized prior infection of the nervous system, leading to muscle weakness, may be a factor in some cases of idiopathic scoliosis.

Subluxation of the head of the radius occurs most commonly in children who are two to five years of age and have been jerked forcibly by the hand. Affected children have pain in the elbow and are unable to supinate the forearm. The diagnosis is established if forcible supination of the forearm, while the elbow is stabilized, easily corrects the subluxation.

66-70. The answers are: 66-A, 67-E, 68-C, 69-E, 70-B. *(Vaughan, ed 11. pp 1831-1837.)* **Achondrogenesis** is a lethal chondrodystrophy which is associated with severe micromelia, a relatively large head, and a narrow trunk. **Diastrophic dwarfism**, another type of short-limbed dwarfism, is distinguishable by the swelling of the pinna that appears within the first three weeks of life and persists for three to four weeks, leaving the ears with thick, firm, deformed cartilage. The disease is inherited as an autosomal recessive trait and intelligence is normal in affected children. **Chondrodystrophia calcificans congenita** (Conradi disease) is frequently associated with cataracts and optic atrophy. These children may also suffer from seborrheic dermatitis or ichthyosiform erythroderma. The radiologic finding of discrete, multiple calcified densities in those bones formed in hyaline cartilage helps to establish the diagnosis. Children with **thanatophoric dwarfism** are born with hypotonia and rapidly develop respiratory distress and asphyxia due to severe narrowing of the thorax. Characteristic x-ray findings include marked flattening of the vertebral bodies. **Chondroectodermal dysplasia** (Ellis-van Creveld syndrome) has an unusually high incidence among the Amish, although cases among non-Amish people have also been reported. Anomalies occur in these children in all the embryonic layers of development. Ectodermal abnormalities include fine, sparse hair, dystrophic nails, and peg-shaped teeth with abnormal spacing. Natal teeth are frequently present. Mesodermal abnormalities are manifested by bone involvement resulting in dwarfism, congenital heart disease, and renal malformations. Polydactylism is usually present in these children, who have normal intelligence. The disease has an autosomal recessive inheritance. Penetrance is variable and may be manifested by polydactyly as an isolated finding.

The Newborn Infant

Marcellina Mian

DIRECTIONS: Each question below contains five suggested answers. Choose the **one best** response to each question.

71. Which of the following patterns noted on continuous fetal heart rate monitoring warrants immediate delivery of the infant?

(A) Baseline variability with periodic acceleration
(B) Increasing baseline variability (saltatory pattern)
(C) Early deceleration pattern
(D) Late deceleration without baseline variability
(E) Variable deceleration with baseline variability

72. An infant weighing 1400 g (3 lb) is born at 32 weeks gestation in a delivery room that has an ambient temperature of 23.9°C (75°F). Within a few minutes of birth, this infant is likely to exhibit all of the following manifestations EXCEPT

(A) pallor
(B) shivering
(C) a fall in body temperature
(D) increased respiratory rate
(E) metabolic acidosis

73. Two infants are born at 36 weeks gestation. Infant A weighs 2600 g (5 lb, 12 oz) and infant B weighs 1600 g (3 lb, 8 oz). Infant B is more likely to have all of the following problems EXCEPT

(A) congenital malformations
(B) low hematocrit
(C) symptomatic hypoglycemia
(D) aspiration pneumonia
(E) future growth retardation

74. In a neonate who has asphyxia, all of the following sequelae can be expected to develop EXCEPT

(A) electrolyte abnormalities
(B) cardiomegaly and heart failure
(C) cerebral edema and seizures
(D) hepatomegaly and jaundice
(E) disseminated intravascular coagulation

75. At 43 weeks gestation a long, thin infant is delivered who is apneic, limp, pale, and covered with "pea soup" amniotic fluid. The first step in the resuscitation of this infant after delivery should be

(A) suction of the trachea under direct vision
(B) artificial ventilation with bag and mask
(C) artificial ventilation with an endotracheal tube
(D) administration of 100 percent oxygen by mask
(E) catheterization of the umbilical vein

76. Which of the following statements about periventricular-intraventricular (intracranial) hemorrhage is true in newborn infants?

(A) Clinical manifestations appear within minutes of a serious hypoxic episode
(B) It most commonly produces sudden severe neurologic deterioration
(C) It is seldom found in infants weighing less than 1500 g
(D) Systemic signs include an acute drop in hematocrit and arterial P_{O_2}
(E) Posthemorrhagic ventricular dilatation cannot be evaluated adequately by CAT scan

77. A one-day-old infant who was born by a difficult forceps delivery is alert and active. However, she does not move her left arm, which she keeps internally rotated by her side with the forearm extended and pronated; she also does not move it during a Moro reflex. The rest of her physical examination is normal. This clinical picture most likely indicates

(A) fracture of the left clavicle
(B) fracture of the left humerus
(C) left-sided Erb-Duchenne paralysis
(D) left-sided Klumpke's paralysis
(E) spinal injury with left hemiparesis

78. Initial examination of a full-term infant weighing less than 2500 g (5 lb, 8 oz) shows edema over the dorsum of her hands and feet. Which of the following findings would support a diagnosis of Turner's syndrome?

(A) A liver palpable to 2 cm below the costal margin
(B) Tremulous movements and ankle clonus
(C) Redundant skin folds at the nape of the neck
(D) A transient, longitudinal division of the body into a red half and a pale half
(E) Softness of the parietal bones at the vertex

79. The infant pictured below is two weeks old. He was delivered at term after a long and difficult labor. He weighed 4200 g (9 lb, 4 oz) at birth. The lesions shown on his arm and back are reddish-purple and indurated. Which of the following diagnoses is most likely to be correct?

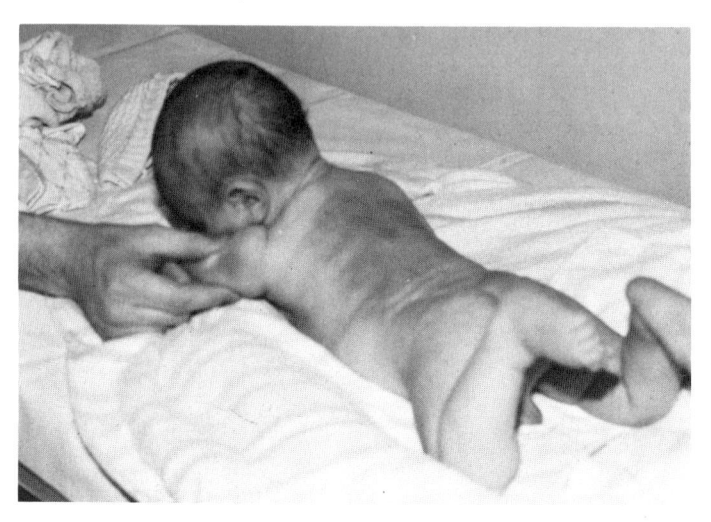

(A) Erythema toxicum neonatorum
(B) Sclerema neonatorum
(C) Subcutaneous fat necrosis
(D) Urticaria pigmentosa
(E) Mongolian spots

---

80. Which of the following statements characterizes the early anemia related to vitamin E deficiency in premature infants?

(A) The platelet count is diminished
(B) The reticulocyte count is elevated
(C) It cannot occur in the presence of a normal serum tocopherol level
(D) It can be prevented by a diet high in polyunsaturated fatty acids
(E) It is partially treated by oral iron supplements

81. The diagnosis of congenital dislocation of the hip in a newborn infant can best be established by which of the following clinical findings?

(A) Shortening of the upper leg (Galeazzi's sign)
(B) Asymmetry of thigh skin folds
(C) Limitation of hip abduction in flexion
(D) Click on hip abduction in flexion (Ortolani's sign)
(E) Pain on hip abduction in flexion

Newborn Infant

82. A three-day-old infant born at 32 weeks gestation and weighing 1700 g (3 lb, 12 oz) has three episodes of apnea, each lasting 20 to 25 seconds and occurring after a feeding. During these episodes the heart rate drops from 140 to 100 beats per minute and the child remains motionless; between episodes, however, the child displays normal activity. Blood sugar is 50 mg/100 ml and serum calcium is normal. The child's apneic periods most likely are

(A) due to an immature respiratory center
(B) a part of periodic breathing
(C) secondary to hypoglycemia
(D) manifestations of seizures
(E) evidence of underlying pulmonary disease

83. If a healthy infant who weighs 2000 g (4 lb, 6 oz) is fed a commercial cow's milk formula that provides 20 cal/30 ml (1 oz), daily intake for good nutrition and growth should be

(A) 240 ml with multiple vitamin supplements
(B) 240 ml without vitamin supplements
(C) 360 ml with multiple vitamin supplements
(D) 360 ml with supplemental vitamin E only
(E) none of the above

84. A primiparous woman whose blood type is O-positive gives birth at term to an infant who has A-positive blood and a hematocrit of 55%. A serum bilirubin level obtained at 36 hours of age is 12 mg/100 ml. Which of the following laboratory findings would be most characteristic of this infant's disease?

(A) An elevated reticulocyte count
(B) A strongly positive direct Coombs' test
(C) Fragmented red blood cells in the blood smear
(D) Nucleated red blood cells in the blood smear
(E) Spherocytes in the blood smear

85. A full-term infant is born after a normal pregnancy; delivery, however, is complicated by marginal placental separation. At 12 hours of age the child, although appearing to be in good health, passes a bloody meconium stool. For determining the etiology of the baby's melena, which of the following diagnostic procedures should be performed first?

(A) A barium enema
(B) An Apt test
(C) Gastric lavage with normal saline
(D) An upper gastrointestinal series
(E) A platelet count, prothrombin time, and partial thromboplastin time

Questions 86-88

After an uneventful labor and delivery, an infant is born at 32 weeks gestation weighing 1500 g (3 lb, 5 oz). Respiratory difficulty develops immediately after birth and increases in intensity thereafter. The child's mother (gravida 3, para 2, no abortions) previously lost an infant because of hyaline membrane disease.

86. At six hours of age the child's respiratory rate is 60 per minute. Examination reveals grunting, intercostal retraction, nasal flaring, and marked cyanosis in room air. Physiologic abnormalities compatible with these data include

(A) decreased lung compliance, reduced lung volume, left-to-right shunt of blood
(B) decreased lung compliance, reduced lung volume, right-to-left shunt of blood
(C) decreased lung compliance, increased lung volume, left-to-right shunt of blood
(D) normal lung compliance, reduced lung volume, left-to-right shunt of blood
(E) normal lung compliance, increased lung volume, right-to-left shunt of blood

87. At eight hours of age the infant described is given 70 percent oxygen. Arterial blood gases are as follows: pH, 7.30; P_{O_2}, 40 mm Hg; and P_{CO_2}, 40 mm Hg. Which of the following therapeutic courses of action would be most appropriate?

(A) Elevation of the inspired oxygen concentration
(B) Initiation of continuous positive airway pressure
(C) Elevation of the inspired oxygen concentration and administration of sodium bicarbonate
(D) Initiation of continuous positive airway pressure and administration of sodium bicarbonate
(E) Initiation of mechanical ventilation and administration of sodium bicarbonate

88. At 48 hours of age and after proper therapy has been instituted, the infant described is much improved. With the child breathing 70 percent oxygen (without any ventilatory assistance), arterial blood gases are as follows: pH, 7.36; P_{O_2}, 210 mm Hg; P_{CO_2}, 40 mm Hg. On evaluating this information, the child's physician should

(A) lower the inspired oxygen concentration to 40 percent and, one hour later, repeat arterial puncture for blood gas values
(B) lower the inspired oxygen concentration to 40 percent and, four hours later, repeat arterial puncture for blood gas values
(C) lower the inspired oxygen concentration to 60 percent and, one hour later, repeat arterial puncture for blood gas values
(D) lower the inspired oxygen concentration to 60 percent and, four hours later, repeat arterial puncture for blood gas values
(E) leave the inspired oxygen concentration at 70 percent and, one hour later, repeat arterial puncture for blood gas values

89. Very shortly after birth, an infant develops abdominal distension and begins to drool constantly. When she is given her first feeding, formula runs out the side of her mouth and she coughs and chokes. Physical examination a few hours later reveals tachypnea, intercostal retractions, and bilateral pulmonary rales.

The esophageal anomaly that most commonly causes the signs and symptoms exhibited by this infant is illustrated by

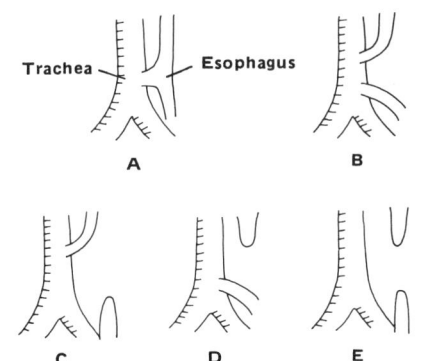

(A) figure A
(B) figure B
(C) figure C
(D) figure D
(E) figure E

90. Failure to administer vitamin K prophylactically to a newborn infant is associated with which of the following?

(A) A deficiency of factor V
(B) A prolonged prothrombin time
(C) Development of hemorrhagic manifestations within 24 hours of delivery
(D) Manifestations that are more severe in male than female infants
(E) A greater likelihood of developing symptoms if the infant is fed cow's milk rather than breast milk

91. A newborn infant who is cyanotic at rest but pink when crying most likely has which of the following malformations?

(A) A double aortic arch
(B) A laryngeal web
(C) Laryngomalacia
(D) Bilateral choanal atresia
(E) Deviation of the nasal septum

92. Which of the following drugs given during the last two weeks of pregnancy may have deleterious effects on the fetus?

(A) Chlorothiazides
(B) Chloramphenicol
(C) Heparin
(D) Hydantoin
(E) Insulin

93. At the time of delivery of her child, a woman is noted to have a large volume of amniotic fluid. At six hours of age her baby begins regurgitating small amounts of mucus and bile-stained fluid. Physical examination of the infant is normal, and an abdominal x-ray is obtained (shown below). The most likely diagnosis of this infant's disorder is

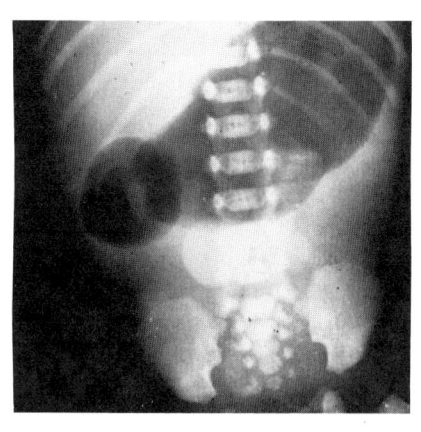

(A) esophageal atresia
(B) pyloric stenosis
(C) gastric duplication
(D) duodenal atresia
(E) midgut volvulus

94. A woman (gravida 3, para 0, 2 abortions) who is in early labor comes to her community hospital at 34 weeks gestation. The hospital, which has an excellent obstetric service but no intensive-care nursery, is located 25 miles from the nearest referral perinatal center. To maximize the child's chances for survival without causing unnecessary hardship to the woman, which of the following courses of action would be most advisable?

(A) Transfer the woman immediately to the referral perinatal center
(B) Transfer the infant to the referral perinatal center immediately after birth
(C) Transfer the infant to the referral perinatal center at the first sign of illness
(D) Transfer the infant to the referral perinatal center only if a severe illness develops
(E) Keep the woman and her infant at the community hospital

95. An infant is born at term to a primigravid woman who has diabetes mellitus. The infant, whose physical examination at birth is normal, is noted at 20 hours of age to be pale and lethargic and to void grossly bloody urine. Physical examination at this time reveals a left flank mass that is firm, lobulated, and about 10 cm in diameter; the mass is opaque on transillumination. The most likely diagnosis is

(A) acute adrenal hemorrhage
(B) retrorenal hematoma
(C) Wilms' tumor
(D) renal vein thrombosis
(E) polycystic kidney

96. A two-week-old premature infant is found to have several milliliters of formula still present in the stomach two hours after being fed. Also noted are gastric distension and the passage of blood-streaked stools. Which of the following historical factors would best support a tentative diagnosis of necrotizing enterocolitis for this infant?

(A) Passage of a thick tenacious meconium plug at 24 hours of age
(B) Severe hyaline membrane disease with anoxic episodes in the first week of life
(C) Hypocalcemia requiring oral calcium supplementation in the first week of life
(D) A maternal history of severe ulcerative colitis
(E) A history of milk-protein allergy in family members

97. A diagnosis of neonatal necrotizing enterocolitis is confirmed by finding air in the bowel wall (pneumatosis intestinalis) on plain x-ray of an infant's abdomen. Which of the following therapeutic approaches would most likely be recommended?

(A) Immediate surgical resection of affected loops of bowel
(B) Reduction of the volume of feedings and administration of oral and systemic antibiotics
(C) Reduction of the volume of feedings, administration of oral and systemic antibiotics, and careful observation for bowel perforation
(D) Discontinuation of feedings, administration of intravenous fluids and oral and systemic antibiotics, and careful observation for bowel perforation
(E) Discontinuation of feedings, administration of intravenous fluids and oral and systemic corticosteroids, and careful observation for bowel perforation

98. Hypocalcemia that is refractory to the continued administration of calcium chloride may be due to a low serum level of

(A) phosphorus
(B) bicarbonate
(C) magnesium
(D) zinc
(E) potassium

99. Which of the following statements about the infant pictured below is true?

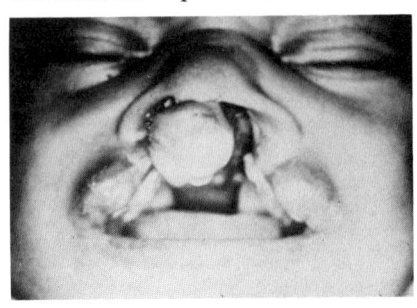

(A) Parenteral alimentation is recommended to prevent aspiration
(B) Surgical closure of the palatal defect should be done before three months of age
(C) Good anatomic closure will preclude the development of speech defects
(D) Recurrent otitis media and hearing loss are likely complications
(E) The chance that a sibling also would be affected is 1 in 1000

Newborn Infant

DIRECTIONS: Each question below contains four suggested answers of which **one** or **more** is correct. Choose the answer:

A	if	1, 2, and 3	are correct
B	if	1 and 3	are correct
C	if	2 and 4	are correct
D	if	4	is correct
E	if	1, 2, 3, and 4	are correct

100. Correct statements concerning breast-fed infants as compared to bottle-fed infants include which of the following?

(1) Their survival rate in lower socioeconomic groups is higher
(2) They tend to be emotionally more stable
(3) They have fewer gastrointestinal disturbances
(4) Their serum bilirubin level during the newborn period is lower

101. Normal full-term newborn infants can demonstrate which of the following reflex reactions?

(1) Stepping reflex
(2) Palmar grasp
(3) Placing reflex
(4) Parachute reaction

102. An infant born to a heroin addict who has received no prenatal care is likely to exhibit

(1) prematurity and low birth weight
(2) onset of symptoms within the first two days of life
(3) hyperirritability and coarse tremors
(4) vomiting and diarrhea

103. A 28-year-old primigravid woman, who is unsure of her dates, gives birth to a girl weighing 1900 g (4 lb, 3 oz); this weight is at the 50th percentile for infants born at 33 weeks gestation. Which of the following findings on physical examination would support a gestational age of 33 weeks for this child?

(1) The clitoris is almost hidden by the labia majora
(2) The ear recoils slowly from folding
(3) The elbow can be brought up to the opposite shoulder
(4) The sole has one or two creases over the anterior third

104. Examination shows that a neonate has a large bulge on the left side of the head; the bulge is sharply demarcated by the coronal, sagittal, and lambdoid sutures. Correct statements concerning this situation include which of the following?

(1) There is a small chance of an underlying skull fracture
(2) Needle aspiration of the swelling is indicated
(3) Anemia may be a complicating factor
(4) If the infant is untreated, a prominent lump will probably persist for many months

SUMMARY OF DIRECTIONS

A	B	C	D	E
1, 2, 3 only	1, 3 only	2, 4 only	4 only	All are correct

105. Recent studies on close mother-infant contact in the early postpartum period have yielded findings which include

(1) higher IQs in infants who had close early contact with their mothers
(2) more divorces by mothers who were separated from their premature infants for three weeks or longer
(3) higher incidence of child abuse and failure-to-thrive in infants not receiving close early contact with their mothers
(4) prolonged breast-feeding in the early-contact group

106. A four-day-old infant has a plasma phenylalanine level greater than 20 mg/100 ml (normal: 0.4 to 2.0); tyrosine levels are normal. Correct statements about this infant include which of the following?

(1) Dietary therapy is needed to prevent mental retardation
(2) Physical examination would be expected to be normal
(3) Both parents are heterozygous carriers for phenylketonuria
(4) Urine would be positive for phenylpyruvic acid

107. Correct statements concerning retinoblastoma in a newborn infant include which of the following?

(1) One parent may be a carrier for retinoblastoma
(2) Bilateral involvement occurs in 5 percent of cases
(3) If affected infants are treated, the mortality rate is 25 percent
(4) Diagnosis of retinoblastoma typically is made in the neonatal period

108. Physicians using phototherapy to treat an infant who has hyperbilirubinemia secondary to hemolysis should monitor which of the following clinical signs or laboratory values at regular intervals during the 48 hours after initiation of treatment?

(1) Hematocrit
(2) Skin color
(3) Serum bilirubin level
(4) Scleral color

109. In the management of an infant who has hyperbilirubinemia, factors to be considered in assessing the risk of kernicterus include the presence of

(1) acidosis
(2) hypoxia
(3) hypoalbuminemia
(4) cold stress

110. Correct statements about hypocalcemia in neonates include which of the following?

(1) It is less likely to occur in breast-fed infants
(2) It is less likely to occur in infants of diabetic mothers
(3) It may be precipitated by obstetric difficulty and asphyxia
(4) It may be partially caused by poor maternal nutrition

111. A boy is born at term after an uncomplicated pregnancy, labor, and delivery. Immediately after birth, however, he is noted to be in severe distress, making gasping respiratory efforts accompanied by intercostal retractions. His abdomen is concave, and he is cyanotic. A chest x-ray obtained at this time is shown below. Treatment of this child, whose condition is deteriorating rapidly must include

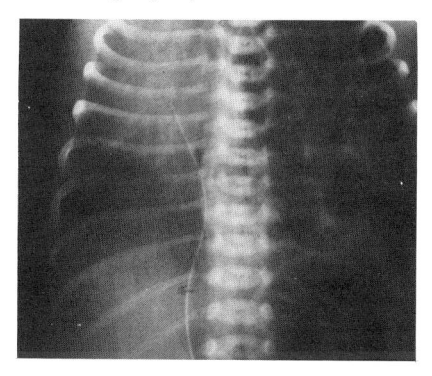

(1) emergency surgical correction
(2) prompt correction of metabolic acidosis
(3) intermittent nasogastric suction
(4) vigorous positive pressure ventilation

112. Pulmonary dysmaturity (Wilson-Mikity syndrome) and bronchopulmonary dysplasia are very similar in which of the following respects?

(1) Characteristic pulmonary pathology
(2) Early clinical course
(3) Known etiologic factors
(4) Radiographic findings

113. The diagnosis of meconium ileus in a neonate who has signs of intestinal obstruction is supported by

(1) a family history of cystic fibrosis
(2) palpation of several doughy masses throughout the abdomen
(3) the radiographic presence of unevenly dilated, granular-looking loops of bowel
(4) a greenish discoloration of the abdominal wall

114. A woman pregnant with twins wonders if such pregnancies are associated with an increased risk of infant morbidity or mortality. She should be told that

(1) second-born twins have a higher mortality rate than first-born twins
(2) twins are more likely to be born prematurely or to be small for dates
(3) dichorionic twins have a higher perinatal mortality rate than monochorionic twins
(4) twins have a fourfold increase in perinatal mortality as compared to singletons

Pediatrics

SUMMARY OF DIRECTIONS				
A	B	C	D	E
1, 2, 3 only	1, 3 only	2, 4 only	4 only	All are correct

115. A woman gives birth to twins at 38 weeks gestation. The first twin weighs 2800 g (6 lb, 3 oz) and has a hematocrit of 70%; the second twin weighs 2100 g (4 lb, 10 oz) and has a hematocrit of 40%. Correct statements concerning these infants include which of the following?

(1) The first twin is at risk for developing respiratory distress, cyanosis, and congestive heart failure
(2) The first twin may have hyperbilirubinemia and convulsions
(3) The second twin may be pale, tachycardic, and hypotensive
(4) The second twin probably had hydramnios of the amniotic sac

116. Correct statements describing hypoglycemia affecting infants of diabetic mothers include which of the following?

(1) It is less frequently symptomatic in these infants than in small-for-dates infants
(2) It usually develops in the second day of life
(3) It is believed to be caused by hyperinsulinism
(4) It is best prevented by rapid infusion of a 25 percent glucose solution

117. A full-term infant has apneic episodes during the third day of life. There appears to be no underlying organic cause. Treatment measures should include

(1) low (2 to 4 cm H_2O) nasal continuous positive airway pressure
(2) intravenous or oral theophylline
(3) increased inspired oxygen to maintain arterial P_{O_2} between 50 and 60 mm Hg
(4) increased vestibular stimulation

Newborn Infant

DIRECTIONS: The groups of questions below consist of lettered choices followed by several numbered items. For each numbered item select the **one** lettered choice with which it is **most** closely associated. Each lettered choice may be used once, more than once, or not at all.

Questions 118-121

For each infant described below, select the lettered curve on the graph that best represents the expected course of that infant's jaundice.

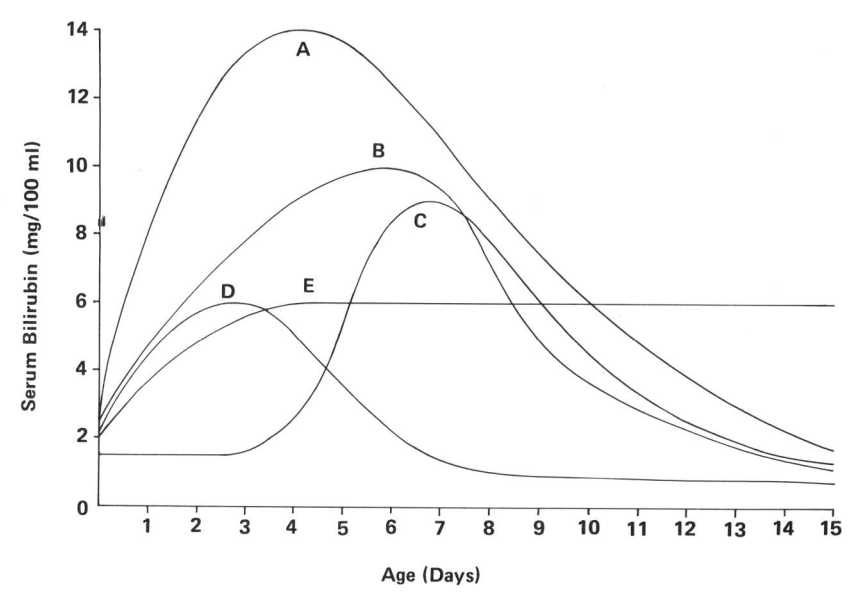

118. A jaundiced premature neonate who is otherwise normal
119. A jaundiced full-term neonate who has septicemia
120. A jaundiced full-term neonate who has hypothyroidism
121. A jaundiced full-term neonate who has erythroblastosis fetalis

Questions 122-125

For each description of congenital anomalies that follows, select the major abnormality with which it is most likely to be associated.

(A) Deafness
(B) Seizures
(C) Wilms' tumor
(D) Congestive heart failure
(E) Optic glioma

122. Nonfamilial bilateral absence of the iris (aniridia)

123. Heterochromia of the iris, broad nasal root, fusion of the eyebrows, and white forelock

124. Flat capillary hemangioma over the anterior scalp and one side of the face

125. Hypopigmented oval macules on the skin of the trunk and extremities

The Newborn Infant

Answers

71. **The answer is D.** *(Behrman, ed 2. pp 86-90.)* Baseline variability with or without periodic acceleration of the fetal heart rate is a sign of fetal well-being. Increasing baseline variability (saltatory pattern) may represent early compromise of fetal oxygenation. The early deceleration pattern is due to pressure of the anterior fontanel on the cervix and is not a sign of fetal distress. The variable deceleration pattern indicates umbilical cord compression. The late deceleration pattern signifies fetal hypoxemia. Both of these patterns in association with loss of baseline variability are signs of severe fetal compromise and warrant immediate delivery of the infant.

72. **The answer is B.** *(Schaffer, ed 4. pp 23-24.)* A room temperature of 24°C (approximately 75°F) provides a cool environment for preterm infants weighing less than 1500 g (3 lb, 4 oz). Aside from the fact that these infants emerge from a warm 37.6° (99.5°F) intrauterine environment, at birth they are wet, have a relatively large surface area for their weight, and have little subcutaneous fat. Within minutes of delivery the infants are likely to become pale or blue and their body temperatures will drop. In order to bring body temperature back to normal they must increase their metabolic rate; ventilation, in turn, must increase proportionally to insure an adequate oxygen supply. Because a preterm infant is likely to have respiratory problems and be unable to oxygenate adequately, lactate can accumulate and lead to a metabolic acidosis. Infants rarely shiver in response to a need to increase heat production.

73. **The answer is B.** *(Klaus, ed 2. pp 82-84.)* Small-for-dates infants are subject to a different set of complications than preterm infants whose size is appropriate for gestational age. The small-for-dates infants have a higher incidence of major congenital anomalies and are at increased risk for future growth retardation, especially if length and head circumference as well as weight are small for gestational age. They also are at greater risk for neonatal asphyxia and the meconium aspiration syndrome, which can lead to pneumothorax, pneumomedi-

astinum, or pulmonary hemorrhage. These, rather than hyaline membrane disease, are the major pulmonary problems in these infants. Because neonatal symptomatic hypoglycemia is commonly found in small-for-dates infants, careful blood glucose monitoring and early feeding are appropriate precautions. Elevated central hematocrit is common in these infants for reasons that are unknown.

74. The answer is D. *(Klaus, ed 2. p 40.)* During a period of asphyxia, hypoxemia and acidosis can damage a neonate's brain, heart, kidneys, and lungs. The resulting clinical abnormalities include cerebral edema, irritability and seizures, cardiomegaly and heart failure, urinary abnormalities or renal shutdown, and the respiratory distress syndrome (even in infants of more than 37 weeks gestation). Hyperkalemia and serum sodium abnormalities are the result of cellular and renal damage. Disseminated intravascular coagulation is not an unusual complication. Liver damage, however, has not been described as one of the sequelae of asphyxia.

75. The answer is A. *(Klaus, ed 2. pp 82-83, 190.)* Infants who are postmature (more than 42 weeks gestation) and show evidence of chronic placental insufficiency (low birth weight for gestational age and wasted appearance, even with good length) have a higher than average chance of being asphyxiated during delivery. Asphyxia leads to the passage of meconium into the amniotic fluid and thus places these infants at risk for meconium aspiration. To prevent or minimize this risk, these infants should have immediate nasopharyngeal suction as their heads are delivered. Immediately after delivery and before initiation of respiration their tracheas must be carefully and thoroughly suctioned through an endotracheal tube under direct vision with a laryngoscope. Afterwards, appropriate and vigorous resuscitative measures should be undertaken to establish adequate ventilation and circulation. Artificial ventilation performed before tracheal suction could well force meconium into smaller airways.

76. The answer is D. *(Oski, 1979. pp 38-42.)* Periventricular-intraventricular hemorrhage is the most common type of intracranial hemorrhage in newborn infants; it occurs in approximately 45 percent of premature infants weighing less than 1500 g. Clinical manifestations occur 24 to 48 hours after a serious hypoxic episode. In contrast to previous beliefs, this type of hemorrhage is not uniformly catastrophic but, in fact, more commonly produces a more subtle neurologic deterioration. Systemic symptoms include an acute drop in hematocrit and arterial P_{O_2}. The lumbar puncture reveals bloody fluid and the CAT scan reveals a high-density cast of the ventricular system. In the more severely affected infants posthemorrhagic ventricular dilatation often occurs; prompt detection and careful follow-up via serial CAT scans are required to initiate appropriate therapy.

Newborn Infant 47

77. The answer is C. *(Vaughan, ed 11. pp 420-422.)* In a difficult delivery in which traction is applied to the head and neck, several injuries, including all those listed in the question, may occur. Erb-Duchenne paralysis affects the fifth and sixth cervical nerves; the affected arm cannot be abducted or externally rotated at the shoulder, and the forearm cannot be flexed or supinated. Injury to the seventh and eighth cervical and first thoracic nerves (Klumpke's paralysis) results in palsy of the hand and also can produce symptoms of Horner's syndrome. Fractures in the upper limb are not associated with a characteristic posture, and passive movement usually elicits pain. Spinal injury causes complete paralysis below the level of injury.

78. The answer is C. *(Vaughan, ed 11. pp 390, 392, 1690.)* Turner's syndrome is a genetic disorder characterized by a 45,XO karyotype. At birth affected infants have low weights, short stature, edema over the dorsum of the hands and feet, and loose skin folds at the nape of the neck. Coarse tremulous movements accompanied by ankle clonus; vascular instability as evidenced, for example, by a harlequin color change (a transient, longitudinal division of a body into red and pale halves); softness of parietal bones at the vertex (craniotabes); and a liver that is palpable down to 2 cm below the costal margins—all of these findings often are demonstrated by normal infants and are of no diagnostic significance in the clinical situation presented in the question.

79. The answer is C. *(Avery, p 902. Schaffer, ed 4. pp 968, 975-977.)* Subcutaneous fat necrosis is found in large infants who suffer a long or difficult labor and delivery. Lesions usually appear at about one week of age over cheeks and extensor surfaces. They vary in size, may be colorless or reddish-purple, and feel firm with a sharp border; in addition, they usually produce no symptoms and regress gradually over a period of weeks. Hypercalcemia may be present. The other diagnoses listed in the question have very different clinical appearances.

80. The answer is B. *(Klaus, ed 2. pp 354-356.)* The premature infant's red blood cell membranes are high in polyunsaturated fatty acids and low in glutathione and enzymes involved in the antioxidant system. Deficiency of vitamin E (tocopherol) increases their susceptibility to peroxidant activity with resulting cell leakage and hemolysis. The infants develop an anemia with reticulocytosis and thrombocytosis; the latter probably represents a nonspecific increase in bone marrow productivity. The susceptibility to peroxidation is aggravated by the administration of peroxidants, such as iron, and a diet high in polyunsaturates; in these circumstances even normal serum levels of tocopherol may not prevent hemolysis. Therefore, pharmacologic amounts of vitamin E should be given to premature infants to maintain high serum levels, and iron should not be administered before three to four weeks of age.

81. The answer is D. *(Avery, p 719.)* Ortolani's sign is the best clinical criterion for diagnosing congenital dislocation of the hip. As the hip of an affected infant is adducted in flexion with the knees fully flexed, the femoral head is dislocated; as the hip is abducted in the same position, a click is felt as the femoral head is lifted into the acetabulum. These movements are painless. Apparent shortening of the upper leg (Galeazzi's sign), limitation of hip abduction in flexion, and asymmetry of thigh skin folds are not present in newborn infants; these signs, which are secondary to migration of the femoral head laterally and superiorly, usually develop by six weeks of age if the dislocated hip is left untreated.

82. The answer is A. *(Klaus, ed 2. pp 195, 366.)* Apneic spells are characterized by an absence of respirations for more than 20 seconds or by bradycardia and cyanosis (or by both). Periods of apnea are thought to be secondary to an incompletely developed respiratory center and are associated most commonly with prematurity. Although seizures, hypoglycemia, and pulmonary disease accompanied by hypoxia all can lead to apnea, these etiologies are unlikely in the infant described, given that no unusual movements occur during the apneic spells, that the blood sugar level is more than 40 mg/100 ml, and that the child appears well between spells. Periodic breathing, a common pattern of respiration in low-birth-weight babies, is characterized by periods of rapid respiration, lasting 10 to 15 seconds, that alternate with periods of apnea, lasting 5 to 10 seconds.

83. The answer is C. *(Klaus, ed 2. pp 116, 120.)* On the average, a normal low-birth-weight infant requires a daily intake of 120 calories per kilogram of body weight in order to grow. Some infants, especially those whose intrauterine growth was retarded, may require 150 to 180 calories per kilogram per day for normal growth. Intake of commercial formulas necessary to satisfy these caloric requirements will provide about 4 g of protein per kilogram per day. Because they would need to drink a quart of formula daily in order to receive adequate amounts of vitamins, small infants, who could not possibly tolerate such a high intake, should receive vitamin supplements.

84. The answer is E. *(Vaughan, ed 11. p 455.)* If a mother has O-positive blood and her baby has A-positive blood, the baby has a 10 percent chance of developing hemolytic disease. Infants who have hemolytic disease due to a major blood-group incompatibility usually are only mildly affected; hyperbilirubinemia is the most frequent complication. The most characteristic laboratory finding is marked spherocytosis in the peripheral blood smear. Although the hematocrit of affected infants usually is normal, elevation of the reticulocyte count and the presence of nucleated red blood cells in the blood smear provide evidence of hemolysis. In contrast to hemolytic disease due to Rh incompatibility, major blood-group incompatibility frequently is associated with a direct Coombs' test that is only weakly positive.

85. The answer is B. *(Schaffer, ed 4. p 317.)* Hematemesis and melena are not uncommon in the neonatal period, especially if gross placental bleeding has occurred at the time of delivery. The diagnostic procedure that should be done first is the Apt test, which differentiates fetal from adult hemoglobin in a bloody specimen. If the blood in an affected infant's gastric contents or stool is maternal in origin, further workup of the infant is obviated.

86. The answer is B. *(Klaus, ed 2. p 184.)* For the child described in the question, prematurity and the clinical picture presented make the diagnosis of hyaline membrane disease all but inescapable. In this disease lung compliance is reduced to as much as 10 to 20 percent of normal; lung volume also is reduced and as much as a 30 to 60 percent right-to-left shunt of blood may be evident. Some of the shunt may result from a patent ductus arteriosus or foramen ovale, and some may be due to an abnormal ventilation-perfusion ratio in the lung. Minute ventilation is higher than normal and affected infants must work harder in order to sustain adequate breathing.

87. The answer is B. *(Klaus, ed 2. pp 177, 186-187, 206-207.)* Continuous positive airway pressure (CPAP) is believed to improve oxygenation by preventing alveolar collapse, thereby improving ventilation and diminishing the intrapulmonary right-to-left shunt. CPAP should be started when the arterial P_{O_2} cannot be maintained above 60 mm Hg without an ambient oxygen concentration greater than 70 percent. Once an affected infant is stabilized on CPAP, the inspired oxygen concentration can be lowered to a value that will maintain arterial P_{O_2} between 60 and 80 mm Hg. Because of the danger of oxygen toxicity to the lungs, concentrations of oxygen greater than 70 percent should, if possible, be avoided. The infant described in the question does not meet the criteria for mechanical ventilation; and because the child's arterial pH is well above 7.25, alkali therapy also is not indicated.

88. The answer is C. *(Klaus, ed 2. pp 176, 187.)* Infants whose gestational ages are less than 36 weeks are at risk for retrolental fibroplasia, especially if they are receiving oxygen therapy at an inspired oxygen concentration of greater than 40 percent and if their arterial P_{O_2} is above 80 mm Hg. Consequently, for the infant described in the question, the ambient oxygen concentration should be decreased as quickly as possible. This decrease can be best achieved by lowering the concentration by 10 percent every hour and monitoring arterial blood gases re-

peatedly. Decreasing the oxygen concentration more radically could provoke the "flip-flop" phenomenon in which the arterial P_{O_2} drops further than expected (when the concentration of inspired oxygen is lowered) and does not return to its previous level when the inspired oxygen is returned to its original higher concentration. Right-to-left shunting may be the cause of "flip-flop."

89. The answer is D. *(Vaughan, ed 11. pp 1041-1042.)* Abdominal distension, choking, the presence of excessive mucus in the oropharynx, and coughing associated with fluid intake all are symptoms of the congenital esophageal anomalies depicted in figures **A** and **D** accompanying the question. However, the anomaly illustrated by figure **D** is the most common and is most likely to produce severe symptoms of regurgitation early in the newborn period; the disorder depicted in figure **A** usually is diagnosed in older children who have repeated episodes of pneumonitis. The anomaly in figure **E** is associated with all of the symptoms of anomaly **D** except abdominal distension, which cannot develop because there is no way for air to enter the gastrointestinal tract. Figures **B** and **C** represent the least common anomalies; because the upper esophageal segment is connected directly to the trachea, massive entry of fluid into the lungs can occur.

90. The answer is B. *(Vaughan, ed 11. pp 1413-1414.)* Failure to give vitamin K prophylactically to newborn infants is associated with a decline in the levels of vitamin K-dependent coagulation factors. In less than 1 percent of infants (but especially those fed human breast milk), the levels reached are low enough to produce hemorrhagic manifestations on the second or third day of life. These manifestations usually include melena, hematuria, and bleeding from the navel; intracranial hemorrhage and hypovolemic shock are serious complications. Diagnosis of this condition is indicated by a prolonged prothrombin time, which reflects inadequate concentrations of factors II, VII, and X in an infant. There is no genetic predisposition to the disease.

91. The answer is D. *(Vaughan, ed 11. pp 936, 955-956, 1170, 1190.)* Newborn infants who are cyanotic at rest when their mouths are closed but become pink when they cry must be suspected of having blockage of both nares. Bilateral choanal atresia is the congenital malformation that most often causes this disturbance. Though some affected neonates are able to breathe by opening their mouths and therefore have respiratory difficulty only during feeding, others are unable to breathe at all through their mouths except during crying, and as a consequence may develop asphyxia severe enough to cause death. Infants who have respiratory obstruction below the pharynx (such as from laryngomalacia, a laryngeal web, or a double aortic arch that impinges on the trachea) are not aided by mouth-breathing; in addition, their condition usually deteriorates with the stress of crying. Deviation of the nasal septum is most commonly an acquired condition that almost never occurs in infants.

92. The answer is A. *(Forfar, Clin Pharm Ther 14:639-641, 1973. Klaus, ed 2. pp 49-50.)* The effect of a drug on the fetus is determined not only by the nature of the drug but also by the timing and severity of exposure in utero. Heparin, insulin, and chloramphenicol have not been shown to produce deleterious effects on the fetus at any time during pregnancy. Hydantoin can produce growth and mental retardation as well as dysmorphic features when given for prolonged periods starting early in pregnancy. When given in the last few weeks of pregnancy, the thiazides produce neonatal thrombocytopenia, which resolves after the newborn infant excretes the transplacentally acquired drug.

93. The answer is D. *(Schaffer, ed 4. pp 86, 352-359.)* The finding of hydramnios can signal the presence in a neonate of high intestinal obstruction, signs of which include abdominal distension and early and repeated regurgitation of intestinal contents. Distension may not be present if the obstruction is very high or if the constant vomiting keeps the intestine decompressed. Because the presence of bile-stained fluid in the vomitus of the infant described in the question places the possible obstruction distal to the ampulla of Vater, esophageal atresia and pyloric stenosis are ruled out. The "double bubble" sign on the accompanying x-ray is characteristic of duodenal atresia, which also is compatible with the infant's history. Midgut volvulus, which usually obstructs the bowel in the area of the duodenojejunal junction, most often produces signs after an affected infant is three or four days old; in addition, several loops of small bowel are typically seen on x-ray. Gastric duplication does not usually produce intestinal obstruction; a cystic mass may be palpated on abdominal examination.

94. The answer is A. *(Klaus, ed 2. pp 27, 30, 382-384.)* The pregnancy of the woman described in the question is considered high-risk by virtue of her history of abortions and the premature onset of labor. The woman's infant will very likely require neonatal intensive care. Statistics show that the mortality rate for low-birth-weight infants is lowest if they are born in centers having facilities for perinatal intensive care (one-third of all deaths of premature infants occur within 24 hours of birth). For this reason, and because a mother's womb is thought to be the best "transport incubator" available, the woman described should be transferred to the referral perinatal center immediately (i.e., before the birth of her child).

95. The answer is D. *(Klaus, ed 2. pp 332-334.)* Nearly three-fourths of abdominal masses in newborn infants involve and stem from the kidney. In the infant described in the question, the presence both of a mass in the flank and of gross hematuria further indicates a renal lesion. A mass not present at birth but discovered at 20 hours of age suggests sudden enlargement of a kidney; this finding makes the diagnosis of renal vein thrombosis most likely in the infant described. Also in support of this diagnosis are the child's pallor and clinical illness and the fact that the mother is diabetic. Evaluation of the infant should include an intravenous pyelogram, coagulation studies, and measurement of the serum creatinine, blood gases, urea nitrogen, and electrolytes.

96. The answer is B. *(Klaus, ed 2. pp 136-137.)* The early clinical signs of neonatal necrotizing enterocolitis include gastric distension, retention of gastric contents between feedings, and the passage of blood-streaked stools. This disorder usually occurs in premature infants who, because of cardiovascular shock or hypoxia (often associated with severe hyaline membrane disease), have had their blood supply preferentially shunted away from the gut to the heart and brain. Intestinal ischemia and invasion of affected bowel by enteric flora are thought to be the two major pathogenetic processes involved in necrotizing enterocolitis. Hypertonic feeding is also believed to play a role. No relationship exists between necrotizing enterocolitis and the meconium plug syndrome, calcium therapy, or maternal bowel disease.

97. The answer is D. *(Klaus, ed 2. p 138.)* If the diagnosis in a neonate of necrotizing enterocolitis either is strongly entertained or is confirmed by finding pneumatosis intestinalis on abdominal x-ray, therapy should consist of gastric drainage, discontinuance of oral feedings, administration of oral and systemic antibiotics, and vigorous administration of intravenous fluids that include vascular volume expanders, as needed, and as high a caloric content as possible. Because bowel perforation, a serious complication, occurs frequently, signs of acute deterioration must be watched for very carefully. Only if intestinal infarction or perforation is believed to be present is surgical intervention generally advocated. Steroids are not a recommended treatment for this disease.

98. The answer is C. *(Behrman, ed 2. pp 741-745.)* Serum magnesium and calcium levels are both affected by a number of factors including parathyroid function and vitamin D and phosphorus levels. Although hypocalcemia is not always accompanied by hypomagnesemia, infants who have hypomagnesemia almost always have hypocalcemia, too. Low serum magnesium interferes with calcium homeostasis by causing failure of parathyroid hormone release and function. Hypocalcemia associated with hypomagnesemia can be corrected by the administration of magnesium alone; calcium administration is of no corrective value. Hypocalcemia usually is associated with high serum phosphorus levels. Alkalosis is likely to precipitate symptoms in hypocalcemic individuals by decreasing the amount of calcium that is ionized; it does not affect the total calcium level. Zinc and potassium levels also are not related to hypocalcemia.

Newborn Infant 53

99. The answer is D. *(Vaughan, ed 11. pp 1027-1028.)* The infant pictured in the question has an obvious bilateral cleft lip and palate. This defect occurs in 4 to 7 percent of the siblings of affected infants; its incidence in the general population, on the other hand, is 1 in 1000. Although affected infants are likely to have feeding problems initially, these problems usually can be overcome by feeding in a propped-up position and using special nipples. Complications include recurrent otitis media and hearing loss as well as speech defects, which may be present in spite of good anatomic closure. Repair of a cleft lip usually is performed within the first two months of life; the palate is repaired later, usually between the ages of six months and five years.

100. The answer is B (1, 3). *(Klaus, ed 2. p 248. Vaughan, ed 11. pp 191-193.)* Human breast milk is fresh, sterile, and always at the right temperature. It is easily digestible, is associated with fewer gastrointestinal disturbances than cow's milk, produces no allergic manifestations, and contains several factors, including antibodies, that are believed to provide protection from infection. However, breast-feeding may be associated with a higher incidence of physiologic jaundice than bottle-feeding. In less than 3 percent of infants, human milk gives rise to significant unconjugated hyperbilirubinemia, which is believed to be caused by a factor in the milk that inhibits conjugation. A brief cessation of breast-feeding is almost always the only treatment necessary. No significant difference in emotional well-being appears to exist between well-nurtured breast-fed and bottle-fed infants.

101. The answer is A (1, 2, 3). *(Vaughan, ed 11. p 1738.)* Normal term neonates demonstrate a large number of reflex patterns that are mediated by the brain stem or spinal cord. These reactions include the Moro (startle) reflex; the sucking and rooting reflexes; the stepping reflex, by which movements of forward progression are elicited on a flat surface; the placing reflex, which produces leg flexion; and the palmar and plantar grasps, which result from slight pressure on the palms and soles. The parachute reaction, which is extension of the arms and hands that occurs when an infant in the prone position is brought sharply towards a firm surface, does not appear until the age of nine months.

102. The answer is E (all). *(Vaughan, ed 11. pp 462-463.)* Infants born to narcotic addicts are more likely than other children to exhibit a variety of problems, including perinatal complications, prematurity, and low birth weight. The onset of withdrawal symptoms commonly occurs during an infant's first two days of life. The most characteristic symptoms in these infants are hyperirritability and coarse tremors. Other symptoms include vomiting, diarrhea, fever, high-pitched cry, and hyperventilation; seizures, respiratory depression, and other symptoms are less common.

103. The answer is C (2, 4). *(Avery, pp 133-135.)* Infants born at 33 weeks gestation are covered with vernix and have smooth skin and fine wooly hair. They have no breast tissue, and because ear cartilage is scant, ears recoil slowly when folded. There are one or two anterior sole creases, and in the female the clitoris is readily visible between widely separated labia majora. At rest, the arms are extended and the hips flexed. There is some resistance in bringing the heel to the ear, and the elbow passes the midline but does not reach to the opposite shoulder. Although sucking, rooting, and the grasp and Moro reflexes are all present, they are not fully developed.

104. The answer is B (1, 3). *(Schaffer, ed 4. pp 694-696.)* On the skull of a newborn infant, a swelling that is sharply demarcated by the margins of one particular bone typically indicates a cephalhematoma. It is reported in 1.5 to 2.5 percent of births, especially those associated with obstetric difficulty at the outlet. Systematic study has shown that 5.4 percent of cephalhematomas are accompanied by a linear skull fracture. The majority of these swellings resorb spontaneously within a few weeks; a few, however, become calcified and persist for a few months as prominent lumps on the head. No treatment is needed in either event. Needle aspiration is contraindicated because of the possibility of introducing infection. Anemia may be found in infants who have very large hematomas.

105. The answer is E (all). *(Klaus, ed 2. pp 154-155.)* Studies in the last ten years have shown several benefits of early close contact between mothers and their newborn infants. The mothers show more affectionate behavior toward their infants and use more descriptive words and questions when talking to them than mothers who have less or late contact with their infants. In the early close contact group there were fewer divorces and mothering disorders, including child abuse, neglect, and abandonment. The infants smiled more, cried less, and in one study were shown to have higher IQs than infants who had late or less contact with their mothers. Breast-feeding was also prolonged in close-early-contact group.

106. The answer is A (1, 2, 3). *(Behrman, ed 2. pp 682-685.)* Phenylketonuria is an autosomal recessive disease that leads to mental and motor retardation in untreated infants. Affected infants appear normal during the perinatal period; clinical signs of the retardation of brain development may first appear at the age of four months. The primary defect is an inability to synthesize tyrosine from phenylalanine, which, as a result, accumulates in the plasma. Phenylpyruvic acid, a metabolite of phenylalanine, is excreted in the urine by older children but not neonates. When the plasma phenylalanine level is 20 mg/100 ml or higher, dietary restriction of this amino acid is indicated.

107. The answer is B (1, 3). *(Avery, pp 984-985.)* Retinoblastomas either occur sporadically or are transmitted as autosomal dominant traits with 80 percent penetrance. They usually are detected at about 18 months of age; in high-risk cases, however, the diagnosis may be made in the neonatal period with careful indirect ophthalmoscopy. The clinical signs of retinoblastoma include leukokoria, strabismus, and ocular phthisis; bilateral involvement occurs in one-third of cases of sporadically occurring retinoblastoma and more frequently in association with the familial variety. The mortality rate among untreated children is almost 100 percent, but among treated children it drops to 25 percent.

108. The answer is B (1, 3). *(Vaughan, ed 11. p 448.)* The presence of anemia must not be overlooked in infants who have hemolytic disease and are being treated for hyperbilirubinemia with, for example, phototherapy. Once phototherapy is started, the skin color of affected infants can no longer be relied upon in an assessment of either jaundice or pallor; similarly, scleral icterus is an unreliable indicator of the degree of hyperbilirubinemia.

109. The answer is E (all). *(Klaus, ed 2. pp 250-252.)* Factors that reduce the amount of unconjugated bilirubin bound to albumin (and therefore cause an increase in free unconjugated bilirubin) increase the risk of kernicterus. Among these factors are the following: hypoalbuminemia; acidosis, which decreases the affinity of bilirubin for albumin; and certain drugs (e.g., salicylates and sulfonamides) and other compounds (such as nonesterified fatty acids, which are elevated during cold stress) that as anions compete with bilirubin for albumin binding sites. Acidosis and hypoxia also are believed to increase brain-cell susceptibility to bilirubin toxicity.

110. The answer is B (1, 3). *(Klaus, ed 2. pp 231-234.)* Because of active transport, calcium stores accumulate in a fetus during the third trimester regardless of the maternal nutritional state. Breast-fed infants have higher calcium and lower phosphorus levels than bottle-fed infants due to the higher calcium:phosphorus ratio in breast milk as compared to cow's milk. Stress associated with asphyxia or a difficult labor or delivery may cause elevations in calcitonin and glucocorticoids, which in turn may cause symptomatic hypocalcemia. The incidence of hypocalcemia is higher than normal among premature infants and infants of diabetic mothers due to immaturity of the parathyroid.

111. The answer is A (1, 2, 3). *(Vaughan, ed 11. pp 1140-1141.)* Severe respiratory distress that is present from birth in an infant who has a scaphoid abdomen suggests the presence of a diaphragmatic hernia. Breath sounds are absent on the affected side of the chest, and the heart sounds are displaced to the unaffected side. A chest x-ray showing intestinal loops in the chest (usually on the left side) and displacement of the mediastinum to the unaffected side is diagnostic of diaphragmatic hernia. Definitive treatment is surgical and must be carried out on an emergency basis. Before surgery, however, affected infants must be resuscitated as effectively as possible. A nasogastric tube with intermittent suction should be placed to minimize the accumulation of air in the herniated intestine. If positive pressure ventilation is required, it should be used with caution in order to avoid a pneumothorax in lungs that are being unevenly ventilated. Metabolic acidosis should be corrected promptly.

112. The answer is D (4). *(Avery, pp 255-263.)* Both pulmonary dysmaturity (Wilson-Mikity syndrome) and bronchopulmonary dysplasia are chronic lung diseases of newborn infants. On chest x-ray both produce evidence of generalized cystic changes, which later resolve into hyperlucency at the lung bases. Bronchopulmonary dysplasia is thought to be due to oxygen toxicity and respiratory therapy; pathologic examination of lung tissue from affected individuals yields distinct evidence of damage to alveolar and bronchiolar epithelium with subsequent bronchiolar metaplasia and peribronchial and interstitial fibrosis. The eitology of Wilson-Mikity syndrome is unknown, and the disease is not associated with characteristic pathologic findings. Infants who have bronchopulmonary dysplasia develop symptoms after exposure to high concentrations of oxygen used as a treatment for hyaline membrane disease or other illnesses. Infants who have Wilson-Mikity syndrome are usually quite premature and appear well until the onset of symptoms, which occurs at the end of the first week.

113. The answer is A (1, 2, 3). *(Vaughan, ed 11. pp 441-442.)* Meconium ileus occurs among newborn infants who have cystic fibrosis, because the absence in these infants of normal pancreatic enzymes makes their meconium abnormally tenacious. Affected neonates present with signs of intestinal obstruction, and numerous, doughy masses of intestine are palpable throughout the abdomen; no discoloration of the abdominal wall occurs. Plain films of the abdomen characteristically show unevenly dilated loops of bowel that, because of a mixture of meconium and air, appear granular. Meconium ileus is often fatal.

114. The answer is C (2, 4). *(Klaus, ed 2. p 71. Vaughan, ed 11. p 403.)* Twin pregnancies are associated with a fourfold increase in perinatal mortality as compared to single pregnancies; this increase is particularly notable among monochorionic twins. As a rule, the mortality rate is the same for first- and second-born twins. Twins are likely to be born prematurely, and if born after 35 weeks gestation, they are likely to be small for dates. Monoamniotic twins have an increased incidence of asphyxia because of the greater likelihood of cord entanglement. Twin pregnancies also have an increased incidence of severe congenital malformations, bleeding during labor, and twin-to-twin transfusions as well as maternal complications.

115. The answer is A (1, 2, 3). *(Behrman, ed 2. p 352. Schaffer, ed 4. pp 623-625.)* Twin-to-twin transfusion occurs in about 15 percent of monochorionic twins and commonly causes intrauterine death. This disorder should be suspected when the hematocrits of twins differ by more than 15 percent units (e.g., 45% and 61%). The donor twin is likely to have oligohydramnios, anemia, and hypovolemia with evidence of shock; the recipient twin is likely to have hydramnios and plethora and to be larger than the donor twin. As the central venous hematocrit rises above 65 percent, blood viscosity increases exponentially, putting affected infants at risk for several complications, including respiratory distress, hyperbilirubinemia, hypoglycemia, hypocalcemia, renal vein thrombosis, cyanosis, congestive heart failure, and convulsions.

116. The answer is B (1, 3). *(Klaus, ed 2. pp 228-229. Vaughan, ed 11. pp 464-467.)* Infants of diabetic mothers have a very rapid drop in blood glucose levels after delivery and are often hypoglycemic within six hours of birth. Hyperinsulinism, either alone or in combination with diminished epinephrine and glucagon responses, is believed to be the major cause of the hypoglycemia, macrosomia, and other metabolic abnormalities seen in these infants. Hypoglycemia in infants of diabetic mothers is less frequently symptomatic than in small-for-dates infants. Hypoglycemia is best prevented by frequent blood sugar monitoring and early feeding of affected infants. If necessary, a constant intravenous infusion of a 10% to 15% glucose solution may be given. Rapid infusion of glucose at high concentrations may result in rebound hypoglycemia after initial hyperglycemia.

117. The answer is E (all). *(Klaus, ed 2. pp 195-196, 198.)* Apnea secondary to abnormalities such as hypoglycemia, sepsis, or anemia should be managed by treating the underlying cause. Idiopathic apnea itself requires therapy, because untreated, it can lead to death or anoxic brain damage. The several methods used include (1) increased vestibular, cutaneous, or proprioceptive stimulation; (2) low (2 to 4 cm H_2O) nasal continuous positive airway pressure; (3) intravenous or oral theophylline; (4) increased inspired oxygen to maintain arterial P_{O_2} between 50 and 60 mm Hg; and (5) artificial ventilation.

118-121. The answers are: 118-B, 119-C, 120-E, 121-A. *(Vaughan, ed 11. pp 443-444.)* In premature infants who have physiologic jaundice (curve **B**), serum bilirubin levels reach a peak of 8 to 12 mg/100 ml at five to seven days of age; jaundice disappears after the tenth day of life. Physiologic jaundice in full-term neonates (curve **D**), on the other hand, appears at two to three days of age; peak bilirubin levels of about 5 to 6 mg/100 ml appear at two to four days of age. Bilirubin levels drop below 2 mg/100 ml within a few days.

Jaundice in infants who have hypothyroidism (curve **E**) initially appears to be physiologic. However, jaundice associated with these infants (as well as infants who have pyloric stenosis) can persist for several weeks.

In neonates born with erythroblastosis fetalis (curve A), jaundice is apparent in the first 24 hours of life. Bilirubin accumulates rapidly, reaching a peak level (up to 20 mg/100 ml) that varies with the degree of hemolysis. The duration of jaundice is also dependent on the severity of the disease.

Curve C on the graph presented is compatible with a diagnosis of septicemia. In this disorder jaundice appears between the fourth and seventh days of life; as the infection is treated, bilirubin levels return to normal.

122-125. The answers are: 122-C, 123-A, 124-B, 125-B. *(Smith, ed 2. pp 124-125. Vaughan, ed 11. pp 1447, 1764-1765.)* Sporadic aniridia is found in 1 to 2 percent of children with Wilms' tumor. Genitourinary anomalies and hemihypertrophy are associated with this tumor in 13 percent of patients.

Waardenburg's syndrome is inherited as an autosomal dominant trait with variable penetrance. It includes, in decreasing order of frequency, the following anomalies: lateral displacement of the medial canthi; broad nasal bridge; medial hyperplasia of the eyebrows; partial albinism commonly expressed by a white forelock or heterochromia (or both); and deafness in 20 percent of cases.

A flat capillary hemangioma in the distribution of the trigeminal nerve is the basic lesion in the Sturge-Weber syndrome. The malformation also involves the meninges and results in anoxic damage to the underlying cerebral cortex. The damage is manifested clinically by grand mal seizures, mental deficiency, and hemiparesis or hemianopia on the contralateral side. The etiology is unknown.

Infants who have tuberous sclerosis often are born with hypopigmented oval or irregularly shaped skin macules. Cerebral sclerotic tubers are also present from birth and become visible radiographically during the second year of life. Myoclonic seizures, present in infancy, may convert to grand mal seizures later in childhood. Adenoma sebaceum appears at two to five years of age. The disease, which also affects the eyes, kidneys, heart, bones, and lungs, is inherited as an autosomal dominant trait with variable expression; new mutations are very common.

The Cardiovascular System

Harvey L. Chernoff

DIRECTIONS: Each question below contains five suggested answers. Choose the **one best** response to each question.

126. A four-year-old child presents with a grade III/VI ejection systolic murmur over the pulmonic area. The pulmonic component of the second sound is accentuated. Electrocardiography reveals right ventricular hypertrophy, and chest x-rays show normal pulmonary vascular markings with mild prominence of the pulmonary artery segment. The most likely diagnosis is

(A) atrial septal defect
(B) partial anomalous pulmonary venous return
(C) valvular pulmonic stenosis
(D) supravalvular pulmonic stenosis
(E) none of the above

127. The presence of endocardial cushion defects is most likely to be associated with

(A) Turner's syndrome
(B) Noonan's syndrome
(C) Down's syndrome
(D) Marfan's syndrome
(E) Hunter-Hurler syndrome

128. A three-day-old infant has had progressively deepening cyanosis since birth but no respiratory distress. Chest radiography demonstrates no cardiomegaly and normal pulmonary vasculature. An electrocardiogram shows an axis of 120 degrees and right ventricular prominence. The congenital cardiac malformation most likely responsible for the cyanosis is

(A) tetralogy of Fallot
(B) transposition of the great vessels
(C) tricuspid atresia
(D) total anomalous pulmonary venous return below the diaphragm
(E) pulmonary atresia with intact ventricular septum

129. A four-year-old girl is brought to the pediatrician's office. Her father reports that she suddenly became pale and stopped running while he had been playfully chasing her. During play she had been very excited, laughing to the point at which "she almost lost her breath." After 30 minutes, she was no longer pale and wanted to resume the game. She has never had a previous episode nor ever been cyanotic. Her physical examination was normal as were her chest x-ray and echocardiogram. An electrocardiogram showed the patterns seen in figures A and B below. The most likely cause of the episode is

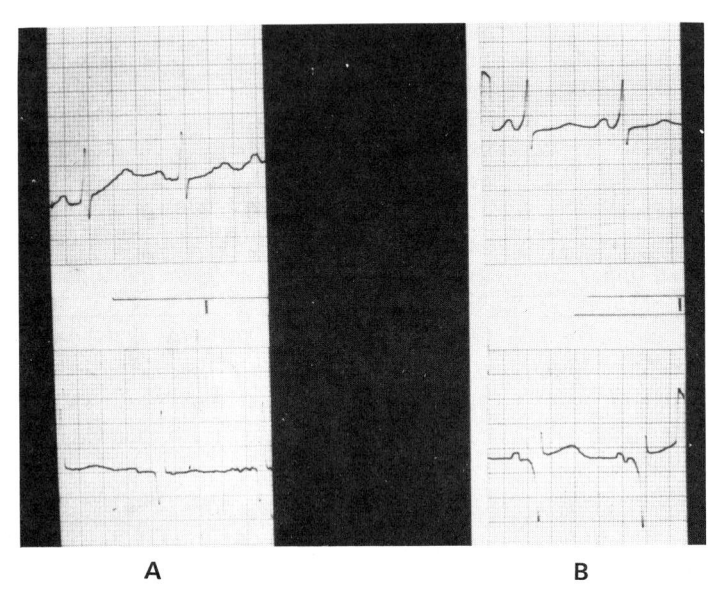

A   B

(A) paroxysmal ventricular tachycardia
(B) paroxysmal supraventricular tachycardia
(C) Wolff-Parkinson-White syndrome
(D) an unsuspected congenital heart defect
(E) excessive stress during play

130. A child has a history of spiking fevers, which have been as high as 40°C (104°F). She has spindle-shaped swelling of finger joints and complains of upper sternal pain. She had streptococcal pharyngitis two weeks before her fevers began. The most likely diagnosis is

(A) rheumatic fever
(B) rheumatoid arthritis
(C) toxic synovitis
(D) septic arthritis
(E) osteoarthritis

131. Examination of a newborn infant reveals a heart rate of 60 beats per minute. At no time during the next three days does the rate rise above 68 beats per minute. Electrocardiography would be most likely to demonstrate

(A) second-degree atrioventricular block
(B) complete atrioventricular block
(C) complete atrioventricular block and atrial fibrillation
(D) sinus arrest with an idioventricular rhythm
(E) sinus bradycardia

132. The major electrocardiographic abnormality in children who have ostium primum atrial septal defects (endocardial cushion defects) is

(A) right axis deviation
(B) left axis deviation
(C) incomplete right bundle-branch block
(D) first-degree atrioventricular block
(E) second-degree atrioventricular block

133. A two-year-old child with minimal cyanosis has a quadruple rhythm, a systolic ejection murmur in the pulmonic area, and a pansystolic murmur along the lower left sternal border. An electrocardiogram is obtained and shows P pulmonale and a ventricular block pattern in the right chest leads. The child most likely has

(A) tricuspid regurgitation and pulmonic stenosis
(B) pulmonic stenosis and a ventricular septal defect (tetralogy of Fallot)
(C) an atrioventricular canal
(D) Ebstein's anomaly
(E) Wolff-Parkinson-White syndrome

134. A child with an atrial septal defect has an accentuated pulmonic closure sound; electrocardiography shows right ventricular hypertrophy. These findings suggest that the child most likely has

(A) valvular pulmonic stenosis
(B) infundibular pulmonic stenosis
(C) pulmonary hypertension
(D) congestive heart failure
(E) pulmonic regurgitation

135. Congestive heart failure due to congenital heart disease is encountered most frequently in which of the following age groups?

(A) Less than six months of age
(B) Six to twelve months of age
(C) One to five years of age
(D) Six to fifteen years of age
(E) Sixteen to twenty-one years of age

136. A five-year-old boy presents with a grade V/VI harsh ejection systolic murmur in the second interspace at the right sternal border. The murmur radiates to the neck and upper left sternal border. The right brachial pulse is brisk, the left diminished. Blood pressures are right arm 110/60 mm Hg, left arm 100/60 mm Hg, and right leg 120/60 mm Hg. He has a small chin, full lips, open mouth, upturned nose, and wide-set eyes. An electrocardiogram shows left ventricular hypertrophy. The most likely defect would be

(A) bicuspid aortic valve
(B) valvular aortic stenosis
(C) discrete subvalvular aortic stenosis
(D) supravalvular aortic stenosis
(E) aortic coarctation

137. The most common congenital heart lesion is

(A) pulmonic stenosis
(B) patent ductus arteriosus
(C) atrial septal defect
(D) ventricular septal defect
(E) tetralogy of Fallot

138. A neonate born at term presents in the first day of life with cyanosis and progressive dyspnea. A chest x-ray reveals a heart of normal size but a significant increase in pulmonary vascular and interstitial markings. This infant most likely is suffering from

(A) transposition of the great vessels
(B) infracardiac total anomalous pulmonary venous return
(C) pulmonic atresia
(D) hyaline membrane disease
(E) mitral stenosis

139. A three-year-old child has had two episodes of syncope. On examination, blood pressure is normal in the arms and legs; no murmurs are heard. Prior neurologic evaluation revealed no neurologic abnormalities. The study most likely to aid in diagnosing this child's condition would be

(A) electrocardiography
(B) vectorcardiography
(C) echocardiography
(D) isotope angiography
(E) cardiac catheterization

140. Individuals who have chronic hypoxia have an increased hematocrit. Although the precise metabolic pathways are not yet clear, most authorities attribute the stimulation of red blood cell production to release of erythropoietin by the

(A) spleen
(B) liver
(C) kidneys
(D) bone marrow
(E) lungs

141. A newborn infant has mild cyanosis, diaphoresis, poor peripheral pulses, hepatomegaly, and cardiomegaly. Respiratory rate is 60 per minute, and heart rate is 230 per minute. The child most likely has congestive heart failure due to

(A) a large atrial septal defect and valvular pulmonic stenosis
(B) a ventricular septal defect and transposition of the great vessels
(C) atrial flutter and partial atrioventricular block
(D) hypoplastic left heart syndrome
(E) paroxysmal atrial tachycardia

142. The agent most frequently employed in preventing the recurrence of paroxysmal supraventricular tachycardia is

(A) propranolol
(B) quinidine
(C) procainamide
(D) digitalis
(E) diphenylhydantoin

143. A newborn infant has a history of occasional cyanosis. On examination, a grade III/VI harsh pansystolic (holosystolic) murmur is heard along the lower left sternal border. Radiography of the chest shows a normal cardiothoracic ratio, normal pulmonary vascular markings, and a right aortic arch. The most likely diagnosis is

(A) a ventricular septal defect
(B) a ventricular septal defect and transposition of the great vessels
(C) tetralogy of Fallot
(D) truncus arteriosus
(E) anomalous pulmonary venous return

144. Of the combined ventricular output of a normal fetal heart, the placenta receives about 45 percent and the fetal lungs only about 8 percent. This distribution is determined primarily by which of the following factors in a fetus?

(A) P_{O_2}
(B) P_{CO_2}
(C) pH
(D) Blood pressure
(E) Vascular resistance

145. A two-year-old boy is brought into the emergency room with a complaint of fever for six days and development of a limp. On examination he is found to have mild erythematous macular exanthem over his body, ocular conjunctivitis, dry, cracked lips, a red throat, and considerable cervical lymphadenopathy. The skin around his fingernails is peeling. There is a grade II/VI vibratory systolic ejection murmur at the lower left sternal border. He refuses to bear weight on his left leg. On questioning, his mother relates that a cousin who visited a week earlier had been taking penicillin for a sore throat. A white blood cell count and differential show predominantly neutrophils with increased platelets on smear and a sedimentation rate of 100 mm.

The most likely diagnosis of this boy's condition is

(A) scarlet fever
(B) rheumatic fever
(C) Kawasaki disease
(D) juvenile rheumatoid arthritis
(E) infectious mononucleosis

146. Pulmonary vascular resistance in an infant begins to diminish rapidly following delivery. This physiologic change is thought to be regulated primarily by

(A) a rise in arterial P_{O_2}
(B) a decrease in intrathoracic pressure
(C) a reduction in the tortuosity of the pulmonary vasculature
(D) closure of the ductus arteriosus
(E) release of humoral factors after cessation of placental circulation

147. A three-month-old infant has a history of short episodes during feeding of apparent abdominal pain associated with diaphoresis, duskiness, and rapid pulse and breathing. A pansystolic murmur that was not present when the child was examined two months earlier is heard over the cardiac apex. Which of the following studies would be most likely to aid in reaching the correct diagnosis?

(A) Chest x-ray
(B) Angiocardiography
(C) Electrocardiography
(D) Phonocardiography
(E) Dye dilution study

148. An eight-month-old infant has a one-week history of increasing shortness of breath and fatigue. Examination of the infant reveals evidence of severe congestive heart failure; radiography of the chest shows marked cardiomegaly, and electrocardiography reveals left ventricular hypertrophy with negative T waves in the left chest leads. No other physical abnormalities are noted.

The most likely diagnosis for this child is

(A) an aberrant left coronary artery
(B) idiopathic hypertrophic subaortic stenosis
(C) Pompe's disease (glycogen storage disease, type II)
(D) acute myocarditis
(E) endocardial fibroelastosis

149. A child presents with tall stature, long fingers and toes, and scoliosis. Cardiac examination would be most likely to demonstrate

(A) aortic stenosis
(B) mitral stenosis
(C) mitral regurgitation
(D) pulmonary incompetence
(E) none of the above

150. A three-day-old infant has developed tachypnea and tachycardia. Initial examination shows hepatomegaly, cardiomegaly, and peripheral pulses present in the upper extremities and the femoral arteries. A few hours later, however, the pulses in the femoral arteries have disappeared. The infant is minimally cyanotic. The most likely diagnosis is congestive heart failure, patent ductus arteriosus, and

(A) postductal aortic coarctation
(B) preductal aortic coarctation
(C) ventricular septal defect
(D) tetralogy of Fallot
(E) none of the above

151. A five-day old infant presents with rapid respiration, wheezing, and stridor; in addition, the child has gagged on occasion while being fed. During the physical examination the child becomes agitated and develops marked retractions. The noninvasive procedure most likely to provide a definitive diagnosis would be

(A) electrocardiography
(B) vectorcardiography
(C) M-mode echocardiography
(D) sector-scan echocardiography
(E) esophagography

152. A two-day-old infant is in congestive heart failure. Cardiac catheterization and angiography reveal a hypoplastic left ventricle and aortic atresia. Which of the following statements about this child is true?
(A) Aortic valvuloplasty, if performed early, will be of help
(B) The child's condition should improve dramatically with treatment of the congestive heart failure
(C) Digitalization should be an effective medical treatment
(D) The child is unlikely to benefit from surgery
(E) The average survival time of infants like the one described is two months

153. A three-month-old child has a pansystolic murmur along the lower left sternal border. Chest x-ray shows a mild increase in pulmonary vascular markings as well as in left atrial size. Electrocardiography suggests mild left ventricular hypertrophy. These findings persist during the first year of life; when the child, who is in good health, is examined at 18 months of age, a continuous murmur is heard along the left sternal border. Radiographic and electrocardiographic findings remain unchanged.
  This child most likely has a
(A) patent ductus arteriosus
(B) coronary arteriovenous fistula
(C) ventricular septal defect with mitral insufficiency
(D) ventricular septal defect with aortic insufficiency
(E) ventricular septal defect with rupture of an aneurysmal sinus of Valsalva

154. Electrocardiography of a cyanotic two-day-old infant shows a suggestion of right ventricular enlargement. The child's chest x-ray is presented below. The most likely diagnosis is

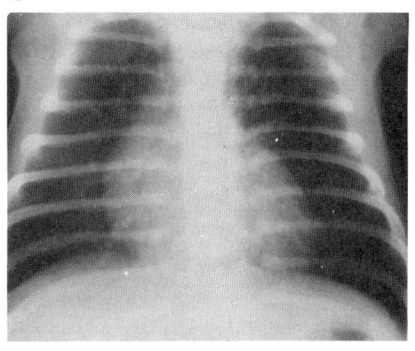

(A) tetralogy of Fallot
(B) transposition of the great vessels
(C) tricuspid atresia
(D) pulmonic valve atresia
(E) Ebstein's anomaly

155. In an infant the major clinical manifestation of digitalis toxicity would be
(A) headache
(B) dizziness
(C) vomiting
(D) visual disturbances
(E) anorexia

156. A 15-year-old girl of short stature who has neck webbing and sexual infantilism is found to have coarctation of the aorta. The most likely diagnosis is
(A) Marfan's syndrome
(B) Down's syndrome
(C) Turner's syndrome
(D) Ellis-van Creveld syndrome
(E) an unrelated group of findings

DIRECTIONS: Each question below contains four suggested answers of which **one** or **more** is correct. Choose the answer:

A	if	1, 2, and 3	are correct
B	if	1 and 3	are correct
C	if	2 and 4	are correct
D	if	4	is correct
E	if	1, 2, 3, and 4	are correct

157. Maldevelopment of the endocardial cushions may result in

(1) an atrial septal defect
(2) a ventricular septal defect
(3) deformity of the mitral valve
(4) deformity of the tricuspid valve

158. Cardiac catheterization shows that a child has a partial anomalous pulmonary venous return to the right atrium with an intact atrial septum. Pulmonary artery and right ventricular pressures are not elevated. Physical examination might be expected to reveal

(1) pulmonic ejection systolic murmur
(2) fixed wide splitting of the second heart sound
(3) right ventricular heave
(4) accentuated pulmonic valve closure sound (P_2)

159. A cyanotic 20-month-old child has a continuous murmur over the precordium and over the back. The child is in no visible distress. This clinical picture can be associated with which of the following disorders?

(1) Truncus arteriosus
(2) Total anomalous pulmonary venous return
(3) Tetralogy of Fallot
(4) Patent ductus arteriosus

160. A newborn infant weighing 2000 g (4 lb, 6 oz) presents with cyanosis; there is no evidence of respiratory distress. Cardiac catheterization reveals pulmonic valve atresia and pulmonary flow that derives from the aorta through a patent ductus arteriosus. Maintenance of adequate pulmonary blood flow may be achieved by

(1) aorticopulmonary anastomosis
(2) administration of E-type prostaglandins
(3) formalin infiltration of the ductus arteriosus
(4) pulmonary valvotomy

161. At birth the transition from fetal to extrauterine circulation is associated with a rapid decrease in pulmonary arterial resistance due to

(1) increased oxygen tension producing pulmonary arterial vasodilation
(2) increased oxygen tension stimulating closure of the ductus arteriosus
(3) initial inspiration producing inflation of the lungs
(4) closure of the foramen ovale, producing increased right heart and, therefore, pulmonary arterial blood volume

162. A newborn infant of a diabetic mother presents with signs of congestive heart failure. Laboratory analysis is likely to reveal

(1) hypoglycemia
(2) hyperbilirubinemia
(3) hypocalcemia
(4) anemia

163. Which of the following manifestations of acute rheumatic fever can be relieved by salicylate or steroid therapy?

(1) Carditis
(2) Abdominal pain
(3) Arthritis
(4) Chorea

164. An eight-year-old boy is brought into the hospital with a complaint of a seizure which occurred while chasing a friend. There is a history of recent onset of fatigue and heavier breathing than peers during play. On examination he is thin, in no distress, and without cyanosis, clubbing, edema, thrills, or murmurs. The pulmonic second sound is mildly accentuated. Neurologic examination reveals no abnormalities except for a mild hearing deficit. Further evaluation should be directed toward ruling out the possibility of

(1) long Q-T syndrome
(2) aortic stenosis
(3) primary pulmonary hypertension
(4) paroxysmal atrial tachycardia

165. The hypoplastic left-heart syndrome describes a group of left-sided lesions that can result in underdevelopment of the left ventricle. Among these left-sided lesions may be included

(1) aortic atresia
(2) hypoplasia of the aortic arch
(3) mitral atresia
(4) endocardial fibroelastosis

166. Which of the following lesions, when combined with a ventricular septal defect, frequently can cause cardiac decompensation in newborn infants?

(1) Preductal aortic coarctation
(2) Postductal aortic coarctation
(3) Patent ductus arteriosus
(4) Tetralogy of Fallot

167. A three-year-old boy, who otherwise appears well, presents with a history of pallor and a heart rate that has been persistently rapid for the last 30 minutes. Examination reveals a pansystolic murmur along the lower left sternal border and at the apex. Electrocardiography shows a sinus arrhythmia at a rate of 100 beats per minute, a QR pattern in V_1 with no right bundle-branch block, and a pure R wave in V_6; the P-R interval is questionably prolonged.

These findings may be associated with

(1) atrioventricularis communis
(2) Ebstein's anomaly
(3) an ostium primum atrial septal defect
(4) corrected transposition of the great vessels

SUMMARY OF DIRECTIONS

A	B	C	D	E
1, 2, 3 only	1, 3 only	2, 4 only	4 only	All are correct

168. A fall in arterial P_{O_2} or development of congestive heart failure can lead to a sympathetic response that increases the heart rate and supports myocardial contractility. This response is the result of

(1) constriction of renal vascular beds
(2) an increase in left ventricular end-diastolic volume
(3) stimulation of alpha adrenergic receptors
(4) stimulation of beta adrenergic receptors

169. In a normal fetus there is relative equalization of systolic pressures between the ductus arteriosus and the

(1) right ventricle
(2) left ventricle
(3) pulmonary artery
(4) aorta

170. A single second heart sound in the pulmonic area may be associated with which of the following anomalies?

(1) Persistent truncus arteriosus
(2) Transposition of the great vessels
(3) Tricuspid atresia
(4) Tetralogy of Fallot

171. Onset of diarrhea in a neonate is followed by the sudden development of a high fever, cyanosis, and circulatory collapse. Tachycardia and a gallop rhythm are present, but no murmurs are noted; electrocardiography reveals low voltages and ST and T wave changes. The diagnosis suggested by this clinical picture can be confirmed by

(1) viral cultures of feces and blood
(2) selective angiography
(3) a titer of serum neutralizing antibodies
(4) cardiac catheterization

172. A newborn infant who is in respiratory distress because of congestive heart failure would be likely to exhibit which of the following breathing patterns?

(1) Tachypnea
(2) Grunting
(3) Hyperpnea
(4) Periodic breathing

173. A child who has known valvular pulmonic stenosis (i.e., a pulmonic ejection click and a stenotic systolic murmur) has had increasing narrowing of the pulmonic valve. Auscultatory evidence of this narrowing could include

(1) earlier appearance of the ejection click
(2) increased intensity of the systolic murmur
(3) extension of the systolic murmur beyond the aortic component
(4) increased intensity of the ejection click

174. Many individuals who have ostium secundum atrial septal defects have a wide, fixed splitting of the second heart sound that is thought to be due to

(1) an incomplete right bundle-branch block
(2) delayed emptying of the right ventricle
(3) relative pulmonic stenosis
(4) low pulmonary vascular resistance

175. In children who have persistent truncus arteriosus, the degree of oxygen saturation in arterial blood depends on the

(1) size of the pulmonary arteries
(2) size of the ventricular septal defect
(3) degree of pulmonary resistance
(4) hematocrit

176. Although hypertrophic osteoarthropathy (clubbing of fingers and toes) in the pediatric age group occurs primarily in association with cyanotic congenital heart disease, it occasionally can appear in children who have

(1) lung abscesses
(2) cirrhosis of the liver
(3) subacute bacterial endocarditis
(4) chronic anemia

DIRECTIONS: The group of questions below consists of lettered choices followed by several numbered items. For each numbered item select the **one** lettered choice with which it is **most** closely associated. Each lettered choice may be used once, more than once, or not at all.

Questions 177-180

For each syndrome listed below, select the major cardiovascular abnormality with which it is most likely to be associated.

(A) Atrial septal defect
(B) Ventricular septal defect
(C) Patent ductus arteriosus
(D) Supravalvular aortic stenosis
(E) Peripheral pulmonic stenosis

177. Ellis-van Creveld syndrome

178. Thrombocytopenia-absent radius syndrome

179. Holt-Oram syndrome

180. Cri du chat syndrome

The Cardiovascular System

Answers

126. The answer is D. *(Nadas, ed 3. pp 322-323, 531, 535, 537.)* Valvular pulmonic stenosis, atrial septal defect, partial anomalous pulmonary venous return, and supravalvular pulmonic stenosis all are associated with a pulmonic ejection murmur. The latter three disorders can result in an increase in pulmonary pressure distal to the pulmonic valve and, as a consequence, accentuation of the pulmonic valve closure sound (as in the patient described in the question); valvular pulmonic stenosis, however, causes diminution of the pulmonic closure sound. The pulmonary artery segment may be enlarged in all four disorders, either from increased flow or due to poststenotic eddy currents that dilate the vessel. Peripheral pulmonary arterial markings usually will be normal or slightly decreased in stenotic lesions but increased in the presence of atrial septal defects (due to elevated pulmonary flow) and partial anomalous pulmonic venous return that is sufficient to cause right ventricular hypertrophy. Thus, the presence of normal pulmonary vascular markings in the child described, in conjunction with the other physical findings, points to a diagnosis of supravalvular pulmonic stenosis.

127. The answer is C. *(Nadas, ed 3. p 295.)* Among the wide variety of cardiac defects associated with Down's syndrome, the most common are endocardial cushion defects and atrial septal defects (ostium secundum). Evidence indicates that half of all children affected by trisomy 21 have congenital heart disease; estimates of the percent of Down's syndrome children who have cardiac anomalies range from a low of 7 percent to a high of 70 percent. Some cardiac lesions, such as tetralogy of Fallot and coarctation of the aorta, have been found to occur with less frequency in children who have Down's syndrome than in controls; other anomalies, like transposition of the great vessels, do not seem to be associated at all with the disorder.

128. The answer is B. *(Keith, ed 3. pp 487, 568.)* Transposition of the great vessels with an intact ventricular septum presents with early cyanosis, a normal sized heart, normal or slightly increased pulmonary vascular markings, and an

72   Pediatrics

electrocardiogram showing right axis deviation and right ventricular hypertrophy. In asymptomatic tetralogy of Fallot, cyanosis is unlikely in the first few days of life. Tricuspid atresia, a cause of early cyanosis, causes diminished pulmonary arterial blood flow; the pulmonary fields on x-ray demonstrate a diminution of pulmonary vascularity. There is a left axis and left ventricular hypertrophy by electrocardiogram. Total anomalous pulmonary venous return below the diaphragm is associated with obstruction to pulmonary venous return and a classical radiographic finding of marked fluffy appearing pulmonary venous congestion. In pulmonic atresia with intact ventricular septum, cyanosis appears early, the lung markings are normal to diminished, and the heart is large.

129. The answer is B. *(Keith, ed 3. pp 279, 286-288.)* The child described in the question who has no cyanosis or murmur, no cardiac or pulmonary vascular abnormalities by chest x-ray, and no evidence of structural anomalies by echocardiogram is unlikely to have an underlying gross anatomic defect. The electrocardiographic pattern in figure B shows the configuration of pre-excitation, the pattern seen in the Wolff-Parkinson-White syndrome (WPW). These patients have an aberrant atrioventricular conduction pathway which causes the early ventricular depolarization appearing on the electrocardiograms as a shortened P-R interval. The initial slow ventricular depolarization wave is referred to as the delta wave. Seventy percent of patients with WPW have single or repeated episodes of paroxysmal supraventricular tachycardia, which can cause the symptoms described in the question. The pre-excitation electrocardiographic pattern and WPW can occur in Ebstein's malformation, but this is unlikely in the absence of cyanosis and with a normal echocardiogram. Ventricular tachycardia is unlikely with WPW. If this were present, the symptoms are likely to be more profound. Active play in a healthy four-year-old child rarely causes symptoms such as those described in the question, but in children with WPW it can occasionally precipitate paroxysmal supraventricular tachycardia.

130. The answer is B. *(Nadas, ed 3. pp 148-149.)* Rheumatoid arthritis frequently causes spindle-shaped swelling of finger joints and may involve unusual joints such as the sternoclavicular joint. This disorder can be associated with spiking high fevers, which are not a feature of rheumatic fever, toxic synovitis, septic arthritis, or osteoarthritis. Although septic arthritis may affect any joint, it would not be likely to affect finger joints by causing spindle-shaped swellings; in this respect, septic arthritis resembles acute rheumatic fever. Toxic synovitis usually involves hip joints in boys, and osteoarthritis is not a disease of childhood.

131. The answer is B. *(Schaffer, ed 4. pp 226, 288.)* During the first day of life, an infant's pulse rate can range from 70 to 180 beats per minute (average: 125); during the first week, the rate varies between 100 and 190 beats per minute (average: 140). A heart rate that persistently falls below 70 beats per minute almost invariably indicates congenital atrioventricular block, which is of the complete type in nearly all cases. Affected infants often present only with bradycardia; however, cyanosis, cardiomegaly, and heart failure can ensue, especially if the pulse rate falls below 50 beats per minute; these children would require cardiac pacing.

132. The answer is B. *(Nadas, ed 3. pp 338-339.)* Maldevelopment resulting in ostium primum atrial septal defects also causes displacement of the atrioventricular node. As a result, leftward deviation of the electrocardiographic axis is seen. First-degree atrioventricular block occurs in some patients who have primum atrial defects. Incomplete right bundle-branch block very commonly accompanies secundum atrial septal defects.

133. The answer is D. *(Nadas, ed 3. pp 598-600.)* A quadruple rhythm associated with the murmur of tricuspid regurgitation and pulmonic stenosis is sufficient to make the diagnosis of Ebstein's anomaly (downward displacement of the tricuspid valve). The presence of P pulmonale (tall P waves in leads II and III) and right ventricular conduction defects confirms the diagnosis. Both tricuspid regurgitation with pulmonic stenosis and tetralogy of Fallot give electrocardiographic evidence of right ventricular enlargement. The Wolff-Parkinson-White syndrome, which frequently accompanies Ebstein's malformation, is not associated with murmurs or cyanosis as an isolated entity.

134. The answer is C. *(Nadas, ed 3. pp 322-333.)* Children who have an atrial septal defect also may have right ventricular hypertrophy. A loud pulmonic component of the second sound occurs with development of pulmonary arterial hypertension. This is usually of the reversible variety during childhood.

135. The answer is A. *(Nadas, ed 3. p 262.)* The greatest cause of congestive heart failure in children is congenital heart disease. Congestive heart failure due to congenital heart disease most often occurs in infants during their first weeks of life. Other etiologies of heart failure in young infants include primary myocardial disease and paroxysmal atrial tachycardia; other causes, such as bacterial endocarditis and rheumatic heart disease, are rare in the first year of life.

136. The answer is D. *(Perloff, ed 2. pp 93-96, 119, 137.)* A loud systolic ejection murmur in the aortic area occurs with valvular, discrete subvalvular, and supravalvular aortic stenosis, but only supravalvular aortic stenosis is associated with developmental abnormalities. These patients are described as having elfin faces and very often suffer some degree of mental retardation. A bicuspid valve will more likely be associated with regurgitation and, therefore, a diastolic mur-

74   Pediatrics

mur. A brisk right brachial and weaker left brachial pulse are frequent findings in supravalvular aortic stenosis and are thought to be due to the jet of blood directed into the innominate artery by the supravalvular narrowing, causing the more prominent pulse on the right. For the same reason, the right arm blood pressure is about 10 to 15 mm higher than the left. With coarctation of the aorta, the left arm blood pressure and pulse may be less than in the right arm if the left subclavian artery is narrowed by the coarcted portion of the aorta. However, in aortic coarctation one would expect higher pressure in the right arm than in the leg.

137. The answer is D. *(Braunwald, p 969.)* Ventricular septal defect is by far the most common congenital cardiac defect, constituting about 30 percent of all congenital cardiac anomalies. Atrial septal defect and patent ductus arteriosus each account for about 10 percent of congenital heart abnormalities, and pulmonic stenosis 7 percent. Tetralogy of Fallot, the most common cyanotic lesion, has a 6 percent incidence among neonates with congenital cardiac defects.

138. The answer is B. *(Schaffer, ed 4. pp 134, 249-250, 267.)* Infants born with the infracardiac variety of total anomalous pulmonary venous return have obstruction to the drainage of pulmonary veins. This anomaly results in a marked degree of pulmonary vascular congestion. Despite the presence of heart failure, cardiomegaly does not develop because of the decreased venous return to the heart. Transposition of the great vessels and pulmonic atresia usually produce cardiomegaly; and mitral stenosis can be expected to be accompanied by evidence of a large left atrium. Hyaline membrane disease in a term infant is unlikely.

139. The answer is A. *(Gellis, pp 239, 243-245.)* Syncopal episodes in children are not common. Evaluation of children presenting with syncope should include electrocardiography, because a prolonged Q-T interval can be associated with syncope. It is less likely that syncope in a three-year-old child would be caused by asymmetric septal hypertrophy; echocardiography is the procedure best able to evaluate this disorder.

140. The answer is C. *(Braunwald, p 1783. Friedman, p 106.)* Hypoxic stimulation of the kidneys is thought to cause the release of erythropoietin, a glycoprotein hormone that stimulates production of red blood cells in the bone marrow. A substrate manufactured in the liver is converted into erythropoietin, most likely in a reaction catalyzed by renal erythropoietic factor, an enzyme produced in the kidneys. Aside from inducing production of red blood cells, erythropoietin also increases the rate of erythrocyte production and causes the release of immature reticulocytes into the blood.

141. The answer is E. *(Friedman, pp 107-108.)* Congestive heart failure from any cause can result in mild cyanosis, even in the absence of a right-to-left shunt, and poor peripheral pulses when cardiac output is low. Congestive heart failure usually is associated with a rapid pulse rate (up to 200 beats per minute). A pulse rate greater than 200 beats per minute, however, should suggest the presence of a tachyarrhythmia.

142. The answer is D. *(Keith, ed 3. p 282.)* Digitalis administration is the drug treatment of choice for individuals who have paroxysmal supraventricular tachycardia. Procainamide, propranolol, diphenylhydantoin, and quinidine all have been used to treat patients who have paroxysmal ventricular tachycardia. Use of digitalis generally is contraindicated in this latter disorder, and digitalis toxicity can, in fact, lead to ventricular tachycardia; diphenylhydantoin is one of the drugs used to treat individuals who have digitoxicity. Propranolol and quinidine are employed to prevent recurrence of paroxysmal supraventricular tachycardia in patients not responding favorably with digoxin.

143. The answer is C. *(Schaffer, ed 4. p 260.)* The presence of a pansystolic murmur in the infant described in the question makes a diagnosis of anomalous pulmonary venous return unlikely. A ventricular septal defect that is either an isolated lesion or associated with other defects can cause a pansystolic murmur; isolated ventricular septal defects rarely cause cyanosis. Although truncus arteriosus occasionally causes a pansystolic murmur, it usually causes a continuous murmur. The presence of a right aortic arch is found in 25 percent of children who have tetralogy of Fallot and therefore increases the likelihood of this diagnosis in the situation presented. As the child becomes older, the degree of right ventricular outflow obstruction is likely to increase, causing persistent cyanosis and a change in the murmur to systolic ejection.

144. The answer is E. *(Friedman, p 57.)* In a fetus, aortic and pulmonary arterial pressures are equal because of the large size of the ductus arteriosus. As a result of the equalization of pressures, blood flow to the fetal organs is determined primarily by local vascular resistance. This resistance may, in turn, be affected by pH, P_{CO_2}, P_{O_2}, or circulating vasoactive agents.

145. The answer is C. *(Braunwald, pp 1085-1086.)* All of these conditions can be associated with prolonged fever and a limp due to arthralgia as well as exanthem, adenopathy, and pharyngitis. Conjunctivitis, however, is most likely in Kawasaki disease. The fissured lips, while common in Kawasaki disease, could occur after a long period of fever from any cause if the child became dehydrated. The predominance of neutrophils and high sedimentation rate are common to all. An increase in platelets, however, is found only in Kawasaki disease. Kawasaki disease presents a picture of prolonged fever, rash, epidermal peeling on the hands, especially around the fingertips, ocular conjunctivitis, lymphadenopathy, fissured lips, oropharyngeal mucosal erythema, and arthralgia or arthritis. The diagnosis is still possible in the absence of one or two of these physical findings. The cardiovascular abnormality, if present, involves aneurysms of systemic arteries, especially the coronary arteries.

146. The answer is A. *(Friedman, p 57.)* Although pulmonary arterioles are affected by pH and P_{CO_2} as well as by the presence of vasoactive substances, P_{O_2} is considered to be the major regulating influence on the pulmonary arteriolar resistance. The major smooth-muscle relaxing effect of a high P_{O_2} causes pulmonary vascular resistance to fall. The theory that tortuosity of the pulmonary vasculature causes elevation of pulmonary vascular resistance is now discounted.

147. The answer is C. *(Nadas, ed 3. p 221.)* The clinical picture presented in the question suggests the presence of an aberrant left coronary artery arising from the pulmonary artery. Electrocardiograms of these infants, in addition to showing nonspecific ST-T changes, often reveal deep Q waves in leads I and aVL and QR or Q-S complexes in V_2, V_3, and V_4. These electrocardiographic changes indicate the presence of infarction and can confirm a diagnosis of an aberrant left coronary artery suggested by clinical examination.

148. The answer is E. *(Friedman, pp 192-193, 207. Nadas, ed 3. pp 228-233.)* Endocardial fibroelastosis is a primary myocardial disease that is characterized by hyperplasia of the elastic tissue of the endocardium. Symptoms, which typically include those of congestive heart failure, usually manifest suddenly in children between the ages of four and ten months. In contrast, an aberrant left coronary artery produces symptoms in neonates. Myocarditis does not produce electrocardiographic evidence of hypertrophy; and Pompe's disease characteristically includes large tongue and hypotonia. Heart failure in infancy rarely is due to idiopathic hypertrophic subaortic stenosis.

149. The answer is C. *(Nadas, ed 3. p 287.)* Tall stature, long digits, and progressive scoliosis point to a diagnosis of Marfan's disease, an inherited disorder of collagen metabolism. Affected children frequently suffer from mitral regurgitation caused by papillary muscle dysfunction; aortic regurgitation due to dilatation of the valve rings also is common. Pulmonic regurgitation stemming from pulmonary artery dilatation, though it too can occur, is much less common in children who have Marfan's disease than are disturbances of the aortic or mitral valves.

Cardiovascular System 77

150. The answer is B. *(Nadas, ed 3. pp 462-463.)* Variation in the strength of femoral pulses indicates pressure alterations in the descending aorta, most likely due to a variation in blood flow. In preductal aortic coarctation, blood flow in the descending aorta is affected by a patent ductus arteriosus, which may close intermittently or even permanently. This effect would not occur in a postductal aortic coarctation with a patent ductus arteriosus, because the descending aortic flow is by way of collateral vessels. Due to aortic runoff, pulses in children who have a ventricular septal defect with a patent ductus would be consistently full. The closing of a patent ductus in children with tetralogy of Fallot likely would result in marked cyanosis. Children with preductal aortic coarctation may obtain temporary relief in the situation described in the question by infusion of E-type prostaglandin.

151. The answer is E. *(Nadas, ed 3. pp 496-502. Watson, pp 235-239.)* Symptoms of respiratory obstruction, especially if aggravated by exertion, that occur during the first days of life strongly suggest the presence of a vascular ring. Esophagography is the diagnostic study most likely to demonstrate the disorder, because it can show the characteristic indentation of the esophagus caused by the compressing vessels. Vascular rings are due to anomalous development of the aortic arch and its branches; surgical treatment is recommended.

152. The answer is D. *(Schaffer, ed 4. p 240.)* The majority of infants who have aortic atresia cannot be helped by surgery and at best get only temporary relief from medical therapy. These children usually do not survive to one week of age (the average age attained by one series of affected infants was 4.5 days). The prognosis for infants having hypoplasia of the aortic arch may be somewhat better.

153. The answer is D. *(Watson, pp 264-265.)* The clinical history of the child described in the question is compatible with a diagnosis of ventricular septal defect associated with aortic insufficiency. Evidence of increased pulmonary vascularity and left atrial and ventricular enlargement also could indicate a patent ductus arteriosus sustaining a significant blood flow. This condition, however, would have resulted in a continuous murmur when the infant described first presented at the age of three months. The same is true of the murmur of a coronary arteriovenous fistula, which in addition is unlikely to produce signs of cardiac enlargement. A ventricular septal defect associated with mitral insufficiency would produce a diastolic rumble of relative mitral stenosis in addition to a pansystolic murmur and would be likely to cause considerable heart failure. It is unlikely that rupture of an aneurysmal sinus of Valsalva would occur without sudden and marked symptoms of heart failure.

154. The answer is B. *(Nadas, ed 3. p 26.)* Infants who have transposition of the great vessels classically present with cyanosis during the first few days after birth. Pulmonary vasculature is engorged. The cardiac contour in infants who have transposition often is described as an "egg on a string." The egg-shaped contour is a result of general enlargement of the heart (due to increased cardiac volume) accompanied by a narrowing of the left upper cardiac border because of the "missing" pulmonary artery at that site. The "string" is the narrow superior mediastinal shadow produced by the anteroposterior alignment of the aorta and main pulmonary artery. Cineangiocardiography can establish with certainty the presence of transposition.

155. The answer is C. *(Braunwald, p 980. Nadas, ed 3. pp 271-272.)* The major clinical manifestation of digitalis toxicity in infants is vomiting. Affected infants also exhibit certain electrocardiographic changes, including sinus arrhythmia and a wandering pacemaker, paroxysmal tachycardia, and a heart rate of less than 100 beats per minute. Digitalis intoxication appears to be increasing dramatically in frequency, in part because of the widespread use of more potent preparations of the drug. The commonly used digitalis preparation in infants is digoxin. Digoxin blood levels of 2 ng/100 ml or less are usually therapeutic in adults; in contrast, therapeutic digoxin blood levels in infants range from 1 to 5 ng/100 ml.

156. The answer is C. *(Nadas, ed 3. p 295. Watson, pp 690-691.)* Short stature, neck webbing, sexual infantilism, hyperextensible elbows, and a shieldlike chest with widely spaced nipples are signs of Turner's syndrome, which is associated with an XO genotype. Aortic coarctation and pulmonic stenosis are the cardiovascular defects that occur most frequently in individuals who have this disorder. Down's syndrome most commonly is associated with atrial septal defects and endocardial cushion defects; Marfan's syndrome with dilatation of the pulmonary artery and mitral and aortic regurgitation; and Ellis-van Creveld syndrome with an atrial septal defect or single atrium.

157. The answer is E (all). *(Perloff, ed 2. pp 344-350.)* The embryonic endocardial cushions are responsible for the conjoining of the lower (primum) portion of the atrial septum and the upper portion of the ventricular septum, as well as the development of the anterior mitral leaflet and septal leaflet of the tricuspid valve. Maldevelopment of the cushions can result, depending on degree, in a single or combination of defects: ostium primum atrial septal defect, ventricular septal defect, mitral or tricuspid regurgitation, or when severe, complete atrioventricular canal defect with communication of all four heart chambers.

158. The answer is B (1, 3). *(Perloff, ed 2. pp 299-301.)* As in atrial septal defects, the increased flow across the pulmonic valve due to the shunt causes a pulmonic flow murmur. The increased right ventricular volume results in a prominent right ventricular impulse (heave). The pulmonic second sound (P_2) is accentuated only in the presence of pulmonary hypertension. Wide and fixed splitting of the second heart sound, which classically occurs with atrial septal defects with significant flows, does not occur with the increased flow into the right atrium secondary to partial anomalous venous return with intact atrial septum. The variation in right ventricular and left ventricular filling that normally occurs with inspiration does not occur with atrial septal defect. In atrial septal defect with inspiration, right ventricular volume increases due to caval return. Shunting decreases due to the increase in pulmonary impedance, resulting in increased left ventricular filling. There is thus a delay of both the aortic component of the second sound and the pulmonic second sound. During expiration, right ventricular volume is again increased, but by increase in shunt. The latter results in a smaller left ventricular volume. The result is splitting during inspiration and expiration.

159. The answer is A (1, 2, 3). *(Nadas, ed 3. pp 406-407, 413-414, 417-418.)* The continuous flow of blood through a truncus arteriosus into the pulmonary vessels gives rise to a continuous murmur. Similarly, the continuous blood flow through bronchial collateral vessels can cause a continuous murmur in children who have tetralogy of Fallot. In total anomalous pulmonary venous return, the flow through the pulmonary venous trunk carrying the blood from the pulmonary veins to the right heart may result in a continuous murmur. The murmur associated with patent ductus arteriosus is continuous and affected only to a minor degree by position or respiration, but patients are not cyanotic; in patent ductus arteriosus complicated by pulmonary hypertension, flow through the ductus is not continuous and, therefore, neither is the murmur.

160. The answer is A (1, 2, 3). *(Gellis, pp 235-236.)* Pulmonic stenosis usually is associated with a small-chambered right ventricle that, even following valvotomy, will not allow adequate blood flow into the pulmonary artery. Affected infants require maintenance of their aorticopulmonary shunts. Surgical aorticopulmonary anastomosis, when possible, is the best treatment; infiltration of the ductus arteriosus with formalin has been used for patients who, for anatomical reasons, cannot undergo anastomosis. Prostaglandin (type E) infusion, a temporary emergency measure, can maintain ductal patency until surgery is performed.

161. The answer is A (1, 2, 3). *(Braunwald, p 974.)* The major factor in rapid fall of the pulmonary arterial resistance is pulmonary arterial vasodilation resulting from the increased P_{O_2}, to which vessels are exposed. Inflation of the lungs allows the vessels to expand, which is the initial cause of reduction of the resistance. Ductus arteriosus closure, which is brought about by the increase in P_{O_2} plus the change in local prostaglandin, results in a fall in pulmonary arterial pressure. The pressure, if high, retards vasodilation. The enhanced volume due to foramen ovale closure is noncontributory.

162. The answer is A (1, 2, 3). *(Friedman, p 113.)* Infants born to diabetic mothers commonly have hypoglycemia, hypocalcemia, and hyperinsulinemia; hyperbilirubinemia also is more common in these infants than in infants of nondiabetic mothers. Newborn infants who are severely hypoglycemic may develop profound congestive heart failure. Even without associated cardiac lesions murmurs of tricuspid insufficiency may appear due to marked cardiac dilation and persistent fetal pulmonary circulation.

163. The answer is A (1, 2, 3). *(Braunwald, pp 1737, 1743-1744. Nadas, ed 3. pp 147, 152-155.)* Administration of salicylates and steroids can relieve the inflammatory manifestations of acute rheumatic fever. Salicylates alone usually are sufficient to treat affected children who do not have severe carditis. Neither salicylates nor corticosteroids have an effect on chorea, which is a noninflammatory process.

164. The answer is B (1, 3). *(Keith, ed 3. pp 269, 279-280, 292, 700-701.)* In a child presenting with a seizure, cardiac causes, even though less likely than neurologic causes, must be considered. Ventricular arrhythmia may cause syncope resembling a seizure. Long Q-T syndrome, aortic stenosis, and primary hypertension can all cause ventricular fibrillation with stress. Atrial tachycardia may cause heart failure but does not cause syncope. If aortic stenosis were present, there would be a loud systolic ejection murmur with a thrill. The hearing deficit suggests the possibility of the Jervell-Lange-Nielsen syndrome, the recessive form of the long Q-T syndrome, which is associated with congenital hearing deficit. The mildly accentuated second sound is difficult to evaluate in a child with a thin chest wall, as is the recent onset of fatigue. These two findings, however, may be seen in pulmonary hypertension.

165. The answer is A (1, 2, 3). *(Schaffer, ed 4. pp 238-239, 290-291.)* Reduced blood flow through the left ventricle results in underdevelopment of this chamber of the heart. Aortic atresia, mitral atresia, and hypoplasia of the aortic arch, either individually or in combination, can cause this reduction in flow and lead to endocardial fibroelastosis. Isolated endocardial fibroelastosis, however, is not associated with development of a small left ventricle.

Cardiovascular System 81

166. The answer is A (1, 2, 3). *(Schaffer, ed 4. pp 247-248.)* A large number of newborn infants who have preductal aortic coarctation are symptomatic within a week or two after birth. Development of heart failure is especially likely if this lesion, or postductal aortic coarctation, is associated with a large left-to-right shunt at the ventricular level. Although patent ductus arteriosus alone may cause early failure in the newborn period, the combination of a ductus with a ventricular septal defect is very likely to result in failure due to marked left ventricular volume overload resulting from the combined shunt. Infants who have tetralogy of Fallot have large ventricular septal defects as part of that lesion; they do not, however, have large left-to-right shunts, because right ventricular pressure is elevated due to the pulmonic and subpulmonic stenosis associated with tetralogy of Fallot.

167. The answer is D (4). *(Nadas, ed 3. pp 335, 598, 631-633.)* Atrioventricularis communis, an ostium primum defect, Ebstein's anomaly, and corrected transposition of the great vessels all may be associated with atrioventricular conduction delay. Tachyarrhythmia is associated frequently with Ebstein's malformation and corrected transposition of the great vessels; and a QR pattern may be present in V_1 in either of these conditions. In Ebstein's malformation, however, a right bundle-branch block pattern is frequently present, and the appearance of a pansystolic murmur is unusual. Although a pansystolic murmur also may be present in children who have atrioventricularis communis, these children are in considerable distress before the age of three years. A pansystolic murmur would not be present in children who have an isolated ostium primum atrial septal defect. Thus, the only condition of those listed in the question that would be likely to be compatible with the clinical picture presented is corrected transposition, which is associated with mitral regurgitation and a ventricular septal defect.

168. The answer is D (4). *(Friedman, p 105.)* With hypoxemia and congestive heart failure there is a sympathoadrenal response resulting in stimulation of beta adrenergic receptors. Support of myocardial contractility and increase in heart rate then occur. Stimulation of alpha receptors aids in redistribution of cardiac output to vital organs by causing constriction in renal and skin vascular beds.

169. The answer is E (all). *(Friedman, p 57. Hurst, ed 4. p 815.)* In a fetus, the ductus arteriosus provides circulatory communication between the pulmonary and systemic vascular compartments. This phenomenon, coupled with the fact that the diameter of the ductus arteriosus is as large as that of the descending aorta, results in a relative equalization of the systolic pressures of the pulmonary artery, aorta, and both ventricles. (It should be noted that the systolic pressure in the fetal aorta most likely is a few millimeters less than in the pulmonary artery and right ventricle.)

170. The answer is E (all). *(Robinson, Cardiovasc Clinics 2:89, 1970.)* In children who have persistent truncus arteriosus and only a single semilunar valve, the second heart sound is single. In transposition of the great vessels the placement of the pulmonic valve posterior and inferior to the anteriorly displaced aorta can mask the pulmonic closure sound. Tricuspid atresia and tetralogy of Fallot usually are associated with marked pulmonic stenosis, which results in inaudible pulmonic-valve closure.

171. The answer is B (1, 3). *(Friedman, p 210.)* Myocarditis caused by infection with group B coxsackievirus is the most common type of myocarditis in newborn infants. A history of diarrhea followed by the sudden onset of fever and cardiovascular collapse in a neonate who has an electrocardiogram showing abnormal repolarization suggests coxsackie B viral myocarditis. Confirmation of this diagnosis is by viral culture and serum neutralizing antibody titer. Although the prognosis for affected infants is poor, early diagnosis and prompt initiation of maintenance therapy can be of considerable benefit.

172. The answer is B (1, 3). *(Friedman, p 107.)* Infants who are in congestive heart failure usually are hyperpneic, if they have hypoxemia and acidemia, or tachypneic, if they have volume overload of the pulmonary circuit. Grunting is associated primarily with pulmonary disease, and periodic breathing with disease of the central nervous system.

173. The answer is A (1, 2, 3). *(Watson, p 514.)* With increased obstruction to right ventricular outflow, the pulmonic ejection click of valvular pulmonic stenosis becomes quieter and occurs earlier. On the other hand, increased stenosis causes an increase in the grade of the systolic murmur. Due to prolongation of right ventricular emptying, pulmonic valve closure is extended beyond aortic valve closure.

174. The answer is C (2, 4). *(Watson, pp 379, 389.)* The normal reduction in right ventricular blood volume during expiration does not occur in the presence of an atrial septal defect and a left-to-right shunt. Ventricular emptying is prolonged during expiration and the second heart sound is split. An increase in pulmonary resistance will reduce the degree of shunting. Most patients who have an ostium secundum defect have an incomplete right bundle-branch block pattern, which, however, does not affect auscultation. The murmur of an atrial defect is generated at the pulmonic valve and indicates relative pulmonic stenosis, but it too has no significant effect on the second heart sound.

Cardiovascular System 83

175. The answer is B (1, 3). *(Nadas, ed 3. pp 438-439, 443.)* In truncus arteriosus the magnitude of pulmonary blood flow in relation to systemic blood flow determines the degree of arterial oxygen saturation. High pulmonary vascular resistance or a hypoplastic pulmonary arterial tree can limit this flow and reduce the saturation of arterial blood. A large pulmonary circulation through pulmonary arteries of adequate diameter, on the other hand, will keep saturation of truncus blood high.

176. The answer is A (1, 2, 3). *(Nadas, ed 3. p 307.)* After cyanosis, hypertrophic osteoarthropathy (clubbing) is the most characteristic sign of arterial oxygen unsaturation. Clubbing most often occurs in association with cyanotic congenital heart disease and is a very early indicator of hypoxemia. Other conditions associated on occasion with clubbing include lung abscess, subacute bacterial endocarditis, and hepatic cirrhosis.

177-180. The answers are: 177-A, 178-A, 179-A, 180-B. *(Braunwald, pp 970-971.)* The Ellis-van Creveld syndrome is an autosomal recessive trait. The common cardiac defects occur in 50 to 60 percent of affected individuals, commonly a secundum atrial septal defect. This may be associated with some variant of hypoplastic left heart syndrome. The characteristic skeletal findings are short stature from birth, distal extremity shortening, and bilateral polydactyly. The latter permits an in utero diagnosis.

In thrombocytopenia-absent radius syndrome there is a high occurrence of atrial septal defects. There may also be an associated tetralogy of Fallot. The radius, despite the implication of the syndrome name, may be hypoplastic or absent.

The Holt-Oram syndrome is one of the rare disorders in which a secundum atrial septal defect seems to be the result of a single dominant gene. Ventricular septal defect is the second most common cardiac anomaly. The most common hand/arm defect is a fingerlike appearance of one or both thumbs. First degree relatives of patients with Holt-Oram syndrome have a 50 percent incidence of atrial septal defects, as opposed to a 3 percent occurrence in the sporadically occurring type of atrial septal defect.

Children with cri du chat (literally, cat cry) syndrome have a chromosomal abnormality. The associated cardiac anomaly is a ventricular septal defect. There is microcephaly, an antimongoloid slant of the palpebral fissures, and severe mental retardation.

The Gastrointestinal Tract

John B. Watkins

DIRECTIONS: Each question below contains five suggested answers. Choose the one best response to each question.

Questions 181-183

A 14-month-old infant is admitted to the hospital with a six-month history of irritability, developmental delay, and failure to thrive; malnutrition is suspected.

181. Which of the following growth patterns would be most characteristic of a child with malnutrition?

(A) Subnormal weight, normal height and head circumference
(B) Subnormal weight and height, normal head circumference
(C) Subnormal weight and head circumference, normal height
(D) Subnormal head circumference, normal weight and height
(E) Subnormal weight, height, and head circumference

182. Additional diagnostic tests that should be ordered for the child described include all of the following EXCEPT

(A) 72-hour stool collection for fat
(B) thyroid scan
(C) complete blood cell count
(D) urinalysis
(E) urine culture

183. All of the following findings support a diagnosis of malnutrition in the child described above due to excessive caloric losses from the gastrointestinal tract EXCEPT

(A) a stool fat concentration greater than 10 percent of intake
(B) a sweat chloride concentration of 75 mg/100 ml
(C) increase in serum xylose at one hour of more than 30 mg/100 ml
(D) the presence of iron-deficiency anemia
(E) the presence of multisegmented polymorphonuclear leukocytes

184. All of the following factors can be associated with an increased risk of neurologic damage in a jaundiced newborn EXCEPT

(A) metabolic acidosis
(B) sulfisoxazole therapy
(C) the presence of reducing substances in the urine
(D) maternal ingestion of aspirin during pregnancy
(E) maternal ingestion of phenobarbital during pregnancy

185. A biopsy sample from the small intestine of a child is examined by light microscopy; a photomicrograph is shown below. The diagnosis most compatible with the findings depicted is

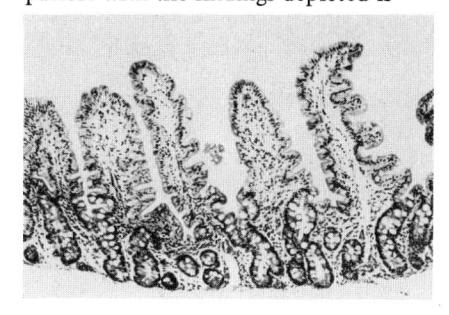

(A) celiac disease
(B) abetalipoproteinemia
(C) Whipple's disease
(D) congenital agammaglobulinemia
(E) sucrase-isomaltase deficiency

186. Which of the following malabsorptive conditions principally influences the intestinal or mucosal phase of digestion?

(A) Zollinger-Ellison syndrome
(B) Enterokinase deficiency
(C) *Giardia lamblia* infestation
(D) Gastrocolic fistula
(E) Biliary atresia

187. The D-xylose tolerance test may be abnormal in individuals with any of the following conditions that are characterized by malabsorption EXCEPT

(A) celiac disease
(B) pancreatic deficiency
(C) bacterial overgrowth syndrome
(D) short bowel syndrome
(E) regional enteritis

Questions 188-189

A three-day-old infant is noted in the newborn nursery to be jaundiced. Total serum bilirubin level is 10.5 mg/100 ml (direct, 0.5 mg/100 ml).

188. Additional physical findings or historical factors that could be associated with this infant include all of the following EXCEPT

(A) breast-feeding
(B) normal-size liver
(C) history of jaundice in a sibling
(D) family history of Rotor's syndrome
(E) family history of hereditary spherocytosis

189. Which of the following laboratory findings would be consistent with the diagnosis of physiologic jaundice in the infant described above?

(A) An elevated peripheral normoblast cell count
(B) An elevated level of hepatic glucuronyl transferase
(C) An elevated level of serum glutamic-oxaloacetic transaminase
(D) Normal excretion of bromsulphalein
(E) None of the above

190. A child who has primary sucrase-isomaltase deficiency would be likely to have

(A) no family history of the disorder
(B) abnormal small-bowel mucosa
(C) reduced lactase activity
(D) reduced glucose absorption
(E) production of hydrogen following a sucrose load

191. All of the following statements concerning the digestion and absorption of medium-chain triglycerides are true EXCEPT that

(A) bile salts are required for their absorption
(B) they are incorporated into chylomicrons only to a minor degree
(C) during transport they are bound to albumin
(D) they are rapidly hydrolyzed by pancreatic lipase
(E) they are metabolized in the liver

192. Findings that are commonly associated with ulcerative colitis include

(A) rectal bleeding
(B) transmural pathology
(C) perianal abscesses
(D) "skip" lesions
(E) anorectal fistulas

193. Which of the following laboratory findings would be consistent with a diagnosis of Reye's syndrome?

(A) Hypoammonemia
(B) Cellular spinal fluid
(C) Leukopenia
(D) Diffusely abnormal electroencephalogram
(E) Shortened prothrombin time

194. A three-week-old infant who is still at birthweight has bloody diarrhea. The child had delayed passage of meconium while in the newborn nursery. All of the following disorders should be strongly considered in the differential diagnosis EXCEPT

(A) necrotizing enterocolitis
(B) cystic fibrosis
(C) Hirschsprung's disease
(D) hypothyroidism
(E) salmonellosis

Questions 195-196

A three-year-old girl who has a prominent abdomen and lymphedema of the right arm is admitted to the hospital for investigation of her abdominal distension and persistent diarrhea. Initial laboratory findings include a total serum protein concentration of 3.2 g/100 ml (albumin, 1.2 g/100 ml).

195. Based on these symptoms and laboratory findings, the most likely diagnosis for this child would be

(A) Menetrier's disease
(B) cystic fibrosis
(C) tropical sprue
(D) intestinal lymphangiectasia
(E) severe pulmonic stenosis with heart failure

196. The child described above would be expected to display which of the following laboratory findings?

(A) An elevated serum calcium level
(B) A peripheral lymphocyte count of more than 3000/ml
(C) A 72-hour stool fat content greater than 10 g
(D) Normal intestinal excretion of chromium-labeled albumin
(E) Normal delayed hypersensitivity

197. Which of the following clinical or laboratory findings would be associated with worsening or fulminating hepatitis?

(A) Hyperalbuminemia
(B) Heightened gag reflex
(C) Progressive liver enlargement
(D) Markedly depressed levels of serum glutamic-oxaloacetic transaminase
(E) Prothrombin time increase that is resistant to vitamin K therapy

198. Cirrhosis, complicated by portal hypertension, can occur in association with all of the following disorders EXCEPT

(A) cystic fibrosis
(B) alpha$_1$-antitrypsin deficiency
(C) congenital hepatic fibrosis
(D) Wilson's disease
(E) fructose intolerance

199. A six-week-old dehydrated child is admitted to a hospital following ten days of vomiting. Pyloric stenosis is suspected. Which of the following findings would be most consistent with this diagnosis?

(A) Jaundice and indirect hyperbilirubinemia
(B) Hyponatremia with a hyperchloremic metabolic acidosis
(C) An elevated serum potassium level
(D) A urine specific gravity of 1.005
(E) A urine pH of 4.5

200. All of the following medications are associated with drug-induced liver disease EXCEPT

(A) aspirin
(B) acetaminophen
(C) oxacillin
(D) prednisone
(E) azathioprine

201. A child who has undergone an ileal resection would be likely to exhibit all of the following findings EXCEPT

(A) iron-deficiency anemia
(B) renal oxalate stones
(C) an abnormal Schilling test with intrinsic factor
(D) a positive response to cholestyramine therapy
(E) an increase in glycine-conjugated bile acids

202. In a child who has long-standing cholestasis, the laboratory finding LEAST likely to be exhibited would be
(A) an elevated serum cholesterol level
(B) an elevated serum lipoprotein X level
(C) an elevated serum carotene level
(D) an elevated serum alkaline phosphatase level
(E) a normal prothrombin time

203. Which of the following clinical and pathologic findings is most characteristic of Crohn's disease?
(A) Rectal bleeding
(B) Granuloma formation
(C) Pericholangitis
(D) Toxic megacolon
(E) Small bowel involvement

Gastrointestinal Tract

DIRECTIONS: Each question below contains four suggested answers of which **one** or **more** is correct. Choose the answer:

A	if	1, 2, and 3	are correct
B	if	1 and 3	are correct
C	if	2 and 4	are correct
D	if	4	is correct
E	if	1, 2, 3, and 4	are correct

204. An 18-month-old girl was evaluated for poor weight gain and growth during the prior six months, iron deficiency anemia, irritability, decrease in appetite, and diarrhea. An upper gastrointestinal series and small bowel biopsy were performed, the results of which are illustrated below. The possible pathogenic mechanisms operating in this child include which of the following?

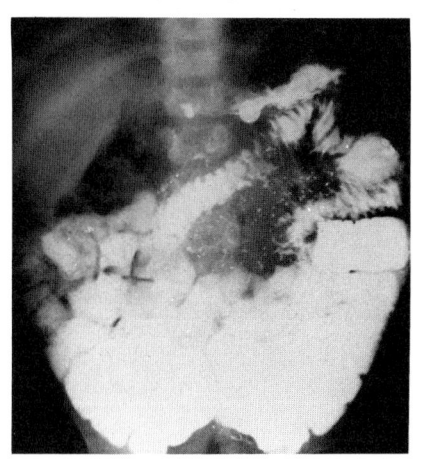

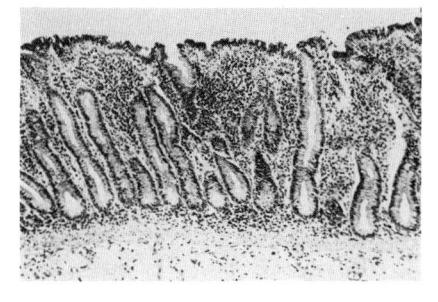

(1) Viral infection
(2) Peptidase deficiency
(3) Endocrine disorder
(4) Immunologic disorder

SUMMARY OF DIRECTIONS

A	B	C	D	E
1, 2, 3 only	1, 3 only	2, 4 only	4 only	All are correct

205. A six-week-old infant is admitted to a hospital because of jaundice. Which of the following disorders could be responsible for obstructive jaundice in this infant?

(1) Cystic fibrosis
(2) Gilbert's disease
(3) Alpha$_1$-antitrypsin deficiency
(4) Hypothyroidism

206. Factors thought to be involved in nonhemolytic hyperbilirubinemia of newborn infants include

(1) shortened life span of fetal red blood cells
(2) decreased hepatic uptake of bilirubin
(3) enterohepatic recycling of bilirubin
(4) deficiency of glucuronyl transferase

207. Which of the following conditions that are characterized by malabsorption are associated with abnormal function of the intestinal mucosa?

(1) Dermatitis herpetiformis
(2) Hartnup disease
(3) Folic acid deficiency
(4) Cystic fibrosis

208. Lactose intolerance can be diagnosed by which of the following laboratory studies?

(1) Blood glucose levels before and after oral administration of lactose
(2) Hydrogen excretion in breath after oral administration of lactose
(3) Stool pH and reducing substances
(4) Small intestinal biopsy and enzyme (lactase) assay

209. Clinical findings in children who have congenital sucrase-isomaltase deficiency usually include

(1) stool positive for reducing substances
(2) chronic diarrhea
(3) rectal bleeding
(4) normal growth and development

210. Correct statements about Menetrier's disease include which of the following?

(1) It causes excessive gastrointestinal loss of protein
(2) It is associated with hyposecretion of stomach acid
(3) It may be caused by infection with cytomegalovirus
(4) Stomach x-ray characteristically shows normal rugae

211. A 30-hour-old male infant, the product of a pregnancy complicated by polyhydramnios, presents with abdominal distension, poor feeding, and recurrent vomiting, the vomitus being bile stained. The infant has passed one meconium-stained stool. There is no evidence of fever, diarrhea, or melena. The physical examination is normal except for abdominal distension, mild jaundice, and hypotonic bowel sounds. A barium enema (see x-ray below) was obtained and reveals a small-diameter colon. A diagnostic and treatment regimen for this infant should consist of

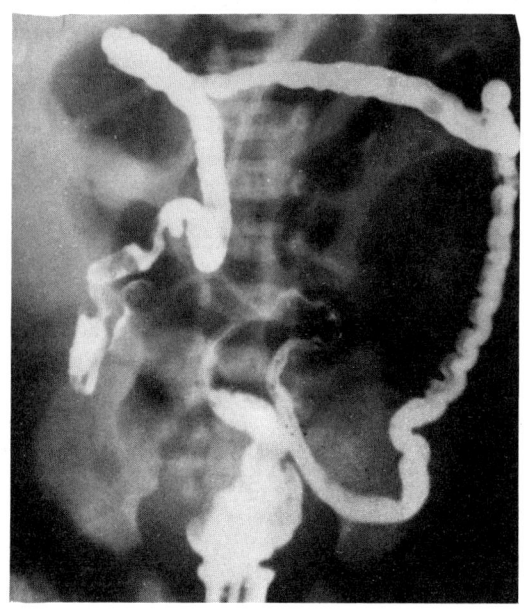

(1) diatrizoate methylglucamine (Gastrografin) enemas
(2) small-bowel surgery
(3) pancreatic enzyme supplements
(4) rectal biopsy for ganglion cells

---

212. Which of the following disorders can be associated with disease of the terminal ileum?

(1) Crohn's disease
(2) Schönlein-Henoch purpura
(3) Tuberculosis
(4) *Yersinia enterocolitica* infection

213. Gastrointestinal manifestations of cystic fibrosis include

(1) portal hypertension and varices
(2) an ileocecal mass
(3) abnormal gallbladder function
(4) constipation and obstruction

SUMMARY OF DIRECTIONS				
A	B	C	D	E
1, 2, 3 only	1, 3 only	2, 4 only	4 only	All are correct

214. Sulfasalazine (Azulfidine) is a commonly used treatment for children who have inflammatory bowel disease. In regard to this drug it is true that

(1) it contains two pharmacologically active ingredients
(2) it is converted into its active form principally by colonic bacteria
(3) it is excreted after being acetylated in the liver
(4) it is extremely effective in treating children who have Crohn's disease isolated in the small bowel

215. True statements about Reye's syndrome include which of the following?

(1) Microvesicular hepatic steatosis is characteristic
(2) A viral etiology recently has been confirmed
(3) Mitochondrial lesions occur in the brain and liver
(4) Uric acid metabolism is markedly abnormal

216. Correct statements concerning Crohn's disease include which of the following?

(1) It typically produces transmural lesions
(2) It can be associated with aphthous stomatitis in children
(3) It is associated with an increased incidence of colonic cancer
(4) It rarely spares the rectum

217. Factors associated with human hepatitis B infection include which of the following?

(1) Oral-fecal exposure and transmission
(2) Dane particles
(3) Migratory arthritis
(4) Surface antigen

218. Correct statements concerning lactase deficiency include which of the following?

(1) Lactase deficiency appears to be an inherited condition
(2) There is a higher incidence of this condition among blacks, orientals and American Indians
(3) Acquired lactase deficiency is often seen in association with bacterial infections of the gastrointestinal tract
(4) Ingestion of lactose followed by the detection of hydrogen in the breath is diagnostic for lactose malabsorption

219. The x-ray shown below can suggest which of the following diagnoses?

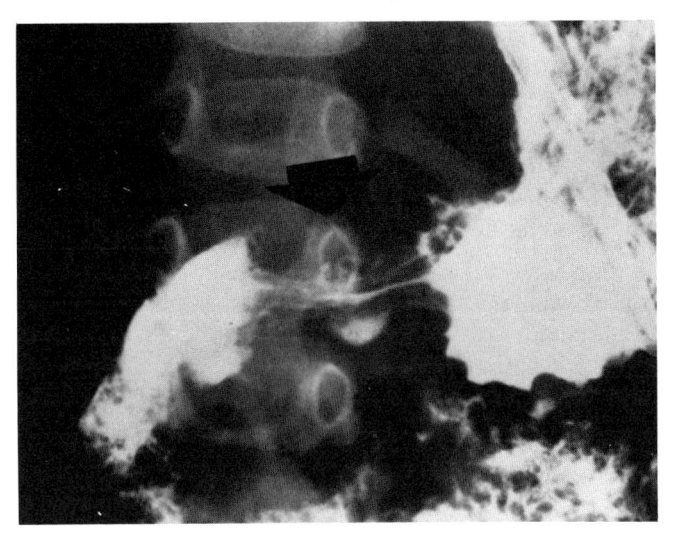

(1) Chronic granulomatous disease
(2) Eosinophilic gastroenteritis
(3) Lymphoma
(4) Crohn's disease

220. Findings associated with Hirschsprung's disease can include

(1) relaxation of the internal sphincter
(2) colonic dilatation
(3) presence of ganglion cells in a rectal biopsy sample
(4) an area of rectal narrowing

Pediatrics

DIRECTIONS: The groups of questions below consist of lettered choices followed by several numbered items. For each numbered item select the **one** lettered choice with which it is **most** closely associated. Each lettered choice may be used once, more than once, or not at all.

Questions 221-225

For each description that follows, select the disorder with which it is most likely to be associated.

(A) Peutz-Jeghers syndrome
(B) Gardner's syndrome
(C) Juvenile polyps
(D) Juvenile polyposis of the colon
(E) Lymphoid polyposis

221. Commonly shows malignant degeneration

222. Is associated with soft-tissue masses

223. May be related to *Giardia lamblia* infection

224. Is definitely not inherited

225. Is associated with adenomatous polyps

Questions 226-230

Match the following.

(A) Wilson's disease
(B) Alpha$_1$-antitrypsin deficiency
(C) Both
(D) Neither

226. Symptoms often appear in the first year of life

227. Inherited as an autosomal recessive trait

228. Can be associated with pulmonary emphysema

229. Causes postnecrotic cirrhosis

230. Can be associated with hemolytic episodes

The Gastrointestinal Tract

Answers

181. The answer is A. *(Silverman, ed 2. pp 4-5.)* Most children who are failing to thrive due to malnutrition have a normal head circumference, normal or near-normal height, but a weight that is less than expected given the height. Common causes of malnutrition include inadequate caloric intake, excessive gastrointestinal losses, peripheral disease impairing caloric metabolism, or a combination of these and other causes. Social and cultural factors often are implicated to some extent in the development of malnutrition.

182. The answer is B. *(Silverman, ed 2. pp 7-8.)* In the workup of a child suspected of having malnutrition, a complete nutritional history should be elicited. Furthermore a complete blood cell count, urinalysis, urine culture, and examination for fat in a 72-hour stool sample are essential tests in evaluating nutritional function. Children whose failure to thrive can be traced to thyroid dysfunction or an endocrine disorder would have a different growth pattern (i.e., subnormal weight and height for their age) than the child described in the question.

183. The answer is C. *(Silverman, ed 2. pp 685-686.)* D-Xylose is a poorly absorbed sugar that is not metabolized in the body and thus is excreted intact in the urine. Measurement of xylose concentration in a 5-hour urine sample or measurement of blood levels at 0, 30, 60, and 90 minutes provides a good indication of the integrity of the mucosa of the small intestine. For a 14-month-old child, a D-xylose excretion greater than 20 percent or a rise in serum levels of 30 mg/100 ml (dose 0.5 g/kg body weight or 14.5 g/m^2) indicates good mucosal function. A sweat chloride level of 75 mg/100 ml indicates cystic fibrosis; iron deficiency anemia and a stool fat concentration exceeding 10 percent of intake indicate malabsorption; and the presence of multisegmented polymorphonuclear leukocytes indicates a deficiency of folic acid or vitamin B$_{12}$ absorption, either primary or secondary to mucosal dysfunction.

96   Pediatrics

184. The answer is E. *(Silverman, ed 2. pp 451-465.)* Unconjugated, unbound bilirubin levels above 20 to 25 mg/100 ml in full-term newborn infants can lead to diffusion of bilirubin into brain tissue and thus to neurologic complications. Sulfisoxazole and salicylates compete with bilirubin for binding sites on albumin; therefore, the presence of these drugs can cause serum unbound bilirubin levels to rise. Metabolic acidosis also reduces binding of bilirubin, and the finding of reducing substances in an infant's urine can suggest galactosemia. Administration of phenobarbital has been used to induce glucuronyl transferase in newborn infants and thus can reduce, rather than exacerbate, neonatal jaundice.

185. The answer is E. *(Silverman, ed 2. pp 208-209. Trier, N Engl J Med 285: 1470, 1973.)* When examined by light microscopy, a biopsy sample from the small intestine of an individual who has sucrase-isomaltase deficiency will appear normal. In the other disorders listed in the question, however, histologic examination of the small bowel reveals the presence of diagnostic or at least highly characteristic lesions. In sucrase-isomaltase deficiency, analysis of the intestinal disaccharidase enzymes demonstrate normal lactase activity with an absence of the sucrase enzyme. Therapy should include removal of the offending sugar from the diet.

186. The answer is C. *(Silverman, ed 2. pp 215-222.)* The intraluminal phase of digestion involves the hydrolysis and solubilization of fats, proteins, and complex carbohydrates. Acid hypersecretion in individuals who have Zollinger-Ellison syndrome results in the inactivation of pancreatic enzymes and the precipitation of bile salts. Enterokinase deficiency restricts the activation of trypsin. Biliary atresia prevents the excretion of bile salts, and a gastrocolic fistula can lead to bacterial overgrowth of the small intestine. Unlike these disorders, which interfere with the intraluminal phase of digestion, infestation by *Giardia lamblia* causes malabsorption by damaging the intestinal mucosa.

187. The answer is B. *(Silverman, ed 2. p 685.)* D-Xylose absorption is a measure of mucosal function of the small intestine. Diseases such as gluten-induced enteropathy (celiac disease) and regional enteritis that damage small bowel intestinal mucosa will cause abnormal D-xylose absorption values. Because pancreatic insufficiency disrupts the intraluminal phase of digestion, the mucosal transport is not altered. Patients with short bowel syndrome have decreased absorption due to decreased absorptive surface area.

188. The answer is D. *(Silverman, ed 2. p 464.)* All of the physical and historical items listed in the question except Rotor's syndrome can be associated with the jaundice of the infant described. A chronic familial disease that is diagnosed only rarely in children, Rotor's syndrome produces elevated levels of serum conjugated bilirubin due to a defect in liver-cell excretion of conjugated bilirubin into the biliary system. It is not a cause of unconjugated hyperbilirubinemia in newborn infants.

189. The answer is E. *(Schaffer, ed 4. pp 641-642.)* The transient elevation of unconjugated bilirubin levels commonly found in newborn infants (physiologic jaundice or hyperbilirubinemia of the newborn) is caused by a temporary deficiency of the hepatic enzyme bilirubin glucuronyl transferase. Aside from an elevation in serum bilirubin levels, infants who have physiologic jaundice typically demonstrate normal laboratory findings. In full-term infants, liver function studies are normal. Defects in coagulation are not observed, and complete blood cell counts are within normal limits. Examination of urine would not show the presence of bile. Tests such as bromsulphalein excretion study, which evaluates conjugation, would be prolonged.

190. The answer is E. *(Silverman, ed 2. pp 208-209.)* Sucrase-isomaltase deficiency is an inherited condition characterized by a reduction in or absence of this disaccharidase. As in other disaccharidase deficiencies, such as lactase deficiency, intestinal mucosa is normal on histologic examination of a biopsy sample. Malabsorption of sucrose results in bacterial metabolism of carbohydrate and production of hydrogen. The mechanism of glucose absorption is independent of—and thus unaffected by a deficiency in—sucrase-isomaltase activity.

191. The answer is A. *(Greenberger, N Engl J Med 280:1047, 1969.)* Medium-chain triglycerides consist of fatty acids that contain from 8 to 12 carbon atoms. They are rapidly hydrolyzed by pancreatic lipase; and because the fatty acids and monoglycerides are water soluble, bile salts are not necessary for solubilization or absorption. Medium-chain triglycerides, which bypass the usual mucosal pathway of triglyceride resynthesis, are transported (albumin-bound) principally in the portal blood; in the liver they undergo nearly complete metabolism.

192. The answer is A. *(Isselbacher, ed 9. pp 1424-1431. Sleisenger, ed 2. pp 1602-1605.)* Ulcerative colitis characteristically is associated with a continuous lesion involving the superficial mucosal tissue of the colon. Rectal bleeding and, especially, bloody diarrhea are major symptoms; however, the severity of the symptoms, the clinical course, and the prognosis are highly variable. Sigmoidoscopic examination typically shows increased mucosal friability and decreased mucosal detail. Anorectal fistulas and perianal abscesses are much more common in individuals who have Crohn's disease. Extraintestinal manifestations, such as skin lesions and liver disease, are not uncommon in association with ulcerative colitis.

193. The answer is D. *(Silverman, ed 2. pp 490-501.)* Reye's syndrome is an idiopathic syndrome that usually begins as a mild, nonspecific illness that worsens suddenly, leading to marked abnormalities of the central nervous system, encephalopathy, coma, and hepatic dysfunction. Serum levels of ammonia, amino acids, and glutamic-oxaloacetic transaminase are elevated in affected children; white blood cell count also is higher than normal. Other laboratory findings include hypoglycemia, prolonged prothrombin time, and acellular cerebrospinal fluid. Electroencephalographic examination is diffusely abnormal and typically demonstrates high-voltage, slow-wave activity.

194. The answer is D. *(Schapiro, pp 217-236. Silverman, ed 2. p 721.)* Delayed passage of meconium occurs in a high percentage of children who have Hirschsprung's disease. These children may develop enterocolitic complications, poor weight gain, and diarrhea—rather than constipation—in the first few months of life. Infections including salmonellosis may cause bloody diarrhea in a neonate and occur frequently in association with Hirschsprung's disease. Dilatation, necrosis, perforation, and intramural pneumatosis of the ileum and colon, often with bloody diarrhea, are characteristics of necrotizing enterocolitis, an idiopathic complication of prematurity, exchange transfusions, and severe neonatal infection. Other conditions associated with delayed passage of meconium include a meconium plug, inspissated meconium accompanying cystic fibrosis, and hypothyroidism. An infant who has hypothyroidism, however, usually is constipated; diarrhea rarely occurs in association with this disorder.

195. The answer is D. *(Silverman, ed 2. pp 259-265.)* The child described in the question has abnormally low levels of serum albumin and total serum protein. Intestinal lymphangiectasia is a type of protein-losing enteropathy that probably results from a congenital abnormality of the lymphatic system. It is frequently associated with chronic lymphatic obstruction and lymphedema in various parts of the body, such as the hands, the arms, and especially the legs; this chronic lymphedema is called Milroy's disease. Although severe right-sided heart disease and Menetrier's disease both may cause protein loss in the gastrointestinal tract, they rarely are associated with lymphatic aberrations. Diarrhea and growth problems are common to tropical sprue and cystic fibrosis, both of which also can lead to protein loss from the bowel.

196. The answer is C. *(Isselbacher, ed 9. p 1409. Silverman, ed 2. pp 262-265.)* Children who have intestinal lymphangiectasia have hypoproteinemia as a result of protein loss from the small bowel. These children also have lymphocytopenia, which is caused by the loss of lymphocytes by way of the lymph. Other associated findings include abnormal delayed hypersensitivity, hypocalcemia, malabsorption, edema, and occasionally pleural effusions. Treatment with a low-fat diet, supplemented by medium-chain triglycerides often reduces lymph flow and may be beneficial.

197. The answer is E. *(Silverman, ed 2. pp 507-509. Zieve, Arch Intern Med 118:211-223, 1966.)* Diminished gag reflex is an important indicator of deterioration in neurologic status in an individual who has fulminating hepatitis. Physical examination also is likely to reveal rapid shrinkage in the size of an affected patient's liver. Laboratory findings include hypoalbuminemia, hyperbilirubinemia, and a markedly elevated serum glutamic-oxaloacetic transaminase level; prothrombin time is prolonged and does not respond to vitamin K therapy.

198. The answer is C. *(Kerr, Q J Med 30:91-117, 1961. Silverman, ed 2. pp 594-598.)* All of the conditions listed in the question are associated with portal hypertension, and all but congenital hepatic fibrosis are associated with cirrhosis as well. Children who have congenital hepatic fibrosis usually present with portal hypertension and upper gastrointestinal bleeding; their portal hypertension is due to a presinusoidal block, and they have normal liver function. The findings of associated renal lesions and a positive family history help confirm the diagnosis of congenital hepatic fibrosis. In the other disorders listed in the question, liver disease is a primary or associated finding which can be complicated by cirrhosis.

199. The answer is A. *(Scharli, J Pediatr Surg 4:108-114, 1969.)* Symptoms of children who have pyloric stenosis include vomiting, dehydration, constipation, moderate jaundice (indirect hyperbilirubinemia), and a palpable mass in the right upper quadrant. The differential diagnosis, particularly in male infants, should include salt loss due to one type of the adrenogenital syndrome; infants with this disorder characteristically are acidotic and have an elevated serum potassium level. In contrast, infants who have pyloric stenosis have metabolic alkalosis and an alkaline, concentrated urine.

200. The answer is D. *(Mathis, J Pediatr 90:864-880, 1977.)* The administration of certain medications commonly causes iatrogenic liver disease (including hepatocellular dysfunction) by toxic as well as idiosyncratic mechanisms. Aspirin and acetaminophen, for example, are direct hepatotoxins; how oxacillin and azathioprine lead to liver disease is less clear. Although prednisone is not associated with drug-induced liver disease, it can exacerbate existing hepatic cirrhosis.

201. The answer is A. *(Isselbacher, ed 9. pp 1521-1522. Sleisenger, ed 2. pp 278-279.)* Functions of the ileum include vitamin B_{12} absorption and absorption of bile salts by an active transport mechanism to complete the enterohepatic circulation of bile salts. Loss of ileal absorption of vitamin B_{12} can lead to the development of pernicious anemia. Excessive loss of bile salts, which can occur in association with ileal resection, may cause diarrhea, which is responsive to cholestyramine therapy, and an increase in glycine-conjugated bile acids. Malabsorption of fat and calcium secondary to bile-salt deficiency may result in increased oxalate absorption and the formation of calcium oxalate renal stones.

202. The answer is C. *(Mathis, J Pediatr 90:864-880, 1977.)* Absorption of carotene, a lipochrome, is decreased in children who have malabsorption from cholestatic syndromes. Obstructive liver disease causes elevation of serum cholesterol and alkaline phosphatase levels; the serum level of lipoprotein X, an abnormal lipoprotein that accumulates in the absence of proper amounts of lecithin-cholesterol acyltransferase, also is increased. Lipoprotein X is characteristic of cholestatic syndromes. Although prothrombin time is vitamin K-sensitive, it often remains normal until deficiency of this lipid-soluble vitamin becomes severe.

203. The answer is E. *(Schiff, ed 4. pp 1373-1378. Sleisenger, ed 2. pp 1660-1663.)* Small bowel involvement differentiates ulcerative colitis from Crohn's disease: in the latter any area of the small intestinal tract may be affected, whereas in ulcerative colitis only the colon is involved. Granulomas are characteristic of Crohn's disease but are not found in all cases or on all biopsy specimens. Rectal friability and bleeding are commonly associated with both ulcerative colitis and Crohn's disease, whereas toxic megacolon and pericholangitis are more often complications of ulcerative colitis. Isolated small bowel disease should be differentiated from lymphoma or infection by the appropriate diagnostic procedures before assuming Crohn's disease as the etiology.

204. The answer is C (2, 4). *(Silverman, ed 2. p 224. Vaughan, ed 11. pp 1083-1087, 1094-1101.)* Symptoms of celiac disease, which include chronic vomiting and diarrhea, irritability, and failure to grow, most commonly present during the first two years of life. Small-bowel x-rays of affected children often show thickened and coarse mucosal folds and dilatation of the intestine; small-bowel biopsy can show severely abnormal morphology. Celiac disease, an inherited condition in which the symptoms of malabsorption may occur sporadically within a family, is characterized by an intolerance to gluten. Treatment of affected children with a gluten-free diet is effective; however, removal of the offending agent is insufficient to establish the diagnosis. Histological recovery after removal of gluten is required, and on occasion it may be necessary to demonstrate recurrence of injury with gluten challenge. Proposed mechanisms for the initiation of injury include the absence of an intracellular or brush border peptidase, which renders the individual unable to digest gluten, and an immunologically mediated mechanism which involves the recognition of gluten as an offending agent. Histological features include an abnormal surface epithelium with loss of columnar cells, shortened villi, and elongation of crypts. While these are not specific for gluten-sensitive enteropathy, they are histologically consistent. Granuloma formation is not seen in celiac disease, nor is a pronounced eosinophilic inflammatory component. Treatment always involves gluten withdrawal and may also include a lactose-free diet if sufficient mucosal damage has occurred. Corticosteroids are reserved for use in acute celiac crises and in supportive management.

The histopathology of some other diarrheal diseases is as follows: ulcerative colitis does not involve the small intestine, and the small bowel biopsy in cystic fibrosis is normal. In lymphangiectasia the biopsy shows dilated lymphatics with a normal mucosa. In primary agammaglobulinemia there is an absence of plasma cells and a variety of histological abnormalities, particularly when complicated by giardiasis, malnutrition, or both. In congenital lactase deficiency, the small bowel biopsy is normal, and the diagnosis is established by enzyme analysis.

205. The answer is B (1, 3). *(Silverman, ed 2. pp 21-22, 399-401.)* Obstructive jaundice (i.e., a direct-reacting bilirubin greater than 15 percent of the total) requires investigation in all infants. Cystic fibrosis and alpha$_1$-antitrypsin deficiency should be considered in the diagnostic evaluation of any child with these presenting findings. Other diseases to be excluded include galactosemia, tyrosinemia, and urinary tract or other infections, including toxoplasmosis, cytomegalovirus, rubella, syphilis, and herpesvirus. Ultrasound examination to rule out choledochal cyst may be included with an ^{131}I rose bengal or ^{99}technetium hepatic iminodiacetic acid (HIDA) scan to assess the patency of the biliary tree. Liver biopsy may show evidence of hepatitis and giant cell transformation both in cystic fibrosis and alpha$_1$-antitrypsin deficiency. These findings may differentiate these diseases from extrahepatic obstruction or biliary atresia, but they are not pathognomonic in themselves. The presence of diastase-resistant, periodic acid schiff (PAS) positive granules is reported but is not specific in alpha$_1$-antitrypsin deficiency alone. In contrast, infants who have Gilbert's syndrome or hypothyroidism present with an indirect hyperbilirubinemia and have normal liver biopsies.

206. The answer is E (all). *(Silverman, ed 2. p 451.)* Nonhemolytic hyperbilirubinemia in newborn infants can result from a number of factors, among which are decreased hepatic uptake of bilirubin and delayed conjugation secondary to reduced levels of intrahepatic binding proteins and glucuronyl transferase. Conditions contributing to these deficiencies include a shortened life span of fetal red blood cells and, most probably, an increased enterohepatic circulation of bilirubin.

207. The answer is A (1, 2, 3). *(Silverman, ed 2. pp 215-222, 363-364, 370.)* Hartnup disease, folic acid deficiency, and dermatitis herpetiformis all disrupt the intestinal phase of digestion. Hartnup disease is an inborn defect in the absorption by intestinal epithelial cells of the amino acids tryptophan and phenylalanine. Folate deficiency, either as a congenital disorder or in association with the malabsorption syndrome, is a sign of jejunal mucosal dysfunction. Dermatitis herpetiformis, which may be associated with celiac sprue, can lead to patchy distribution of flat areas of intestinal mucosa. Cystic fibrosis is principally a defect of pancreatic function and lipolysis; thus, it interferes with the intraluminal phase of digestion.

208. The answer is E (all). *(Silverman, ed 2. pp 206, 209-212.)* Lactase is a disaccharidase localized in the brush border of the intestinal villous cells. It hydrolyzes lactose to its constituent monosaccharides, glucose and galactose. Sucrose, also a disaccharide, is a nonreducing sugar composed of glucose and fructose that is hydrolyzed by the brush border enzyme sucrase. Lactase activity is not readily increased by the oral administration of substrate or the inclusion of lactose in the diet. The clinical symptoms of lactose malabsorption are due to the presence of osmotically active undigested lactose which may act to increase intestinal fluid volume, alter transit time, and produce the symptoms of abdominal cramps, distension, and, occasionally, watery diarrhea. Bacterial metabolism of the nonabsorbed carbohydrates in the colon to carbon dioxide and hydrogen may contribute to the clinical symptoms.

Diagnostic techniques for lactose intolerance include removal of the offending sugar with a reproduction of symptoms following an oral load (2 g/kg, maximum 50 g). This should be accompanied by the failure to demonstrate a rise in blood sugar of more than 30 mg/100 ml. Since the glucose level can be influenced by gastric emptying or by abnormalities in glucose utilization, the recent demonstration of a breath hydrogen rise after lactose administration has proven to be a noninvasive and diagnostic test for lactose malabsorption. Similarly, an acidic stool pH in the presence of reducing substances would be diagnostic. Direct measurement of enzyme levels combined with histologic evaluation helps to differentiate an acquired (secondary versus primary) lactase deficiency in which the intestinal histology is normal.

209. The answer is C (2, 4). *(Silverman, ed 2. pp 205-219.)* Sucrase-isomaltase deficiency is a familial condition inherited as an autosomal recessive trait. Diarrhea, bloating, and cramps are frequent symptoms and disappear when sucrose is removed from the diet. Affected children generally have normal growth and development. Because these children usually do not have an accompanying lactase deficiency, they are able to tolerate milk well. Sucrose is not a reducing sugar and thus requires hydrolysis with hydrochloric acid in order for reducing activity to be exposed.

210. The answer is A (1, 2, 3). *(Isselbacher, ed 9. p 1390.)* Children who have Menetrier's disease lose protein through abnormally hyperplastic gastric mucosa; increased protein loss can be demonstrated by assaying the concentration of labeled albumin. Possible etiologies of this disease include infection, particularly with cytomegalovirus, and gastrointestinal allergy; however, the exact cause is unknown. Mucosal biopsy of the stomach of affected individuals characteristically shows glandular hypertrophy, and x-ray examination reveals giant rugal folds. Gastric secretion of hydrochloric acid is scant. Presenting symptoms include epigastric pain, anorexia, nausea, weight loss, vomiting, diarrhea, and occasionally bleeding.

211. The answer is A (1, 2, 3). *(Silverman, ed 2. pp 66-71, 81-85.)* The x-ray presented in the question shows a microcolon (disuse microcolon), which is characteristic of fetal intestinal obstruction; it requires prompt diagnosis and therapeutic management. Films of the abdomen are the first step in establishing the diagnosis and possible level of obstruction in an infant with abdominal distension and clinical evidence of obstruction. With meconium ileus or meconium peritonitis a characteristic "soap bubble" appearance in the right lower quadrant or evidence of intestinal perforation might be evident. Barium enema is then often required to establish the presence of microcolon and to differentiate between a volvulus and other less common abnormalities. Ileal atresia secondary to meconium inspissation, intestinal perforation, and meconium peritonitis, with its associated intra-abdominal calcifications, are frequently associated with cystic fibrosis. These begin in utero and are accompanied by a secondary microcolon. Occasionally, a microcolon may be present when acute intestinal obstruction due to malrotation and volvulus occurs very early in life. Evidence by barium enema of abnormal placement or lack of fixation of the cecum can suggest this diagnosis. Obstruction in Down's syndrome (trisomy 21) infants also can be caused by jejunoileal atresia, which may be accompanied by malrotation.

Tracheoesophageal fistula with esophageal atresia is associated with polyhydramnios secondary to a failure to reabsorb swallowed amniotic fluid in utero. It does not lead to microcolon unless there is a complete intestinal obstruction. Hirschsprung's disease presents in the newborn period with a delayed passage of meconium but with a normal or increased diameter of the colon; occasionally, there is evidence of enterocolitis. A transition zone may be seen by barium enema, often with failure to clear the barium over the next 24 hours.

Surgery is almost always required to correct meconium ileus. However, occasionally a diatrizoate methylglucamine (Gastrografin) enema or infusion of mucolytic agents such as *N*-acetylcysteine (5 to 10 percent solution) has been useful to relieve the obstruction, thus alleviating the need for an intestinal resection. Enzyme replacement is required in the therapy of the pancreatic insufficiency associated with cystic fibrosis.

212. The answer is E (all). *(Silverman, ed 2. pp 190-191, 193, 291, 314.)* Crohn's disease is a granulomatous disorder that can affect any area of the small or large intestine; another granulomatous disorder, cavitary pulmonary tuberculosis, can lead to ileocecal disease. Intestinal lesions of Schönlein-Henoch purpura can be caused by hemorrhage into the mucosal wall; almost any area of the gastrointestinal tract, however, can be similarly affected. *Yersinia enterocolitica* infection causes an acute gastroenteritis or a more persistent, localized disease involving the colon and distal ileum, often mimicking inflammatory bowel disease. Diagnosis may be confirmed by culture, serological titers, or both.

213. The answer is E (all). *(Silverman, ed 2. p 621. Sleisenger, ed 2. pp 1475-1480.)* Children who have cystic fibrosis can exhibit a wide range of gastrointestinal disorders: indeed, malabsorption in children is more likely to be due to cystic fibrosis than to any other cause. Hepatic lesions associated with cystic fibrosis include portal hypertension (often accompanied by varices and ascites), cirrhosis, and fatty disease. Among affected newborn infants, meconium ileus can lead to intestinal obstruction; obstruction in older children can occur for a variety of reasons. Gallbladder disorders associated with cystic fibrosis include congenital microgallbladder and cholelithiasis.

214. The answer is A (1, 2, 3). *(Goldman, N Engl J Med 293:20-23, 1975.)* Sulfasalazine (Azulfidine) is converted by bacteria in the colon into two active ingredients: 5-aminosalicylate and sulfapyridine. The mechanism for the drug's therapeutic action is unknown. It is most efficacious in the treatment of individuals who have ulcerative colitis and is currently of unproven efficacy in cases of Crohn's disease involving the small bowel. Adverse reactions can occur in patients who are slow acetylators of sulfapyridine and thus develop toxic levels of this drug in their sera.

215. The answer is B (1, 3). *(Isselbacher, ed 9. pp 1487-1488. Partin, N Engl J Med 285:1139-1143, 1971. Reye, Lancet 2:749-757, 1963.)* Although the defect causing Reye's syndrome is unknown, specific biochemical deficiencies, including deficiency of ornithine transcarbamylase, have been suggested. Epidemiology points to a viral etiology, but this association too is unproven. The urea cycle does not seem to be primarily involved. Mitochondrial lesions predominate in the brain and liver; and, in the proper clinical setting, microvesicular hepatic steatosis is diagnostic for the disorder. Presenting symptoms include vomiting, liver damage, hypoglycemia, and central nervous system damage. Girls and boys up to 15 years of age are affected, and a mortality rate of 50 percent has been reported.

216. The answer is A (1, 2, 3). *(Isselbacher, ed 9. pp 1431-1432. Sleisenger, ed 2. pp 1658-1662.)* Crohn's disease (granulomatous colitis) characteristically is associated with transmural, granulomatous intestinal lesions that are discontinuous and can appear in both the small and large intestine. Although Crohn's disease first may appear as a rectal fissure or fistula, the rectum often is spared. Aphthous stomatitis is a common complaint in affected children. In relation to the general population, the risk of colonic carcinoma in affected individuals is increased, but not nearly to the degree associated with ulcerative colitis.

217. The answer is E (all). *(Alpert, N Engl J Med 285:185-189, 1971. Sabesin, N Engl J Med 290:944-950, 996-1002, 1974.)* Human hepatitis B (serum hepatitis) is associated with the hepatitis B antigen and can be identified by the presence of surface antigens, core antigens, or Dane particles, which are thought to be intact hepatitis B viruses. A prodome of migratory arthritis or skin rash recently has been recognized and presumably is due to surface antigen-antibody immune complexes. Although traditionally associated with hepatitis A, oral-fecal transmission also has been linked to hepatitis B.

218. The answer is E (all). *(Isselbacher, ed 9. pp 1406-1407. Silverman, ed 2. pp 202-212.)* Intestinal lactase levels are usually normal at birth in all populations; however, lactase deficiency is a common genetically predetermined condition with an incidence reported to be 5 to 15 percent of the adult white population and 80 to 90 percent of adult blacks and orientals. Acquired lactase deficiency is often associated with conditions of the gastrointestinal tract, which cause intestinal mucosal injury (e.g., sprue and regional enteritis). While the ingestion of even small amounts of lactose can be diagnostic if gastrointestinal symptoms occur, the measurement of breath hydrogen is more specific as it is not affected by glucose metabolism or gastric emptying.

219. The answer is E (all). *(Greseon, Pediatrics 54:456, 1974. Sleisenger, ed 2. pp 740-742.)* The x-ray presented in the question shows antral narrowing, an unusual finding in children. This finding should not be considered as indicating only an ulcer, as it can be associated with all of the disorders listed in the question. Hence, the confirmed diagnosis of these conditions can not be made on the basis of x-ray alone. An intestinal gastric biopsy is necessary in order to differentiate one from the other.

220. The answer is C (2, 4). *(Suzuki, Pediatrics 51:188-191, 1973. Swensen, J Pediatr Surg 8:587-594, 1973.)* Hirschsprung's disease is characterized by an absence of ganglion cells on rectal biopsy; errors in diagnosis can occur if the biopsy is performed at the anal verge or if it is too superficial. Manometric recordings in the rectum of affected infants show a failure of the internal sphincter to relax during rectal dilatation. Radiographic findings characteristically include colonic dilatation followed by an aganglionic transition zone that is narrow and has irregular margins.

221-225. The answers are: 221-B, 222-B, 223-E, 224-C, 225-B. *(Silverman, ed 2. pp 373-383.)* All of the disorders listed in the question cause gastrointestinal polyposis. Peutz-Jeghers syndrome, which is inherited as an autosomal dominant trait, is characterized by the presence of hamartomatous polyps, especially in the small intestine but also occasionally in the stomach and colon. The most striking extraintestinal manifestation of this disorder is lip or buccal pigmentation, which usually develops during infancy. Peutz-Jeghers polyposis rarely leads to carcinoma.

Gardner's syndrome, on the other hand, is characterized by adenomatous polyps that frequently undergo malignant degeneration. This autosomal dominant disorder occurs mainly in the colon. In affected children under the age of ten years, the condition may appear first as a fibromatous mass or epidermoid cyst involving skin or soft tissue.

Isolated juvenile polyps occur as a benign, nonheritable condition typically associated with pedunculated inflammatory polyps that usually occur within 25 cm of the anus. Juvenile polyposis of the colon, in contrast, is an inherited condition (the mode of inheritance is unknown) causing large numbers of juvenile polyps to appear in the intestine. Neither disorder is associated with malignant degeneration. Although children having juvenile polyposis of the colon may have other congenital anomalies, children with juvenile polyps usually do not.

Lymphoid polyposis (nodular lymphoid hyperplasia) can affect both the small and the large intestine. In cases where the appearance of the submucosal nodules, which are composed of lymphoid follicles, is confined to the small intestine, infection with *Giardia lamblia* may be an etiologic factor. Lymphoid polyposis is associated neither with intestinal carcinoma nor with extraintestinal manifestations. Whether this condition is inherited is not known.

226-230. The answers are: 226-B, 227-A, 228-B, 229-C, 230-A. *(Silverman, ed 2. pp 567-580.)* Wilson's disease, an autosomal recessive genetic disorder, is characterized by the defective metabolism of copper. Copper deposition particularly affects the brain—causing tremors, dystonia, and personality changes—and the liver—causing portal hypertension and postnecrotic cirrhosis among other conditions. Hemolysis can lead to recurrent jaundice and anemia. Renal defects, which are associated with glycosuria and aminoaciduria, often occur. Wilson's disease usually appears clinically in individuals between the ages of 6 and 20 years. Administration of D-penicillamine (Cuprimine) has been therapeutically helpful.

Alpha$_1$-antitrypsin deficiency, which has an autosomal codominant mode of inheritance, can cause chronic liver disease in infants and may give rise in adults to gradually developing dyspnea as a result of panacinar emphysema, early symptoms of which can appear in childhood. Jaundice can develop in affected infants during the first weeks of life; histologic examination of the liver shows intralobular bile stasis, perilobular fibrosis, and other abnormalities. Postnecrotic cirrhosis develops later. Management includes symptomatic treatment and genetic counseling.

The Urinary Tract

Julie R. Ingelfinger

DIRECTIONS: Each question below contains five suggested answers. Choose the **one best** response to each question.

231. A ten-year-old boy comes to the emergency room complaining of flank pain. A flat-plate x-ray taken at that time is shown below. The findings exhibited by the x-ray could represent all of the following types of urinary stones EXCEPT

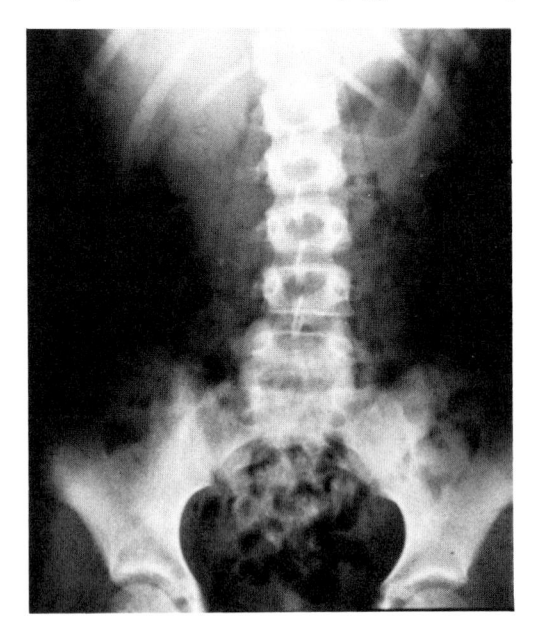

(A) cystine
(B) xanthine
(C) calcium phosphate
(D) calcium oxalate
(E) magnesium ammonium sulfate

232. A five-year-old girl is brought to a hospital because of dysuria. A clean-voided urine sample contains more than 10^6 *Escherichia coli* per mm^3 sensitive to all antibiotics tested. This is the girl's first known episode of dysuria. All of the following steps would be appropriate in the management of her illness EXCEPT

(A) administration of ampicillin
(B) administration of sulfisoxazole
(C) repetition of the urine culture bimonthly after stopping antibiotic therapy
(D) repetition of the urine culture seven days after stopping antibiotic therapy
(E) performing voiding cystourethrography one week hence

233. A previously healthy six-year-old white boy develops acute renal failure. The pathologic processes in his illness may include all of the following EXCEPT

(A) obstructive uropathy
(B) acute papillary necrosis
(C) renal arterial occlusion
(D) myoglobinuria
(E) acute glomerulonephritis

234. Progressive glomerular disease may occur in association with all of the following diseases EXCEPT

(A) lupus erythematosus
(B) anaphylactoid purpura
(C) diabetes mellitus
(D) porphyria
(E) polyarteritis

235. A seven-year-old boy has crampy abdominal pain and a rash on the back of his legs and buttocks as well as on the extensor surfaces of his forearms. Laboratory analysis reveals proteinuria and microhematuria. He is most likely to be affected by

(A) systemic lupus erythematosus
(B) anaphylactoid purpura
(C) poststreptococcal glomerulonephritis
(D) polyarteritis nodosa
(E) dermatomyositis

236. An exogenous substance that is used to measure glomerular filtration rate should be

(A) physiologically active
(B) capable of binding with plasma proteins
(C) freely filterable at the glomerulus
(D) secreted by the renal tubule
(E) reabsorbed by the renal tubule

237. During the first year of a child's life, all of the following parameters of renal function increase EXCEPT

(A) glomerular filtration rate
(B) nephron number
(C) renal plasma flow
(D) tubular reabsorptive capacity
(E) tubular secretory capacity

238. The child shown in the photograph below most likely has

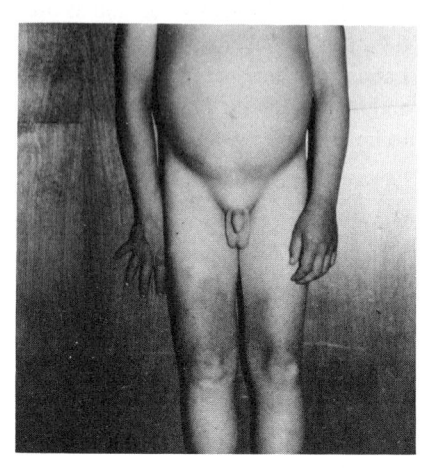

(A) cystinosis
(B) polycystic kidneys
(C) diabetes insipidus
(D) acute poststreptococcal glomerulonephritis
(E) nephrosis

239. A diagnosis of Alport syndrome is made in the case of a six-year-old boy who presents with all of the following abnormalities EXCEPT

(A) sensorineural deafness
(B) patellar abnormalities
(C) glomerular hyalinization
(D) cataracts
(E) renal disease

240. A blood pressure of 120/80 mm Hg is within normal values for children of all of the following ages EXCEPT

(A) 4 years
(B) 7 years
(C) 10 years
(D) 12 years
(E) 15 years

241. The photomicrograph shown below of a urine specimen from a seven-year-old child is LEAST likely to support a diagnosis of

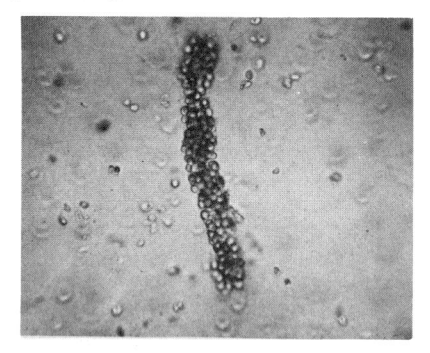

(A) systemic lupus erythematosus
(B) acute poststreptococcal glomerulonephritis
(C) Berger disease
(D) membranous glomerulopathy
(E) mesangiocapillary glomerulonephritis

242. An eight-year-old girl has a glomerular filtration rate of 100 ml/min/1.73 m². Her urine specific gravity has never exceeded 1.010. These laboratory values could be associated with all of the following conditions EXCEPT

(A) diabetes insipidus
(B) sickle cell anemia
(C) childhood nephrosis
(D) nephrocalcinosis
(E) pyelonephritis

243. A ten-month-old child has diarrhea and is dehydrated by an estimated 10 percent. Laboratory analysis reveals a serum sodium level of 162 mEq/L. The clinical sign or symptom that would be LEAST likely to accompany these findings would be

(A) increased reflexes
(B) impaired mental status
(C) marked thirst
(D) marked loss of circulatory volume
(E) doughy skin

244. A six-year-old child develops acute renal failure. A nonhemolyzed serum potassium level, which is determined as soon as the lab receives a blood sample, is reported back as 7.8 mEq/L. The child's physician should now

(A) start peritoneal dialysis
(B) administer sodium polystyrene sulfonate (Kayexalate)
(C) administer intravenous bicarbonate
(D) administer intravenous furosemide
(E) administer intravenous mannitol

245. A three-year-old boy develops edema and proteinuria. His serum cholesterol level is 322 mg/100 ml, and his serum albumin level is 1.9 g/100 ml. The likelihood that he has minimal-change nephrotic syndrome is about

(A) 10 percent
(B) 25 percent
(C) 40 percent
(D) 65 percent
(E) 80 percent

246. A renal biopsy is performed on a patient who has acute onset of renal disease; a sample of the biopsied tissue is shown below. The most likely diagnosis is

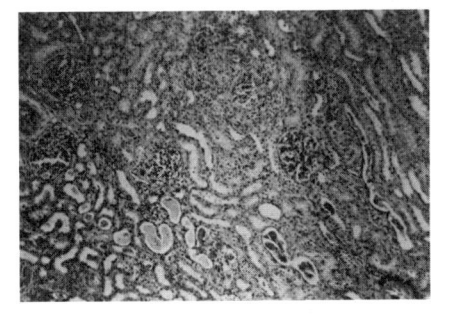

(A) minimal-change nephrotic syndrome
(B) poststreptococcal glomerulonephritis
(C) membranoproliferative glomerulonephritis
(D) rapidly progressive nephritis
(E) segmental glomerulosclerosis

247. Funduscopic examination of a 13-year-old girl shows general and focal arteriolar narrowing. A hemorrhage is observed in the left retina, and sclerosis is present. Her blood pressure is 180/110 mm Hg. This girl would be likely to exhibit all of the following symptoms or signs EXCEPT

(A) isolated facial nerve palsy
(B) headache
(C) hyporeflexia
(D) nocturnal wakening
(E) left ventricular hypertrophy

248. An *Escherichia coli* colony count of $2000/mm^3$ would be definite evidence of a urinary tract infection if the sampled urine

(A) has a specific gravity of 1.008
(B) has been taken from a catheterized bladder and has a specific gravity of 1.022
(C) is from an ileal-loop bag
(D) is from a suprapubic tap
(E) is the first morning sample

249. A seven-year-old boy suffers multiple injuries as a result of blunt abdominal trauma. All of the following statements concerning the proper assessment and treatment of the injury are true EXCEPT that

(A) most renal injuries can be managed nonoperatively
(B) major vascular injuries require rapid surgical intervention
(C) rupture of a full bladder is uncommon
(D) traumatic hematocele requires surgical exploration and repair
(E) prompt surgical repair is needed for most ureteral injuries

250. The presence of drug-induced nephrotic syndrome should be suspected in a proteinuric patient who has received which of the following drugs?

(A) Tetracycline
(B) Streptomycin
(C) Trimethadione
(D) Diazepam
(E) Chlorambucil

251. A child who has vomited and had diarrhea for two days is brought to the emergency room for evaluation. No blood loss has occurred. Serum sodium level is reported to be 138 mEq/L. This child, who weighed 10 kg (22 lb) last week, now weighs 9 kg (19.8 lb). The best therapy would be infusion of

(A) Ringer's lactate, 100 ml over two hours, followed by normal saline with 40 mEq/L of potassium, 500 ml over sixteen hours, and 5% dextrose in quarter-normal saline, 1400 ml over the next eight hours
(B) Ringer's lactate, 200 ml over one to two hours, followed by 5% dextrose in quarter-normal saline, 800 ml over the next eight hours, and 1000 ml over the following sixteen hours
(C) whole blood, 100 ml over 30 minutes, followed by 5% dextrose in quarter-normal saline, 1800 ml over the following 20 to 24 hours
(D) plasma, 100 ml, followed by 5% dextrose in one-sixth-normal saline, 1900 ml over 16 hours
(E) plasma, 200 ml, followed by 5% dextrose in water, 1800 ml over 18 hours

Urinary Tract 113

252. The cells shown below were seen on microscopic examination of a bacteriologically sterile urine specimen. The differential diagnosis should include all of the following conditions EXCEPT

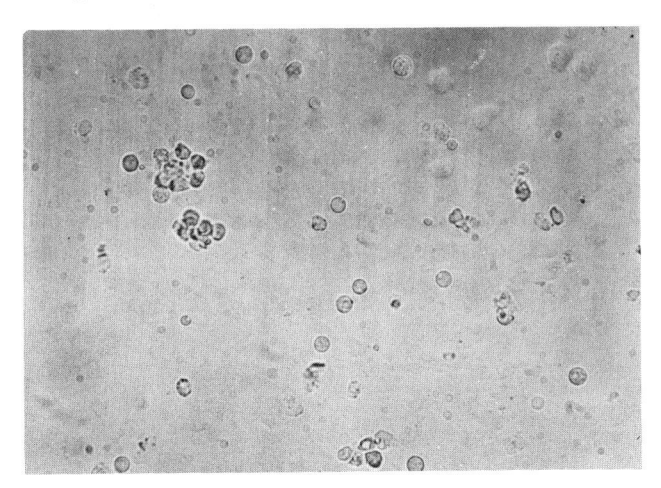

(A) renal tuberculosis
(B) systemic lupus erythematosus
(C) interstitial nephritis
(D) Potter's syndrome
(E) Kawasaki disease

253. All of the following statements about cryptorchidism are true EXCEPT that

(A) 3 to 4 percent of term infants have undescended testes
(B) 10 percent of men who have undergone childhood orchidopexy are oligospermic
(C) 30 percent of low-birth-weight infants have undescended testes
(D) seminoma develops 14 times more frequently in patients with undescended testes
(E) elective orchidopexy should be performed before four years of age

254. All of the following statements about enuretic children are true EXCEPT that

(A) about 1 percent of normal children are enuretic at age 15
(B) about 12 percent of five-year-old boys are bedwetters
(C) a familial pattern is common
(D) organic renal disease is more prevalent in enuretic children
(E) operant conditioning is often therapeutically helpful

114 Pediatrics

DIRECTIONS: Each question below contains four suggested answers of which **one** or **more** is correct. Choose the answer:

A	if	1, 2, and 3	are correct
B	if	1 and 3	are correct
C	if	2 and 4	are correct
D	if	4	is correct
E	if	1, 2, 3, and 4	are correct

255. An arteriogram of an eight-year-old girl who has hypertension is shown below. Findings illustrated in the arteriogram could be the result of

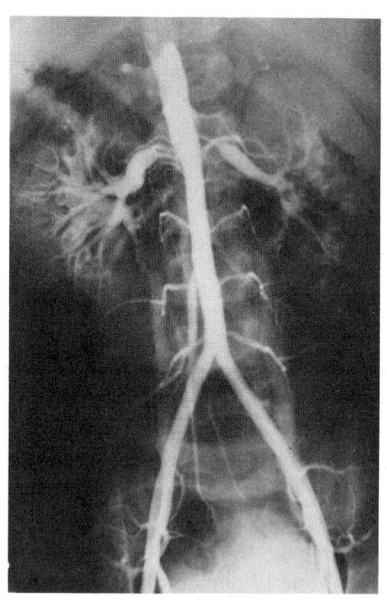

(1) fibromuscular dysplasia
(2) von Recklinghausen's disease
(3) tumorous impingement
(4) arteriovenous malformation

256. For the last three months, a child, whose x-ray is shown below, has been treated with dihydrotachysterol, 0.25 mg/day. The condition depicted in this child's x-ray would be compatible with which of the following conditions?

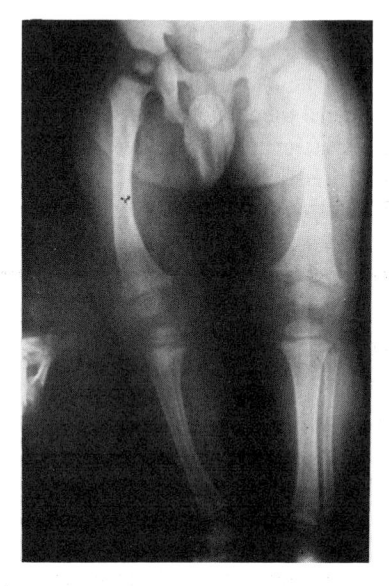

(1) Acidemia
(2) A serum phosphate level of 2.1 mg/100 ml
(3) A blood urea nitrogen level of 150 mg/100 ml
(4) A positive family history

257. Distal renal tubular acidosis (RTA) can occur in association with exposure to which of the following substances?

(1) Lithium salts
(2) Outdated tetracycline
(3) Toluene (by sniffing)
(4) Cadmium

258. A percutaneous kidney biopsy of a child who has steroid-dependent nephrosis should NOT be performed if that child also has which of the following complications?

(1) Single kidney
(2) Pyelonephritis
(3) Dysplastic kidneys
(4) Hypertension

259. A 14-year-old boy who has renal dysplasia develops a urinary tract infection. His serum creatinine is reported to be 6.2 mg/100 ml. Which of the following antibiotics, as possible treatment for the boy's infection, would require dosage alteration in this situation?

(1) Ampicillin
(2) Amoxicillin
(3) Gentamicin
(4) Clindamycin

260. Abdominal ultrasound is a useful diagnostic tool that is able to

(1) localize kidneys for renal biopsy
(2) determine whether or not a renal mass is cystic
(3) differentiate multicystic kidney from hydronephrosis
(4) differentiate hydronephrosis from urinomas, hematomas, or lymphoceles

261. The findings one might expect in a six-year-old boy with brown urine and healing impetigo include which of the following?

(1) Hypertension
(2) Dyspnea
(3) Periorbital edema
(4) Hepatomegaly

262. Hemolytic uremic syndrome can be described by which of the following statements?

(1) It commonly is preceded by infection
(2) It is characterized by development of acute renal failure
(3) Children five years of age or less are most often affected
(4) Blacks are affected more often than whites

263. Congenital nephrosis is characterized by

(1) circulating immune complexes
(2) frequent gross hematuria
(3) responsiveness to steroid therapy
(4) a high familial incidence

264. Hepatorenal syndrome is characterized by

(1) oliguria
(2) azotemia
(3) low urine levels of sodium
(4) high urine specific gravity

SUMMARY OF DIRECTIONS

A	B	C	D	E
1, 2, 3 only	1, 3 only	2, 4 only	4 only	All are correct

265. Correct statements concerning nephrogenic diabetes insipidus include which of the following?

(1) Most North American patients are of common descent
(2) It is probably inherited by an X-linked recessive mode
(3) It is a likely consequence of an enzymatic or biochemical renal tubular abnormality
(4) It is usually diagnosed at birth

266. A six-year-old girl is brought to the emergency room because her urine is red. Examination with Hemastix is negative. Possible causes of the red color of the girl's urine include

(1) ingestion of blackberries
(2) ingestion of beets
(3) phenolphthalein catharsis
(4) presence of myoglobin

267. Hypercalcemia is likely to be associated with which of the following symptoms?

(1) Oliguria
(2) Constipation
(3) Polyphagia
(4) Hypotonia

268. A 16-year-old girl, who has sickle cell disease and red-colored urine, undergoes intravenous pyelography. Her pyelogram, shown below, provides evidence of

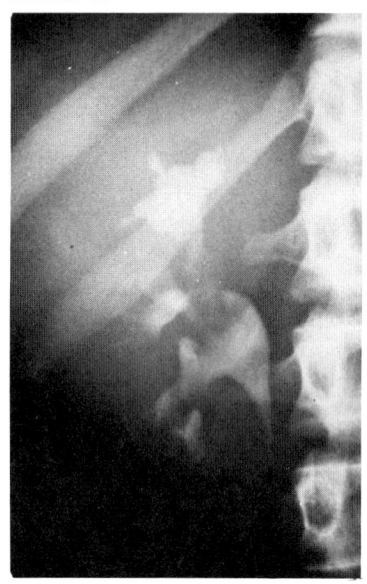

(1) a central papillary filling defect
(2) radiolucent cysts
(3) renal infarction
(4) renal stones

269. A 14-year-old girl who has sickle cell disease presents with red urine. Laboratory examination of her urine would be expected to show

(1) a low specific gravity
(2) proteinuria
(3) red blood cells
(4) oxalate crystals

270. The angiogram below is from a 12-year-old boy who has large kidneys. Findings on the x-ray are consistent with

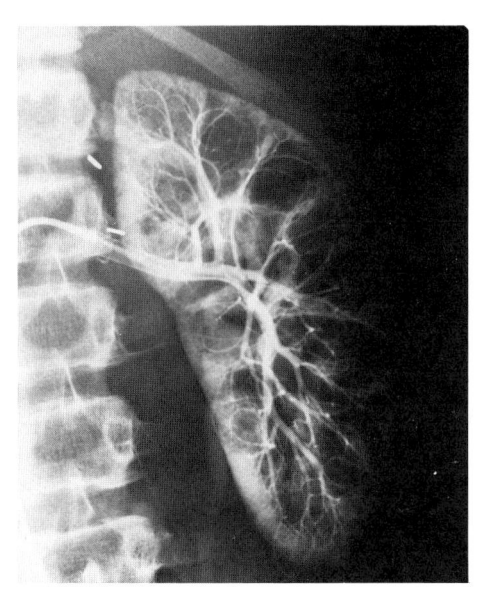

(1) multicystic renal dysplasia
(2) nephronophthisis
(3) megacalyx
(4) adult-type polycystic disease

Pediatrics

DIRECTIONS: The groups of questions below consist of lettered choices followed by several numbered items. For each numbered item select the **one** lettered choice with which it is **most** closely associated. Each lettered choice may be used once, more than once, or not at all.

Questions 271-275

For each diagnosis that follows, select the mode of inheritance with which it is associated.

(A) Autosomal dominant
(B) Autosomal recessive
(C) X-linked dominant
(D) X-linked recessive
(E) None of the above

271. Hypophosphatemic rickets

272. Infantile polycystic disease

273. Systemic lupus erythematosus

274. Nephropathic cystinosis

275. Adult-type polycystic disease

Questions 276-280

For each stage in the development of renal function that follows, choose the age range during which that stage is most likely to be reached.

(A) Newborn
(B) 1 to 2 weeks
(C) 2 to 4 months
(D) 6 to 12 months
(E) 1 to 3 years

276. All glomeruli are present

277. Glomerular filtration rate is comparable to adult

278. Urinary acidification is comparable to adult

279. Filtration fraction is comparable to adult

280. Glomerular filtration rate is twice that at birth

The Urinary Tract

Answers

231. The answer is B. *(Rudolph, ed 16. p 1321.)* Xanthine stones and, to a lesser degree, uric acid stones are radiolucent and therefore do not show up on flat-plate x-rays. When contrast material is used, however, radiolucent stones show up well (as filling defects), whereas radiopaque stones often blend in with the x-ray dye. Although 50 to 60 percent of urinary tract stones in children are idiopathic, a full metabolic workup is indicated to rule out the presence of underlying disease.

232. The answer is E. *(Hoekelman, pp 1620-1621. Vaughan, ed 11. pp 1545-1547.)* Although a positive urine culture in a symptomatic child is good evidence of a urinary tract infection, one or two confirmatory cultures should be performed to document the infection. Either sulfisoxazole or ampicillin can be administered for the management of an acute urinary tract infection provided there is no history of drug allergies that would contraindicate their use. In children, intravenous pyelography is warranted after the first documented urinary tract infection. Voiding cystourethrography, however, is best performed a few months after an infection has been treated, because many children with acute urinary tract infections have a temporary cystoureteral reflux that will disappear spontaneously. Reculturing during and after the course of antibiotic therapy is important in order to ascertain whether resistance has developed during or reinfection has occurred after antibiotic therapy.

233. The answer is B. *(Vaughan, ed 11. p 1532.)* Acute and widespread glomerular injury is a common source of acute renal failure in children. Acute glomerulonephritis, rapidly progressive glomerulonephritis, and hemolytic-uremic syndrome are all associated with widespread glomerular injury. In children, acute tubular necrosis and bilateral cortical necrosis may also occur. In a white child, acute papillary necrosis would be most unlikely.

234. The answer is D. *(Vaughan, ed 11. pp 672, 1536, 1562.)* Although porphyria can cause porphyrinuria and hemolytic anemia and, in a severe attack, lead to oliguria and azotemia, it is not associated with progressive glomerular disease. Anaphylactoid purpura, lupus erythematosus, and polyarteritis can cause a spectrum of proliferative and membranous changes in glomeruli, often culminating in renal failure. Diabetic nephropathy (intercapillary glomerulosclerosis), which eventually develops in most diabetic individuals, also can lead to renal failure.

235. The answer is B. *(Vaughan, ed 11. pp 668, 671.)* The rash of anaphylactoid purpura most often involves extensor surfaces of the extremities; the face, soles, palms, and trunk are rarely affected. Both systemic lupus erythematosus and dermatomyositis often are accompanied by typical facial rashes (butterfly and heliotrope, respectively). Individuals who have polyarteritis usually do not present with a rash. The scarlatiniform rash characteristic of streptococcal infections generally does not coincide with the development of poststreptococcal nephritis; impetiginous lesions, however, may still be present.

236. The answer is C. *(Vaughan, ed 11. pp 1478, 1485.)* If an exogenous substance is capable of being metabolized, bound by plasma proteins, or secreted or reabsorbed by the renal tubule, it will not measure glomerular function adequately. With current radiologic techniques, it is possible to perform glomerular-filtration-rate studies with isotopes such as ^{51}Cr-ethylenediaminotetraacetate (^{51}Cr-EDTA) or ^{125}I-iothalamate. Nonradiolabeled substances such as inulin, cyanocobalamin, and mannitol may also be used.

237. The answer is B. *(Vaughan, ed 11. p 1479.)* The kidneys of a newborn infant already contain their full complement of nephrons. However, glomerular filtration rate and renal plasma flow steadily increase to close to normal adult values (corrected for surface area) by the end of the first year of life. Infants have a relatively low rate of sodium reabsorption, which increases proportionally as body weight increases. The secretion of substances such as paraaminohippuric acid also increases during the first year of life.

238. The answer is E. *(Vaughan, ed 11. pp 1496-1497, 1530-1531.)* Physical findings of individuals who have nephrosis usually stem from edema, which may progress to generalized edema (anasarca). The edema is typically pitting and shifts with position. Although edema may occur in association with acute nephritis, it usually is less marked than in nephrosis. The large abdomens of patients who have polycystic kidney disease are not edematous. Cystinosis and diabetes insipidus do not cause edema.

239. The answer is B. *(Vaughan, ed 11. pp 1523-1525.)* The familial association of sensorineural high-frequency deafness and renal disease, often with ocular abnormalities, such as myopia and cataracts, is called Alport syndrome. Autosomal dominant inheritance, which is more severe in males, is usual. The renal abnormalities include thickening of the glomerular basement membrane, which progresses to glomerular hyalinization, and interstitial fibrosis with tubular atrophy. Microscopic hematuria is the usual presenting clinical feature of renal disease, which leads to azotemia and hypertension. Half of the affected males develop end-stage renal disease by 30 years of age.

240. The answer is A. *(Vaughan, ed 11. p 1354.)* Average blood pressure tends to increase with age. Thus, a value of 120/80 mm Hg, clearly acceptable for most children, is in the hypertensive range for children in the first few years of life. In the newborn period, a systolic pressure above 90 mm Hg is considered hypertensive.

241. The answer is D. *(Vaughan, ed 11. pp 1499, 1502, 1507, 1510.)* The figure accompanying the question depicts a red blood cell cast characteristically found in the urine of patients with glomerular disease. Important exceptions include the minimal lesion form of the nephrotic syndrome (lipoid nephrosis) and membranous glomerulopathy. In these, the urine contains large amounts of protein and hyaline casts but few red blood cells.

242. The answer is C. *(Vaughan, ed 11. pp 1484, 1496, 1520, 1618.)* In individuals affected by childhood nephrosis, there is a reduced ability to excrete a free water load; thus, urine is highly concentrated. Sickle-cell patients have isosthenuria, probably due to the sickling of erythrocytes in the vasa recta. Patients who have diabetes insipidus cannot concentrate their urine, either because of a lack of vasopressin (central diabetes insipidus) or an unresponsiveness to vasopressin (nephrogenic diabetes insipidus). Because patients who have pyelonephritis have interstitial tubular damage, they may not be able to concentrate urine.

243. The answer is D. *(Vaughan, ed 11. pp 290, 294.)* Due to relatively good preservation of circulatory volume, patients who have hypertonic (hypernatremic) dehydration may look stable clinically. However, because the central nervous system is especially liable to insult, therapy must be approached cautiously. Brain edema, for example, can result from the too rapid administration of dilute solution; too much sodium, on the other hand, may increase the danger of brain hemorrhage. Careful and gradual replacement therapy is needed in most cases.

244. The answer is A. *(Vaughan, ed 11. pp 306, 1533-1534.)* Although insulin and glucose, bicarbonate, and calcium gluconate all shift potassium within tissues, they do not remove it. Sodium polystyrene sulfonate (Kayexalate) exchanges sodium for potassium (a resin exchange) but is too slow a treatment when serum potassium levels are higher than 7 mEq/L. Furthermore, diuretic therapy with mannitol or furosemide is not likely to be effective in restoring renal function or inducing kaliuresis at this clinical stage. While temporary measures (such as those mentioned) are underway, prompt peritoneal dialysis should be instituted, because without dialysis, a patient with the laboratory finding of the child described might die.

245. The answer is E. *(Vaughan, ed 11. pp 1495-1496.)* The patient described is of the sex and age most typical for minimal-change nephrotic syndrome, which accounts for about 80 percent of all cases of idiopathic nephrotic syndrome of childhood. The presence of highly selective proteinuria, normal renal function, a normal urinary sediment, and normal blood pressure further increases the likelihood of minimal-change disease. Histologically, the glomeruli of children affected by minimal-change nephrotic disease are normal, except for smudging of epithelial foot processes.

246. The answer is B. *(Vaughan, ed 11. p 1503.)* The exudation and uniform hypercellularity present in the biopsy sample that accompanies the question typify the microscopic pathology associated with poststreptococcal nephritis, which is neither focal nor segmental. Minimal-change nephrotic syndrome is characterized by an essentially normal appearance on light microscopy. Rapidly progressive nephritis is characterized by glomerular crescent formation; and splitting of or deposition in basement membranes is typical of kidneys affected by membranoproliferative glomerulonephritis.

247. The answer is C. *(Vaughan, ed 11. pp 1356-1357.)* Important clinical signs of hypertension in children may include headache, dizziness, visual disturbances, irritability, and nocturnal wakening. Hypertensive encephalopathy may be preceded or accompanied by vomiting, hyperreflexia, ataxia, and focal or generalized seizures. Facial palsy may be the sole manifestation of severe hypertension. When marked fundal changes are present or when there are signs of vascular compromise, emergency treatment of the accompanying hypertension is warranted. Such hypertensive individuals require immediate hospitalization for diagnosis and therapy.

248. The answer is D. *(Vaughan, ed 11. p 1544.)* No bacteria at all should grow in a properly obtained urine sample from a suprapubic tap or from retrograde catheterization of the upper urinary tract. Infected urine of low specific gravity often contains less than 10^5 colonies/mm^3, but a count as low as 2000/mm^3 would be unlikely. First-morning urine usually is concentrated, and a higher colony count thus would be expected. Ileal-loop bags are usually contaminated.

Depending on technique, bladder catheterization of a normal person may produce urine with a low organism count.

249. The answer is C. *(Vaughan, ed 11. pp 1579-1580.)* Because it is an abdominal organ in children, the bladder, especially when full, is often ruptured by blunt trauma and lower abdominal wounds. Though small bladder tears may be treated conservatively by catheter drainage, surgical exploration is likely to be needed. Extensive urethral injuries may require surgical drainage of periurethral hematoma, primary surgical repair, or even urinary diversion procedures. Most ureteral injuries require prompt surgical intervention, though such injuries are rare because of the protected position of the ureter. A retrograde cystourethrogram and intravenous urography may be helpful, especially with pelvic fracture or suspected renal trauma.

250. The answer is C. *(Vaughan, ed 11. pp 1496, 1558.)* Drug-related nephrotic syndrome has been described in connection with the use of trimethadione, penicillamine, tolbutamide, and certain heavy metals. A variety of allergenic causes, including Hymenoptera stings, pollens, insect bites, and snakebites, also have been implicated as etiologic agents. Nephrosis can develop in conjunction with malignancy and diseases such as amyloidosis.

251. The answer is B. *(Vaughan, ed 11. pp 292-295.)* The sodium deficit of the child described in the question is probably 8 to 10 mEq/kg, or a total of 80 to 100 mEq. Sodium maintenance would require the infusion of another 10 to 20 mEq/24 hours. Use of normal saline would provide too much sodium for the child described, whereas one-sixth normal saline would supply too little. Administration of whole blood or packed red blood cells is rarely needed in the absence of blood loss; also, plasma and blood both carry a finite risk of subsequent serum hepatitis. Potassium should not be added to intravenous solutions until adequate urine output has been established.

252. The answer is D. *(Vaughan, ed 11. pp 457, 673, 1544, 1548, 1559.)* In Potter's syndrome, the kidneys are absent; consequently, pyuria cannot be present. Potter's syndrome is a lethal abnormality that may be suspected at birth by the presence of oligohydramnios, a wizened appearance, and a characteristic wide semicircular fold of skin that extends downward and laterally from the inner canthus of both eyes. There may also be pulmonary hypoplasia. Sterile pyuria, as evidenced by the depicted white blood cells, may occur in febrile illnesses, dehydration, acute nephritides, renal cystic disease, toxic nephropathy, and renal transplant rejection, as well as in the other disorders listed in the question.

253. The answer is B. *(Vaughan, ed 11. pp 1571-1572.)* The incidence of cryptorchidism of one or both testes decreases to 0.3 to 0.4 percent by one year of age, and spontaneous descent after that is rare. Proper examination in a warm room and in a relaxed manner is necessary to distinguish retractile from undescended testes. The facts that 30 percent of unilaterally cryptorchid boys who undergo corrective surgery are later oligospermic, that orchidopexy does not appear to reduce the incidence of tumors, and that there is an increased incidence of tumors in the contralateral descended testis suggest the presence of a bilateral end-organ defect. Nevertheless, since orchidopexy makes a testis easier to examine for tumors and may improve fertility, correction should be done.

254. The answer is D. *(Vaughan, ed 11. pp 89-90, 1557.)* Daytime wetting is rare in children who have reached the age of six. However, at this age at least 8 percent of girls and 12 percent of boys are nocturnally enuretic. A careful history should be taken and a physical examination, including urinalysis, should be performed on children whose enuresis has persisted to the age of six. Organic disease is no more prevalent in enuretic than in other children, and blood urea nitrogen and serum creatinine studies and intravenous urography are warranted only if there is evidence of an organic lesion. Treatment, which should attempt to reassure affected children and their parents, can include behavior modification techniques and the use of imipramine (Tofranil).

255. The answer is A (1, 2, 3). *(Vaughan, ed 11. p 1556.)* Causes of renal artery stenosis include abnormalities of the renal vessel wall, external encroachment by tumor or cyst, and embolism. Revascularization by means of arterial repair, vascular grafts, and autotransplantation is essential if hypertension is severe. Renovascular hypertension has been reported in infants as well as in older children.

256. The answer is C (2, 4). *(Vaughan, ed 11. pp 1849-1851.)* Because the obviously rachitic bones revealed in the x-ray accompanying the question do not show hallmarks of renal osteodystrophy, neither an elevated level of blood urea nitrogen nor acidemia would be likely. Although the radiographic findings suggest nutritional rickets, a three-month course of dihydrotachysterol at the given dose would have been sufficient to cure a patient who has this disease. Thus, in view of the radiographic evidence and low serum phosphorus level, the likely diagnosis for the child described is vitamin D-resistant rickets, which also is called familial hypophosphatemic rickets.

257. The answer is B (1, 3). *(Vaughan, ed 11. pp 1515-1519.)* Renal tubular acidosis (RTA) is a syndrome of persistent hyperchloremic acidosis, normal anion gap, and normal overall renal function in which normal plasma bicarbonate levels cannot be maintained because of tubular dysfunction. In proximal RTA

Urinary Tract 125

(type 1) the reabsorption of bicarbonate is impaired, while in distal RTA (type 2) there is defective acidification of urine. Either type may occur as a primary disorder or secondary either to a systemic disease or to a variety of toxins. Secondary proximal RTA occurs with a variety of hereditary tubular disorders and with exposure to heavy metals and outdated tetracycline. Secondary distal RTA may accompany Ehlers-Danlos syndrome or follow renal transplantation, medullary nephrocalcinosis, obstructive uropathy, hyperimmunoglobulinemia, or exposure to amphotericin B, lithium salts, or toluene.

258. The answer is E (all). *(Rudolph, ed 16. pp 1246-1247.)* Hypertension increases the risk of bleeding after a percutaneous kidney biopsy and therefore should be controlled before a biopsy is performed. Patients who have single kidneys or renal dysplasia are at risk for loss of kidney function if they are subjected to closed renal biopsy. Septicemia can result from kidney biopsy of an individual affected by acute pyelonephritis. Although percutaneous kidney biopsy can be performed in the presence of mild edema, patients who have anasarca should first undergo diuresis.

259. The answer is A (1, 2, 3). *(Vaughan, ed 11. p 1541.)* Many antibiotics require dosage alteration when administered to patients in renal failure. For this reason, it is best to avoid use of tetracyclines, methanamine, and nitrofurantoin completely. Major modification is required for gentamicin and other aminoglycosides. Penicillins, including ampicillin and amoxicillin, also require dosage modification. No dosage modification is needed with clindamycin therapy.

260. The answer is E (all). *(Vaughan, ed 11. p 1489.)* Renal ultrasound is noninvasive, and there is no unnecessary radiation exposure. Repeated studies are easily obtained for follow-up of problems. Renal ultrasound is especially helpful when kidneys cannot be visualized urographically. It is helpful in evaluating abdominal masses, especially in the newborn, and in examining transplanted kidneys. For example, renal ultrasound may be helpful in differentiating neoplasms from multicystic kidneys and hydronephrosis.

261. The answer is E (all). *(Vaughan, ed 11. pp 1502-1504.)* The most common form of acute glomerulonephritis involves the deposition of complement, immunoglobulin G, and properdin in glomeruli following a skin or throat infection with certain nephritogenic strains of group A β-hemolytic streptococci. Hematuria often colors the urine dark, and decreased urinary output may result in circulatory congestion and volume overload, which can induce dyspnea, periorbital edema, tachycardia, and hepatomegaly. Acute hypertension is common and may lead to headache, vomiting, and even encephalopathy with seizures. Congestive heart failure may occur.

262. **The answer is A (1, 2, 3).** *(Vaughan, ed 11. pp 1512-1514.)* Hemolytic uremic syndrome typically affects young children five years of age or less. The hallmarks of this disease, which often follows a viral-like gastrointestinal or upper respiratory tract illness, are severe hemolytic anemia, intravascular hemolysis, and platelet consumption that accompany acute renal failure. Hypertension, encephalopathy, and anuria also may occur. The syndrome seems to occur more frequently in whites than blacks.

263. **The answer is D (4).** *(Vaughan, ed 11. pp 1500-1501.)* Congenital nephrosis (infantile nephrosis), which occurs with an increased incidence among families having a history of the disease, is almost totally insensitive to any form of therapy. The characteristic lesion is cystic dilatation of the proximal tubules. Screening for elevated alpha-fetoprotein in maternal serum should be done in at-risk pregnancies.

264. **The answer is E (all).** *(Vaughan, ed 11. pp 1123-1124.)* Renal hypoperfusion can occur in individuals who have severe liver failure, even though their cardiac output is often normal and their plasma volume is normal or increased. The fact that kidneys transplanted from donors who have hepatorenal syndrome function well in recipients whose liver function is unimpaired points to hemodynamic change, and not to intrinsic kidney disease, as the likely etiology. Volume expansion and careful use of dopamine may promote improvement in affected individuals.

265. **The answer is A (1, 2, 3).** *(Vaughan, ed 11. pp 1519-1521.)* Nephrogenic diabetes insipidus is a hereditary congenital disorder in which the urine is hypotonic and produced in large volumes because the kidneys fail to respond to antidiuretic hormone. Most North American patients thus involved are descendants of Ulster Scots who came to Nova Scotia in 1761 on the ship *Hopewell*. Males are primarily affected, apparently through an X-linked recessive mode, though there can be a variable expression in heterozygous females. The defect is unknown, but the disorder is felt to result from primary unresponsiveness of the distal tubule and collecting duct to vasopressin. Although the condition is present at birth, the diagnosis is often not made until several months later when excessive thirst, frequent voidings of large volumes of dilute urine, dehydration, and failure to thrive become obvious. Maintenance of adequate fluid intake and diet and use of saluretic drugs are the bases of therapy of this incurable disease.

266. **The answer is A (1, 2, 3).** *(Vaughan, ed 11. p 1480.)* A number of pH-dependent substances can impart a red color to urine. Use of phenolphthalein, a cathartic agent, or phenindione, an anticoagulant, can cause red urine; inges-

tion of blackberries or beets also may lead to red coloration ("beeturia"). Because myoglobin tests heme-positive in a Hemastix examination, myoglobinuria could not be the source of the red color of the urine of the girl described. Hematuria should be confirmed by dipstick testing as well as by microscopic examination of urinary sediment.

267. The answer is C (2, 4). *(Vaughan, ed 11. p 1657.)* Symptoms of hypercalcemia include muscle weakness, polydipsia, polyuria, anorexia, vomiting, constipation, weight loss, and fever. Development of nephrocalcinosis and renal calculi also is possible. Causes of hypercalcemia include primary and secondary hyperparathyroidism, idiopathic hypercalcemia of infancy, malignancy, sarcoidosis, and thyrotoxicosis.

268. The answer is B (1, 3). *(Rudolph, ed 16. pp 1291-1292. Vaughan, ed 11. p 1529.)* Papillary necrosis, a severe disorder affecting individuals who have sickle cell disease, may appear on an intravenous pyelogram as a central papillary filling defect or as distortion of a papilla. Renal infarction, brought on by bleeding, also can occur. If clots are present, hydronephrosis caused by obstruction may result. Neither stones nor cystic changes are characteristic features of sickle cell disease.

269. The answer is A (1, 2, 3). *(Vaughan, ed 11. p 1529.)* Individuals who have sickle cell disease typically cannot form concentrated urine; this defect usually develops by about the third year of life. Painless gross hematuria, most commonly due to papillary necrosis, also is a frequent symptom; hematuria also can be associated with renal colic caused by the passage of clots. Although some degree of proteinuria normally accompanies gross hematuria, proteinuria due to nephrotic syndrome is relatively uncommon. Crystalluria is not a characteristic feature of sickle cell disease.

270. The answer is D (4). *(Vaughan, ed 11. pp 1526-1528, 1531, 1551.)* The radiograph that accompanies the question shows the splayed-out calyces and large kidneys typical of adult-type polycystic kidneys, which can first appear in childhood. Multicystic kidneys are often unilateral; bilateral involvement in a 12-year-old child would be unlikely to be associated with the level of renal function pictured in the angiogram. Individuals who have nephronophthisis usually have normal or small-sized kidneys. Megacalyx is a rare entity in which the calyces appear large and can be mistaken for cysts; however, the renal cortex is normal.

271-275. The answers are: 271-C, 272-B, 273-E, 274-B, 275-A. *(Vaughan, ed 11. pp 504, 666, 1530-1531, 1849-1851.)* All of the disorders listed in the question are clearly familial except for systemic lupus erythematosus, which appears to result from a combination of environmental and genetic causes. Many current investigators believe that lupus may result from a viral infection in genetically predisposed individuals.

Hypophosphatemic rickets (vitamin D-resistant rickets) is characteristically inherited as an X-linked dominant trait. Affected males usually have a more severe form of this disease than affected females.

Children born with infantile polycystic kidney disease, an autosomal recessive disorder, often die in infancy from pulmonary disease or hypertension. Renal failure also may occur. Liver disease, the main source of later problems, can lead to portal hypertension, which often can be relieved by shunting procedures. Children who have infantile polycystic disease usually do not survive to 20 years of age.

Adult-type polycystic kidney disease, inherited in an autosomal-dominant fashion, is often seen in successive generations of the same family. If adult-type polycystic kidney disease is discovered in a family, siblings and parents should undergo intravenous urography or abdominal ultrasound studies.

Nephropathic cystinosis is an autosomal recessive disease in which affected patients develop renal failure by their early teens. Now that some individuals who have cystine storage disease are receiving renal allografts, the pathologic effects of cystine storage in tissues other than the kidney may become clinically important. Cystinosis should not be confused with cystinuria, which is characterized by nephrolithiasis.

276-280. The answers are: 276-A, 277-E, 278-B, 279-D, 280-B. *(Vaughan, ed 11. p 1479.)* Renal function matures rapidly in the first postnatal months; it is necessary to compare function to age-appropriate standards. The full number of glomeruli are present by the time a fetus is 2100 to 2500 g. The increase in renal size with age is due to tubular mass increase.

Glomerular filtration rate is only 10 to 15 ml/min/m^2 at birth but doubles by two weeks. By six months of age, it is 45 to 50 ml/min/m^2. Only at or after one year of age is it comparable to adult levels when corrected for surface area. Nevertheless, glomerular function is relatively more mature than tubular function—that is, there is glomerular-tubular imbalance. As a probable result, infants excrete a larger percentage than do adults of amino acids, glucose, and phosphates. Acidification of the urine, however, is comparable to that in adults within two weeks of birth, but in contrast to older children, a larger proportion of hydrogen ion is secreted as titratable acid than as ammonium ion.

A higher fraction of renal plasma is filtered in young infants as compared to adults. The filtration fraction (glomerular filtration flow/effective renal plasma flow), is, therefore, high in infants (0.32 to 0.34) compared with adults (0.18 to 0.20). A nearly normal filtration fraction occurs by 6 to 12 months of age.

The Neuromuscular System

Jerome S. Haller

DIRECTIONS: Each question below contains five suggested answers. Choose the **one best** response to each question.

281. A seven-month-old infant develops head-nodding spells, which consist of a series of four to six nods a minute. These episodes are characteristic of which of the following disorders?

(A) Petit mal seizures
(B) Psychomotor seizures
(C) Focal motor seizures
(D) Infantile spasms
(E) Multiple tics

282. A three-year-old child can be expected to do all of the following EXCEPT

(A) undress
(B) copy a square
(C) alternate feet when climbing stairs
(D) name one color
(E) speak in short sentences

283. A ten-year-old child complains of episodic abdominal discomfort; the child's mother says that these episodes are associated with periods of staring and followed by a brief period of lethargy. Which of the following disorders is most likely to be responsible for the child's symptoms?

(A) Psychomotor seizures
(B) Migraine
(C) Petit mal epilepsy
(D) Conversion reaction
(E) None of the above

284. The virus causing subacute sclerosing panencephalitis is presumed to be which of the following?

(A) Rubella
(B) Epstein-Barr
(C) Herpes simplex
(D) Herpes zoster
(E) Measles virus

285. The calcific densities in the skull x-ray shown below are likely to have been caused by

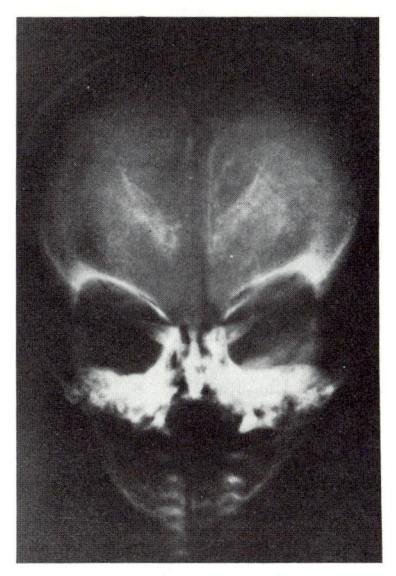

(A) congenital cytomegalovirus infection
(B) congenital toxoplasmosis
(C) congenital syphilis
(D) tuberculous meningitis
(E) craniopharyngioma

286. A subdural effusion most commonly accompanies meningitis caused by

(A) *Escherichia coli*
(B) *Hemophilus influenzae*
(C) *Neisseria meningitidis*
(D) *Pseudomonas aeruginosa*
(E) *Streptococcus (Diplococcus) pneumoniae*

287. The most common central nervous system complication of a mumps infection is

(A) encephalitis
(B) aseptic meningitis
(C) polyneuritis
(D) transverse myelitis
(E) Bell's palsy

288. A growing skull fracture in a 15-month-old infant most likely implies

(A) an enlarging cephalhematoma
(B) an acutely widening fracture line
(C) a subdural effusion beneath the fracture
(D) herniation of the arachnoid membrane
(E) increased intracranial pressure

289. Which of the following signs or symptoms must be present in a child's history in order to support the diagnosis of concussion following a head injury?

(A) Repeated vomiting
(B) Brief unconsciousness
(C) Drowsiness
(D) Seizure activity
(E) None of the above

290. A newborn infant has marked muscular weakness of the extremities and tongue fasciculations. The mother reports her child was relatively inactive in utero. The most likely diagnosis is

(A) infantile spinal muscular atrophy
(B) Duchenne muscular dystrophy
(C) myotonic dystrophy
(D) myasthenia gravis
(E) fiber type I disproportion

291. Children with Bell's palsy can have all of the following symptoms EXCEPT

(A) loss of taste
(B) hyperacusis
(C) weakness of facial muscles on the affected side
(D) inability to open one eye
(E) inability to retract one corner of the mouth when trying to smile

292. Erb's palsy is described best as

(A) weakness of a wrist and ipsilateral Horner's syndrome
(B) weakness of an arm from a fracture of the head of the humerus
(C) weakness of an arm from a traction injury of the upper brachial plexus
(D) total ipsilateral arm weakness resulting from a fracture of a clavicle
(E) pseudoparalysis of an arm due to syphilitic osteochondritis

293. A previously healthy seven-year-old child suddenly complains of a headache and falls to the floor. When examined in the emergency room, he is lethargic and has a left central facial weakness and left hemiparesis with conjugate ocular deviation to the right. The most likely diagnosis is

(A) hemiplegic migraine
(B) supratentorial tumor
(C) Todd's paralysis
(D) acute subdural hematoma
(E) acute infantile hemiplegia

294. The most common location in children for tumors of the nervous system is

(A) subtentorial
(B) supratentorial
(C) intraventricular
(D) in the spinal canal
(E) none of the above

295. In children, the most common type of tumor of the central nervous system is

(A) meningioma
(B) glioma
(C) craniopharyngioma
(D) chordoma
(E) neurinoma

296. A newborn infant has the vascular anomaly shown in the x-ray below. Neonates who have this anomaly most often present with

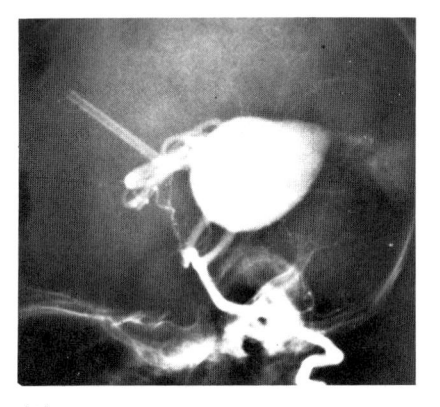

(A) anemia
(B) petechiae
(C) progressive macrocephaly
(D) congestive heart failure
(E) none of the above

297. Following a head injury, seizures are most likely to occur in a child within which of the following time periods?

(A) Immediately
(B) Within one week
(C) Within two years
(D) Between two and four years
(E) None of the above time periods

298. Headache, vomiting, and papilledema are common symptoms and signs in children who have brain tumors. Which of the following signs also is frequently associated with craniopharyngioma?

(A) Sixth-nerve palsy
(B) Unilateral cerebellar ataxia
(C) Unilateral pupillary dilatation
(D) Unilateral anosmia
(E) Bitemporal hemianopia

299. Diagnosis of which of the following lipidoses is confirmed by the absence of hexosaminidase A activity in white blood cells?

(A) Niemann-Pick disease
(B) Infantile Gaucher's disease
(C) Tay-Sachs disease
(D) Krabbe's disease
(E) Fabry's disease

300. Which of the following sets of clinical signs is most likely to be associated with the CAT scan (contrast positive) shown below?

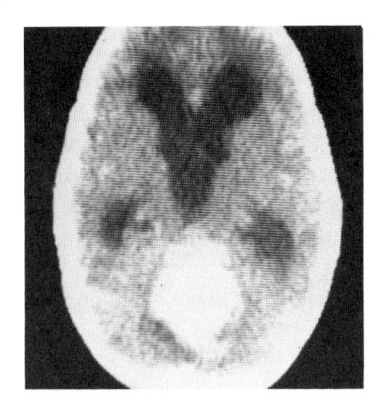

(A) Papilledema, hemiparesis, and ipsilateral sixth-nerve and seventh-nerve palsies
(B) Papilledema, unilateral dysmetria, and falling to the same side
(C) Retinal angiomas, ataxia, and dysmetria
(D) Papilledema and ataxia without dysmetria
(E) None of the above

301. Which of the following aminoacidopathies is associated with acute infantile hemiplegia?

(A) Phenylketonuria
(B) Homocystinuria
(C) Cystathioninuria
(D) Maple syrup urine disease
(E) Histidinemia

302. A ten-year-old child who has acute lymphocytic leukemia is lethargic and unsteady. There is no evidence of hematuria or bleeding into the skin. Neurologic examination shows that the child has a mild spastic hemiparesis and hyperreflexia in all extremities; papilledema, however, is not present. Three months ago, the child was treated with 3000 rads of radiation to the head as well as with intrathecal methotrexate for meningeal leukemia.

The child's current neurologic disturbances most likely are the result of

(A) fungal infection
(B) hydrocephalus
(C) meningeal leukemia
(D) leukoencephalopathy
(E) intracerebral hemorrhage

303. The most frequent complication of congenital rubella is believed to be

(A) cataracts
(B) microcephaly
(C) patent ductus arteriosus
(D) deafness
(E) thrombocytopenia

304. Leigh's syndrome (subacute necrotizing encephalomyelopathy) involves which of the following biochemical abnormalities?

(A) Inhibited conversion of glutamate to glutamine
(B) Inhibited synthesis of thiamine triphosphate
(C) Absence of cystathionine synthetase
(D) Pyridoxine deficiency
(E) Tocopherol deficiency

305. An infant who has achromic skin patches develops infantile spasms. The disorder most likely to be affecting this infant is

(A) neurofibromatosis
(B) tuberous sclerosis
(C) incontinentia pigmenti
(D) pityriasis rosea
(E) psoriasis

306. Viruses that have been associated with Reye's syndrome include all of the following EXCEPT

(A) coxsackievirus
(B) echovirus
(C) varicella-zoster virus
(D) influenza B virus
(E) rubella virus

307. A six-year-old child has an unsteady gait and is irritable. Physical examination reveals a very mild left facial weakness, brisk stretch reflexes in all four extremities, bilateral extensor plantar responses, mild hypertonicity of the left upper and lower extremities, and a somewhat unsteady but nonspecific gait; there is no muscular weakness. The most likely diagnosis is

(A) pontine glioma
(B) cerebellar astrocytoma
(C) right cerebral hemisphere tumor
(D) subacute sclerosing panencephalitis
(E) subacute necrotizing leukoencephalopathy

308. A short nine-year-old boy, who appears physically immature, is seen in an emergency room because of repeated vomiting and headaches. Funduscopic examination reveals papilledema. A skull x-ray (shown below), which was taken immediately, reveals

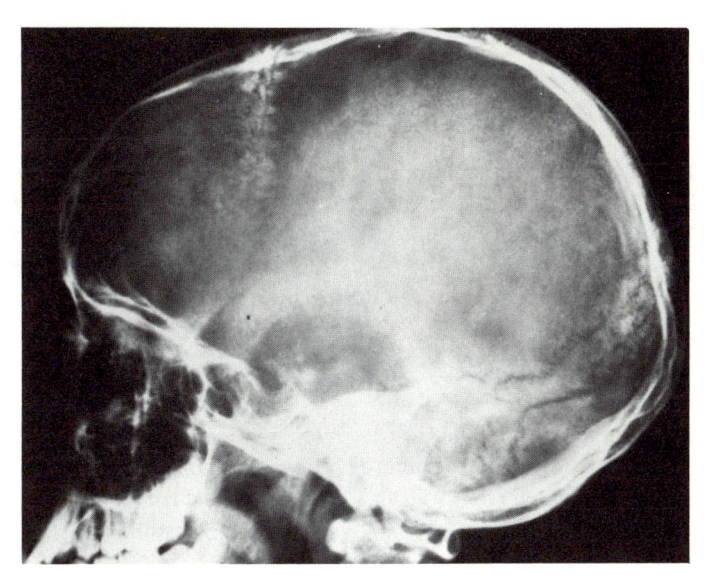

(A) sutural diastasis
(B) an abnormal odontoid process
(C) suprasellar calcification
(D) a widened foramen magnum
(E) chronic hydrocephalus

Pediatrics

DIRECTIONS: Each question below contains four suggested answers of which **one** or **more** is correct. Choose the answer:

A	if	1, 2, and 3	are correct
B	if	1 and 3	are correct
C	if	2 and 4	are correct
D	if	4	is correct
E	if	1, 2, 3, and 4	are correct

309. Intracranial hemorrhage may result from a difficult delivery and from asphyxia or hypoxia. Common sites of bleeding in full-term infants include

(1) intraventricular
(2) posterior fossa
(3) subarachnoid
(4) subdural

310. Bloody cerebrospinal fluid (CSF) produced by a traumatic lumbar puncture can be distinguished from true bloody CSF due to other causes by which of the following methods?

(1) Counting red blood cells in more than one tube
(2) Looking for xanthochromia
(3) Repeating the lumbar puncture at a higher interspace
(4) Observing clotting in the CSF

311. Laboratory findings consistently associated with Reye's syndrome include which of the following?

(1) Prolonged prothrombin time
(2) Elevated levels of serum transaminases
(3) Elevated blood ammonia levels
(4) Elevated blood glucose levels

312. Examination of the cerebrospinal fluid of an eight-year-old, stuporous, mildly febrile child shows the following: white blood cells, 200/mm^3 (all lymphocytes); protein, 150 mg/100 ml; and glucose, 15 mg/100 ml. Blood glucose concentration is 70 mg/100 ml. The differential diagnosis should include

(1) aseptic meningitis
(2) tuberculous meningitis
(3) meningeal leukemia
(4) medulloblastoma

313. The differential diagnosis of acute ataxia of childhood should include

(1) drug intoxication
(2) bacterial meningitis
(3) postinfectious viral syndrome
(4) neuroblastoma

314. Low cerebrospinal fluid (CSF) sugar is commonly associated with bacterial meningitis, but it may also be found in which of the following disorders?

(1) Hypoglycemia
(2) Subarachnoid hemorrhage
(3) Mumps meningitis
(4) Spinal cord tumor

315. A newborn infant is noted to have facial diplegia and difficulty sucking and swallowing. Which of the following disorders should be included in the differential diagnosis?

(1) Infantile spinal muscular atrophy
(2) Myasthenia gravis
(3) Myotonic dystrophy
(4) Duchenne muscular dystrophy

316. Brain abscesses can develop as the result of which of the following infections?

(1) Mastoiditis
(2) Pyoderma
(3) Subacute bacterial endocarditis
(4) Sinusitis

317. Although valproic acid is widely used as an anticonvulsant, particularly for patients with petit mal seizures, there are side effects, which include

(1) hepatotoxicity
(2) hypotension
(3) interference with other anticonvulsants
(4) drug rash

318. A six-year-old child is hospitalized for observation because of a short period of unconsciousness after a fall from a playground swing. Which of the following signs or symptoms would suggest the development of an extradural hematoma?

(1) Unilateral pupillary dilatation
(2) Focal seizures
(3) Recurrence of depressed consciousness
(4) Headache

319. An asymmetric Moro reflex can be elicited at least occasionally from infants who have

(1) a fractured clavicle
(2) infantile hemiplegia
(3) a brachial plexus palsy
(4) neonatal myasthenia gravis

320. Intracranial calcifications can appear in infants who have a congenital infection with

(1) *Treponema pallidum*
(2) *Toxoplasma gondii*
(3) rubella virus
(4) cytomegalovirus

321. Hyperkinetic behavior (hyperactivity), though not a syndrome per se, can be due to which of the following factors?

(1) Deafness
(2) Environmental causes
(3) Progressive neurologic disease
(4) Autism

322. Physical findings characteristic of children who have Sturge-Weber syndrome include

(1) hemiplegia
(2) angiomas of the lips and mouth
(3) a "port wine" nevus on the forehead
(4) an angioma of the retina

SUMMARY OF DIRECTIONS				
A	B	C	D	E
1, 2, 3 only	1, 3 only	2, 4 only	4 only	All are correct

323. By three months of age most normal full-term infants can be expected to
(1) move their heads from side to side 180 degrees while following a moving object
(2) lift their heads from a prone position 45 degrees off the examining table
(3) smile when encouraged
(4) maintain a seated position

324. The calcifications shown on the skull x-ray below can be associated with which of the following?

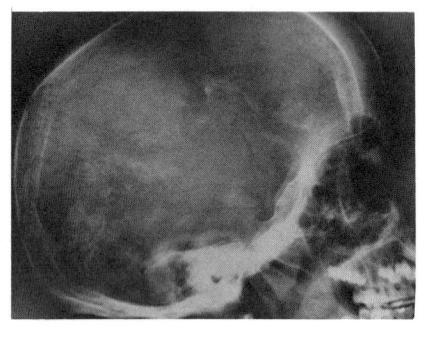

(1) Von Hippel-Lindau disease
(2) Ataxia-telangiectasia
(3) Tuberous sclerosis
(4) Sturge-Weber syndrome

325. A ten-year-old child has pes cavus and scoliosis; other disorders likely to be exhibited by this child include
(1) diminished vibration and position sense
(2) gait and station ataxia
(3) nystagmus
(4) hyperreflexia

326. No precise definition exists for grand mal status epilepticus. This disorder generally can be defined by which of the following criteria?
(1) One seizure lasting no less than a half hour
(2) Continuous tonic-clonic activity for one hour
(3) Repeated seizures with no return to consciousness between them
(4) Several sets of repeated focal seizures occurring in a twenty-four-hour period

327. True statements about febrile seizures include which of the following?
(1) They usually occur in association with infection of the central nervous system
(2) Most last less than 15 minutes
(3) Affected children usually are between three and six years of age
(4) Generalized tonic-clonic activity is typical

328. Gowers' maneuver is used by children who have

(1) pseudohypertrophic muscular dystrophy
(2) limb-girdle dystrophy
(3) late-onset spinal muscular atrophy
(4) congenital myopathy

329. The differential diagnosis for a newborn infant who has multiple joint contractures should include

(1) spinal muscular atrophy
(2) congenital muscular dystrophy
(3) congenital myopathies
(4) myelomeningocele

330. Which of the following intracranial abnormalities can be diagnosed by transillumination during the first year of a child's life?

(1) Acute subdural hematoma
(2) Subdural effusion
(3) Porencephalic cyst
(4) Dandy-Walker syndrome

331. Frontal baldness, cataracts, distal muscle weakness, ptosis, and facial muscle weakness are some of the symptoms of myotonic dystrophy in adults. Children who have this disease commonly exhibit

(1) psychomotor retardation
(2) seizure activity
(3) cardiac arrhythmias
(4) a failure to thrive

332. Neurologic complications that can arise from the acute stage of infectious mononucleosis include

(1) seizures
(2) aseptic meningitis
(3) encephalomyelitis
(4) Guillain-Barré syndrome

333. Neonatal seizures can develop as the result of

(1) hypocalcemia
(2) hypoxia
(3) birth trauma
(4) anomalies of the central nervous system

334. A five-year-old child, who has had slowly progressive ataxia since birth, develops telangiectasia of the conjunctivae, ears, and nose. Physical examination also reveals nystagmus. Which of the following immunoglobulin levels would be likely to be present in this child?

(1) Reduced IgE level
(2) Reduced IgM level
(3) Reduced IgA level
(4) Elevated IgG level

140　　　　　　　　　　　　　　　　Pediatrics

SUMMARY OF DIRECTIONS				
A	B	C	D	E
1, 2, 3 only	1, 3 only	2, 4 only	4 only	All are correct

335. Congenital defects frequently associated with the radiographic findings illustrated below include

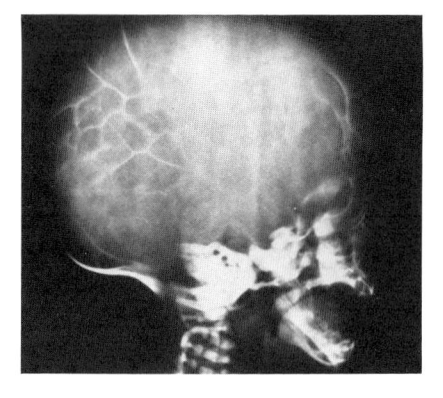

(1) meningomyelocele
(2) cleft lip and palate
(3) encephalocele
(4) craniosynostosis

The Neuromuscular System

Answers

281. The answer is D. *(Menkes, ed 2. pp 558-560. Singer, J Pediatr 96:485-489, 1980.)* The onset of infantile spasms most commonly occurs in children between the ages of three and eight months. The seizures, which occur in clusters, may take the form of head nodding (with or without arm extension) or spasms of more severe flexion ("salaam seizure"). The most effective treatment is administration of adrenocorticotropin; there is no general agreement, however, about the dosage or duration of therapy. Normal intellectual development in any infant who has developed infantile spasms is unlikely if there is evidence of prenatal or perinatal neurologic insults, metabolic disorders, or structural abnormalities of the brain. Petit mal, psychomotor seizures and multiple tics do not occur in infants of this age group. Focal motor seizures may occur at any age but usually involve limbs or facial muscles.

282. The answer is B. *(Illingsworth, ed 7. pp 135, 137, 143, 145, 161.)* Three-year-old children become quite skilled in many areas. Most can say many words and speak in sentences. They are usually toilet trained and can dress and undress themselves with the exception of shoelaces and sometimes buttons. Although they can alternate feet when climbing stairs, they still place both feet on each step when going down stairs. They can identify at least one color by name but have not progressed beyond copying a circle and a crude cross. Only at four to five years of age can a child copy a square.

283. The answer is A. *(Menkes, ed 2. pp 553-556.)* The consecutive appearance of abdominal distress, staring, and sleepiness or lethargy strongly indicates a paroxysmal disorder. Children who have psychomotor seizures often present in this manner. Other symptoms that have been described include stereotyped motor activity (such as buttoning and unbuttoning of clothes), a sensation of unexplained fearfulness, and déjà vu. Affected children frequently have a history of febrile or grand mal seizures.

284. The answer is E. *(Bell, vol 12. p 293.)* The infective agent considered to cause subacute sclerosing panencephalitis is measles virus. This presumption is based on the associated central nervous system pathology, which is consistent with encephalitis and features intranuclear and intracytoplasmic inclusion bodies. In addition, measles (rubeola) antibody titers in serum and cerebrospinal fluid are higher than those found in children recovering from measles, a finding that suggests a continuing infective process.

285. The answer is A. *(Bell, vol 12. pp 228-236.)* Periventricular calcifications are a characteristic finding in infants who have congenital cytomegalovirus infection. The encephalitic process especially affects the subependymal tissue around the lateral ventricles and thus results in the periventricular deposition of calcium. Calcified tuberculomas, if visible radiographically, are present around the base of the brain, the preferential site of tuberculous meningitis. Granulomatous encephalitis caused by congenital toxoplasmosis is associated with scattered and soft-appearing intracranial calcifications, and suprasellar calcifications are typical of craniopharyngiomas. Congenital syphilis does not produce intracranial calcifications.

286. The answer is B. *(Menkes, ed 2. pp 281-282.)* Although subdural effusions can follow all types of acute bacterial meningitis, they most commonly complicate meningitis caused by *Hemophilus influenzae*. How these effusions develop remains uncertain. Abnormal transillumination of the skull as well as certain clinical findings, such as progressive increase in head circumference or occurrence of focal neurologic signs, can suggest the presence of a subdural effusion.

287. The answer is B. *(Bell, vol 12. p 170.)* Aseptic meningitis is the most common central nervous system complication of mumps infection. A mild pleocytosis can be associated with mumps parotitis even in the absence of neurologic signs. Encephalitis, which occurs less frequently than aseptic meningitis in children who have mumps, has a poorer outcome. Transverse myelitis and polyneuritis are encountered infrequently in affected children.

288. The answer is D. *(Menkes, ed 2. pp 419-420.)* A growing skull fracture in a young child results from herniation of the arachnoid membrane through a tear in the dura mater and between the edges of a linear fracture. As a consequence, a leptomeningeal cyst develops; the cyst transmits pulsations from the brain and leads to erosion of the surrounding skull. Skull x-rays, therefore, should be repeated three to six months after a linear fracture to be certain that bony union has been completed.

Neuromuscular System

289. The answer is B. *(Vaughan, ed 11. p 1787.)* Although vomiting and lethargy frequently are associated with a closed head injury, a brief period of unconsciousness always accompanies a concussion. Children old enough to relate their own histories may give evidence of amnesia concerning the events preceding their head injuries (retrograde amnesia) and following their injuries (antegrade amnesia); these historical findings will confirm the diagnosis of concussion. The severity of the injury is generally directly related to the length of time the child was unconscious and the extent of the retrograde amnesia. Children who have had a simple concussion recover fully.

290. The answer is A. *(Brooke, pp 34-36. Dubowitz, p 149.)* Infantile spinal muscular atrophy (Werdnig-Hoffmann disease) is a progressive degenerative disease of anterior horn cells and bulbar motor nuclei. Fasciculations of the tongue can occur in affected infants; however, because tongue fasciculations can accompany crying in normal infants, only the demonstration of fasciculations while a child is at rest will support a diagnosis of infantile spinal muscular atrophy. Some mothers of affected neonates give a history of slowed or arrested fetal movement prior to the onset of labor. Because this disease has an autosomal recessive inheritance pattern, muscle biopsy and examination of histochemically stained specimens should be done to confirm the diagnosis.

291. The answer is D. *(Menkes, ed 2. p 400.)* Bell's palsy is a peripheral neuropathy of cranial nerve VII. All facial muscles on one side of affected children's faces are paralyzed; as a consequence, these children are unable to close one eye, wrinkle their foreheads, or retract one corner of their mouths when trying to smile. Depending on the site of nerve injury, other symptoms of Bell's palsy can include hyperacusis, loss of taste, and impaired salivation.

292. The answer is C. *(Menkes, ed 2. pp 269-270.)* Erb's palsy can be caused by traction on an arm during a breech delivery or on the neck during a vertex delivery. Traction results in injury to the upper brachial plexus, causing weakness of the deltoid, biceps, brachialis, and wrist and finger extensor muscles. Recovery is dependent on the degree of nerve injury. Pain caused by osteochondritis of the humerus in an infant who has congenital syphilis (Parrot's pseudoparalysis) inhibits arm movement.

293. The answer is E. *(Isler, pp 74-102. Menkes, ed 2. pp 264-267.)* The abrupt onset of a hemisyndrome, especially with the eyes looking away from the paralyzed side, strongly indicates a diagnosis of acute infantile hemiplegia. Most frequently this represents a thromboembolic occlusion of the middle cerebral artery or one of its major branches. Hemiplegic migraine commonly occurs in children with a history of migraine headaches. Todd's paralysis follows after a focal or jacksonian seizure and generally does not last more than 24 to 48 hours. The eyes usually look toward the paralyzed side. The clinical onset of a supratentorial brain tumor is subacute with repeated headaches and gradually developing weakness. A history of trauma usually precedes the signs of an acute subdural hematoma. Clinical signs may appear fairly rapidly, but not with the abruptness of occlusive vascular disease.

294. The answer is A. *(Menkes, ed 2. p 498.)* Between 60 and 70 percent of intracranial tumors in children are located below the tentorium. Of these tumors, the two most common types are medulloblastoma and cerebellar astrocytoma. In adults and infants, most intracranial tumors originate above the tentorium; only 25 to 30 percent of brain tumors in adults are subtentorial.

295. The answer is B. *(Rudolph, ed 16. pp 1804, 1807.)* Gliomas—for example, astrocytoma, pontine glioma, and optic glioma—comprise 75 percent of intracranial tumors in children and 45 percent in adults. After leukemia, intracranial tumors are the most common type of neoplastic disease among children. Only about 6 percent of brain tumors in children are metastatic.

296. The answer is D. *(Swaiman, 1975. pp 644-651.)* The x-ray that accompanies the question shows an arteriovenous malformation and a vein of Galen aneurysm. The aneurysm is the result of a high-flow shunt through the malformation; in the newborn period, it results in high-output congestive failure. In older infants, the next most common clinical problem is progressive macrocephaly. Continuing high flow through the vein of Galen causes the vein to become distended, compressing the brainstem and, consequently, the aqueduct; aqueductal stenosis and hydrocephalus develop. The third mode of presentation of this malformation is as a subarachnoid hemorrhage when the aneurysm ruptures, which usually occurs in adolescence and young adulthood.

297. The answer is B. *(Jennett, ed 2. pp 35-39, 68-69, 91, 93.)* Seizures that result from a head injury fall into two categories: early epilepsy and late epilepsy. The former type occurs within the first week following the injury, while the latter does not appear until three months to as much as ten years later. Children, especially those under five years of age, are more likely to have early epilepsy than are adults, in whom late epilepsy is more common.

298. The answer is E. *(Swaiman, 1975. p 529.)* Upward growth of a craniopharyngioma results in compression of the optic chiasm. Particularly affected are the fibers derived from the nasal portions of both retinas (in other words, from those parts of the eyes receiving stimulation from the temporal visual field).

Early in the growth of a craniopharyngioma a unilateral superior quadrantanopic defect can develop; and an irregularly growing tumor can impinge upon the optic chiasm and cause homonymous hemianopia.

299. The answer is C. *(Swaiman, 1975. pp 397, 405, 407, 410.)* Children who have Tay-Sachs disease are characterized by progressive developmental deterioration; physical signs include macular "cherry red" spots and exquisite sensitivity to noise. Diagnosis of this disorder can be confirmed biochemically by the absence of hexosaminidase A activity in white blood cells. Tay-Sachs disease is inherited as an autosomal recessive trait; about 80 percent of affected children are of eastern European Jewish ancestry. The other disorders listed in the question are associated with enzyme deficiencies as follows: Niemann-Pick disease, sphingomyelinase; infantile Gaucher's disease, β-glucosidase; Krabbe's disease (globoid cell leukodystrophy), galactocerebroside β-galactosidase; and Fabry's disease, α-galactosidase.

300. The answer is D. *(Bell, vol 8. pp 359-360, 366-369.)* The CAT scan presented in the question shows dilation of the lateral and third ventricles and a mass filling the fourth ventricle. These findings point to a midline, fourth ventricular tumor, such as a medulloblastoma or ependymoma; clincial signs of these tumors include papilledema and ataxia without dysmetria. The clinical signs of lateralized dysmetria and falling to the same side usually are associated with hemispheric cystic cerebellar astrocytoma; a CAT scan of patients with this disorder can be expected to show a lateralized cystic mass displacing the fourth ventricle to one side. A pontine glioma should be suspected in children who have long-tract signs, either unilaterally or bilaterally, and cranial nerve palsies, especially of the third, sixth, and seventh nerves. Cerebellar hemangioma-blastoma usually occurs in association with a retinal angioma (von Hippel-Lindau syndrome). The clinical signs stemming from bleeding within the tumor depend on the location of the tumor in the cerebellum. Blood can be seen on a CAT scan **without** the use of a contrast agent.

301. The answer is B. *(Menkes, ed 2. pp 1-7, 14-16, 21-25.)* Homocystinuria can cause thromboembolic phenomena in the pulmonary and renal arteries and in the cerebral vasculature; vascular occlusive disease is, in turn, one of the many causes of acute infantile hemiplegia. None of the other disorders listed in the question are associated with acute hemiplegia. Phenylketonuria causes retardation and, on occasion, seizures; maple syrup urine disease, an abnormality of the metabolism of leucine, leads to seizures and rapid deterioration of the central nervous system in newborn infants; histidinemia seems to be associated with speech impairments and other minor neurologic difficulties; and cystathioninuria is most likely a benign aminoaciduria having no effect on the central nervous system.

302. The answer is D. *(Neville, Develop Med Child Neurol 14:75-78, 1972. Price, Cancer 35:306-318, 1975. Rubenstein, Cancer 35:291-305, 1975.)* Acute leukemia in children is associated with a number of complications involving the central nervous system. The child described in the question most likely has necrotizing leukoencephalopathy, a recently recognized complication of combined irradiation and intrathecal methotrexate therapy. It has been suggested that irradiation in excess of 2500 rads permits methotrexate to pass into the white matter, resulting in progressive necrosis. Meningeal leukemia, which has become more common with the advent of improved chemotherapy, can lead to hydrocephalus, presumably by infiltration of the arachnoid membrane and consequent obstruction of the flow and absorption of cerebrospinal fluid. Intracerebral hemorrhages usually occur due to thrombocytopenia and produce evidence of bleeding into the skin and other organs. Because of immunosuppression, leukemic children are prone to infection by fungi and yeast.

303. The answer is D. *(Bell, vol 12. pp 272-273.)* Microcephaly, cataracts, congenital heart defects, vasomotor instability, and developmental retardation are among the many disturbances of the congenital rubella syndrome. Deafness, however, is thought to be the single most common defect associated with this disorder. Although the hearing loss seems to involve the inner ear and result primarily in a sensorineural defect, middle-ear damage also has been suggested as an etiologic factor.

304. The answer is B. *(Montpetit, Brain 94:1-30, 1971. Pincus, Develop Med Child Neurol 14:87-101, 1972.)* Leigh's syndrome (subacute necrotizing encephalomyelopathy) is pathologically similar to Wernicke's encephalopathy; pathologic features include demyelination, gliosis, and increased capillary vascularity in the brain stem, thalamus, and basal ganglia. Because Wernicke's encephalopathy seems to be thiamine-related (inhibited conversion of thiamine pyrophosphate to thiamine triphosphate), the same defect presumably also occurs in association with Leigh's syndrome. An inhibitor substance found in the urine of children who have this disorder prevents conversion into thiamine triphosphate. Signs of Leigh's syndrome, which may appear at any age in children, include hypotonia, nystagmus, strabismus, dysarthria, ataxia, and seizures; although the disorder is progressive, it is somewhat responsive to large doses of thiamine.

305. The answer is B. *(Lacey, pp 30-31.)* In infants, achromic skin patches, especially in association with infantile spasms, are pathognomonic for tuberous sclerosis. Other dermal abnormalities (adenoma sebaceum and subungual fibromata) associated with this disorder appear later in childhood. Although children who have neurofibromatosis may have a few achromic patches, the identifying dermal lesions are café au lait spots. Incontinentia pigmenti also is associated with seizures; the skin lesions typical of this disorder begin as bullous eruptions that later become hyperpigmented lesions. Pityriasis rosea and psoriasis are not associated with infantile spasms.

306. The answer is E. *(Pollack, pp 189-197.)* Various viral agents, including coxsackievirus, echovirus, and reovirus, have been identified either by culture or serologic titer in children who have Reye's syndrome. However, Reye's syndrome consistently has been noted to follow closely an influenza B epidemic or develop shortly after the appearance of chickenpox eruptions. The mechanism of action whereby these viruses provoke hepatoencephalopathy remains obscure.

307. The answer is A. *(Menkes, ed 2. pp 514-516. Pincus, Develop Med Child Neurol 14:87-101, 1972.)* A child who has a subacute disorder of the central nervous system producing cranial-nerve abnormalities (especially of the seventh nerve and the lower bulbar nerves), long-tract signs, unsteady gait secondary to spasticity, and some behavioral changes is most likely to have a pontine glioma. Definitive diagnostic studies would be either pneumoencephalography, which would show enlargement of the pons with posterior displacement of the fourth ventricle, or CAT scan, which also can demonstrate pontine enlargement. Tumors of the cerebellar hemispheres may in later stages produce long-tract signs, but the gait disturbance would be ataxia. Dysmetria and nystagmus also would be present. Supratentorial tumors are quite uncommon in six-year-old children; headache and vomiting would be likely presenting symptoms and papilledema a finding on physical examination.

308. The answer is C. *(Swaiman, 1975. p 528.)* The x-ray presented in the question reveals suprasellar calcification. In children, this finding is the most common radiographic sign of a craniopharyngioma. Changes secondary to increased intracranial pressure include widening of suture lines and erosion of the dorsum sellae and result from obstruction of the third ventricle by an expanding suprasellar tumor. Although hydrocephalus also may cause these secondary changes, it cannot be visualized in plain x-rays of the skull.

309. The answer is C (2, 4). *(Volpe, pp 762-769.)* Intraventricular or germinal matrix hemorrhage with rupture into the lateral ventricle is most commonly seen in hypoxic premature infants. Hypoxia and prematurity are also the common predisposing factors for subarachnoid hemorrhage. In contrast, subdural and posterior fossa hemorrhages are sequelae of difficult deliveries with torsion and tearing of major venous channels. Subdural hemorrhages result from rupture of superficial veins, and posterior fossa hemorrhages from tears of tentorial veins or veins of Galen.

310. The answer is A (1, 2, 3). *(Fishman, pp 171-182.)* When bloody cerebrospinal fluid (CSF) results from a subarachnoid hemorrhage, there will be the same number of red blood cells per mm^3 in the first tube as in the third tube of CSF. With a traumatic lumbar puncture there will be more red blood cells in either the first or the third tube with significantly fewer in all the other tubes. A lumbar puncture in a higher interspace repeated immediately will be free of blood if the first puncture was traumatic. The supernatant of traumatically bloody CSF will be clear while that from a CSF with subarachnoid hemorrhage will demonstrate xanthochromia, usually within two to four hours after the bleeding episode. Because bloody CSF, regardless of cause, rarely clots, observation for clotting will be of no assistance in differentiating the cause.

311. The answer is A (1, 2, 3). *(DeVivo, Pediatr Clin North Am 23:527-540, 1976. Pollack, pp 3-14.)* Reye's syndrome should be suspected when a child begins to vomit unremittingly and appears confused, disoriented, or markedly lethargic. This syndrome generally occurs as a child is recovering from a mild viral illness or on the third to fifth day of a chickenpox infection. Tachypnea and seizures may develop even in the early stages of the disorder. The most characteristic laboratory findings are serum transaminase levels at least two times normal, elevated levels of blood ammonia, and prothrombin times that are two or more seconds longer than in controls. Hypoglycemia also is common, particularly in younger children. Specific treatment remains controversial, but good supportive care and management of brain edema and increased intracranial pressure are essential.

312. The answer is E (all). *(Bell, vol 12. pp 79-80.)* Aseptic meningitis, tuberculous meningitis, meningeal leukemia, and medulloblastoma all can cause pleocytosis as well as elevated protein and lowered glucose concentrations in cerebrospinal fluid. Of the four diseases, tuberculous meningitis is associated with the lowest cerebrospinal fluid glucose levels. The cellular response to viral (aseptic) meningitis will be predominantly lymphocytic. Cells found in the cerebrospinal fluid of a child who has meningeal leukemia most commonly are lymphocytes or lymphoblasts. Children who have a medulloblastoma generally present with the signs and symptoms caused by a mass in the posterior cranial fossa; their pleocytotic cerebrospinal fluid contains unusual-appearing cells of the monocytic variety. The decrease in the cerebrospinal glucose concentration associated with these disorders has been attributed to a disturbance of glucose transport as a result of meningeal irritation.

313. The answer is E (all). *(Bell, vol 12. pp 434-436.)* Cerebellar ataxia in childhood most commonly occurs in association with a mild viral syndrome or viral

exanthem. Ingestion—whether intentional or accidental—of barbiturates, phenytoin, or alcohol also must be considered. Children who have bacterial meningitis can present, though rarely, with acute ataxia. Ataxia, opsoclonus (chaotic eye movements), and myoclonus comprise infantile polymyoclonia, which can occur in association with neuroblastoma.

314. The answer is E (all). *(Fishman, pp 208-214.)* Low cerebrospinal fluid (CSF) sugar (hypoglycorrachia) is found in all of the conditions listed in the question. The amount of glucose in CSF reflects both entry and exit of the glucose in and out of the CSF space as well as its utilization by cellular elements bordering that space. The CSF sugar level tends to be 60 to 80 percent of that in the plasma; therefore, hypoglycorrachia is found in conjunction with hypoglycemia. In bacterial infections of the central nervous system, such as mumps meningitis, low CSF sugar results from increased utilization by the adjacent arachnoid, ependyma, glia, and neurones and, in small part, by the polymorphonuclear leukocytes and impaired transmembranal transport. This also may hold true for subarachnoid hemorrhage, but it does not account for the low CSF sugar below the block caused by a malignant tumor, the cause of which remains unknown.

315. The answer is A (1, 2, 3). *(Brooke, pp 34-36, 131. Dubowitz, pp 139-142, 149, 192-193.)* Spinal muscular atrophy occurring in a neonate is associated with hypotonia and feeding difficulties; a muscle biopsy can confirm this diagnosis. Neonatal myasthenia gravis, though uncommon, must be considered in a newborn infant who has the symptoms described in the question. The symptoms presented also could represent myotonic dystrophy; this diagnosis is confirmed by examination of both parents for percussion and grip myotonia and by electromyographic depiction of myotonic discharges. Duchenne (pseudohypertrophic) muscular dystrophy clinically appears in children who are about two or three years of age.

316. The answer is E (all). *(Vaughan, ed 11. pp 1781-1782.)* Almost half of all brain abscesses in childhood develop secondarily to disease in other locations. For example, some brain abscesses occur from infections, such as mastoiditis and sinusitis, of areas contiguous to the brain, while others result from infections spread hematogenously from other sources, including the lungs, heart, and skin. On occasion, no primary source of infection can be ascertained in affected individuals. Presenting symptoms most often include low-grade fever, headache from increased intracranial pressure, vomiting, and lethargy. The treatment of choice is broad spectrum antibiotic therapy and surgical drainage if that is indicated.

317. The answer is B (1, 3). *(Browne, N Engl J Med 302:661-665, 1980.)* There have been several reported deaths believed due to liver failure in patients being treated with valproic acid. It is necessary to measure a patient's serum aspartate aminotransferase (serum glutamic-oxaloacetic transaminase, SGOT) and alanine aminotransferase (serum glutamic-pyruvic transaminase, SGPT) on a monthly basis when introducing the drug, and at three to six month intervals when the maintenance dosage has been achieved. If elevations of these enzymes occur, they may respond to reduction of dosage; however, if they exceed three times the upper limit of normal or are associated with other indications of altered liver function, the medication should be discontinued. While valproic acid may increase the serum level of phenobarbital and cause signs of toxicity, it also may decrease the total phenytoin level without increasing the free (active) serum phenytoin. This could result in increased seizure activity.

318. The answer is B (1, 3). *(Menkes, ed 2. pp 421-424.)* Compression of the third cranial nerve and distortion of the brain stem, resulting in unilateral pupillary dilatation and depressed consciousness, suggest a progressively enlarging mass, most likely an extradural hematoma. Such a hematoma displaces the temporal lobe into the tentorial notch and presses on the ipsilateral third cranial nerve. Pupillary dilatation occurs before third cranial nerve pareses. Brain stem compression by this additional tissue mass leads to progressive deterioration in consciousness. A CAT scan is the best method to differentiate this problem from an intracerebral hematoma or focal brain swelling. Seizures are not a frequent complication of head injury in children. Headache following a head injury is a common and nonspecific symptom.

319. The answer is A (1, 2, 3). *(Swaiman, 1975. p 19.)* The most common causes of an asymmetric Moro reflex in infants are injuries to the brachial plexus and clavicular fractures. Humeral, radial, and ulnar fractures also may produce an asymmetric response. Infantile hemiplegia, too, is associated, though less commonly than the factors listed above, with an asymmetric Moro reflex.

320. The answer is C (2, 4). *(Menkes, ed 2. pp 307, 309.)* Neonates who have congenital syphilis, rubella, toxoplasmosis, or cytomegalic inclusion disease all have jaundice and hepatosplenomegaly. Only the latter two diseases, however, are associated with intracranial calcification. In infants who have congenital toxoplasmosis, intracranial calcifications occur in scattered locations in the brain. Calcium deposits in infants who have a cytomegaloviral infection, on the other hand, appear in subependymal tissue; as a consequence, these calcifications tend to outline the ventricular system.

Neuromuscular System 151

321. The answer is E (all). *(Swaiman, 1975. pp 888-898.)* There are many causes in children for distractibility and shortened attention span, the most commonly accepted manifestations of hyperactivity. Because neither these characteristics nor restlessness may be evident during physical examination of an affected child, a detailed medical history should be obtained, including the educational and social background of parents and siblings and concise information regarding the setting in which hyperactivity occurs. A careful medical and developmental assessment can uncover unsuspected retardation or environmental reasons for a child's hyperkinesis. Progressive neurologic disease, deafness, and autism also may cause hyperactivity; and the diagnosis of developmental hyperactivity is one of exclusion. Treatment clearly is determined by the etiology of the hyperkinetic behavior.

322. The answer is A (1, 2, 3). *(Caffey, ed 7. pp 239-240. Swaiman, 1975. pp 655-656, 745-747.)* Children who have Sturge-Weber syndrome characteristically can be recognized by the port wine vascular nevus occurring in the distribution of the ophthalmic and maxillary branches of the trigeminal nerve. Angiomas involving the nose, mouth, and lips are not uncommon in these children. Hemiplegia, if present, occurs contralaterally to the port wine stain and leptomeningeal angiomas. Angiomas of the retina, along with cerebellar and spinal cord hemangioblastomas and renal cysts, are characteristic of von Hippel-Lindau disease.

323. The answer is A (1, 2, 3). *(Illingworth, ed 7. pp 133, 140.)* Infants who are developing normally should be able to smile when smiled at or talked to by eight weeks of age. By three months of age, infants should be able to follow a moving toy not only from side to side but also in the vertical plane. When placed on their abdomens, normal three-month-old infants can raise their faces 45 to 90 degrees from the horizontal. Not until infants reach six to eight months of age should they be able to maintain a seated position.

324. The answer is D (4). *(Caffey, ed 7. p 239.)* The parallel linear calcifications ("tram line" calcifications) seen in the skull x-ray presented are typical of Sturge-Weber syndrome. These calcifications lie within the cerebral cortex; they are not associated with the intracranial vascular malformations common in individuals who have this syndrome. Sturge-Weber syndrome is an inherited disorder associated with a high incidence of mental retardation.

325. The answer is A (1, 2, 3). *(Menkes, ed 2. pp 118-122.)* Friedreich's ataxia, a spinocerebellar degenerative disease, is characterized by both cerebellar and posterior column dysfunction. Pes cavus (high arch) and scoliosis are skeletal hallmarks of this disorder, which can be inherited as either an autosomal dominant or an autosomal recessive trait. Neurologic symptoms frequently encountered include abnormal speech, diminished position and vibration sense, nystagmus, hyporeflexia, and gait and station ataxia. There is no curative treatment for children who have Friedreich's ataxia.

326. The answer is A (1, 2, 3). *(Schmidt, pp 176-177.)* Although no exact definition of grand mal status epilepticus now exists, there is general agreement that the term implies either repeated seizures without a lucid, responsive interval or a grand mal seizure lasting at least a half hour. Some neurologists prefer to use the criterion of continuous tonic-clonic activity for one hour. Grand mal status epilepticus occurs more commonly than petit mal or psychomotor status and, if not treated, is the most serious and potentially lethal of the three. It can develop secondarily to a central nervous system infection, a toxic metabolic state, or a primary seizure disorder.

327. The answer is C (2, 4). *(Faerø, Epilepsia 13:279-285, 1972. Nelson, N Engl J Med 295:1029-1033, 1976.)* Febrile seizures generally occur in children between the ages of six months and three years and usually in association with upper respiratory illness, roseola, shigellosis, or gastroenteritis. The generalized seizures are mostly brief (two to five minutes) and the cerebrospinal fluid is normal. Infants who have seizures that are prolonged (longer than 15 minutes), focal, or lateralized or who had neurologic problems before the febrile seizure are at a higher risk than other affected infants for developing an afebrile seizure disorder during the next five to seven years. These children should be treated on a chronic basis with phenobarbital; blood levels of this drug should be maintained at 20 μg/ml.

328. The answer is E (all). *(Brooke, p 41. Dubowitz, pp 24-26.)* Gowers' maneuver is characteristic of individuals who have proximal muscle weakness of the pelvic girdle, regardless of the etiology. These individuals, when wishing to arise after lying down, must become prone and gradually stand by using their hands to "walk" up their legs. Not specific just for Duchenne (pseudohypertrophic) muscular dystrophy, Gowers' maneuver also is used by children who have limb-girdle dystrophy, late-onset spinal muscular dystrophy, and congenital myopathy.

329. The answer is E (all). *(Dubowitz, pp 232-235. Walton, ed 3. p 716.)* Multiple joint contractures in newborn infants are symptoms of diseases of muscle or of disturbances in muscle innervation. The clinical picture associated with these contractures has been called arthrogryposis multiplex congenita. Infants who have a myelomeningocele frequently have contractures of ankle and knee joints as a result of the spinal cord defect and immobilization of the lower extremities in utero.

330. The answer is E (all). *(Haller, Neurol 21:494-506, 1971. Rabe, GP 36: 78, 1967.)* Skull transillumination should be performed on all infants less than one year old being examined for progressive macrocephaly. (Thick, dark hair and darkly pigmented skin can interfere with the interpretation of this procedure; and its usefulness declines in children one year of age or more due to thickening of the scalp and skull.) Skull transillumination can be done with a number of instruments, including a common flashlight equipped with an adapter to confine the light to the skull. The presence of an acute subdural hematoma should be considered if there is an absence of transillumination on one side of the head and a normal pattern on the other. The pattern associated with a unilateral subdural effusion is increased frontoparietal transillumination, the medial border of which is demarcated by the shadow of the sagittal sinus. A focally increased transilluminated area may be caused by a porencephalic cyst lying close to the calvarium. A triangular pattern of transillumination confined to the posterior cranial fossa is diagnostic of Dandy-Walker syndrome, a type of congenital hydrocephalus; this pattern results from a cystically dilated fourth ventricle surrounded by the posterior attachment of the tentorium.

331. The answer is B (1, 3). *(Calderon, J Pediatr 68:423-431, 1966. Dodge, Pediatrics 35:3-19, 1965. Menkes, ed 12. pp 616-619.)* Psychomotor retardation may be the presenting complaint of children who have myotonic dystrophy. Ptosis and facial immobility also are early signs of the disorder, and cardiac arrhythmias are known to occur in about half of affected infants. Not infrequently the mother may have the disease in a mild form, and a careful family history and, at times, examination of the parents may be necessary to elicit the diagnosis in an affected infant. Seizures and failure to thrive are not prominent features of myotonic dystrophy.

332. The answer is E (all). *(Bell, vol 12. pp 243-247.)* Infectious mononucleosis can involve the nervous system at any level. Seizures as a manifestation of encephalitis can precede the usual clinical signs of lymphadenopathy, splenomegaly, and the presence of atypical lymphocytes in the peripheral smear. Infectious mononucleosis also can lead to aseptic meningitis, encephalomyelitis, and the Guillain-Barré syndrome.

333. The answer is E (all). *(Rose, Pediatrics 45:404-425, 1970. Swaiman, 1975. pp 863-870.)* The most frequent causes of neonatal seizures are tetany and birth trauma associated with anoxia. It is not clear in the case of hypocalcemia-related seizures whether the metabolic abnormality acts alone or in addition to brain injury caused by hypoxia to lower the threshold for seizure activity. Anomalies such as porencephaly and agenesis of the corpus callosum may be found in neonates who are having seizures.

334. The answer is B (1, 3). *(Menkes, ed 2. pp 535-537.)* In a child, ataxia that develops in infancy and the appearance of telangiectasias of the conjunctivae, ears, and nose later in life suggest ataxia-telangiectasia. Nystagmus and choreoathetosis also may be present in affected children, who may have a history of recurrent upper and lower respiratory tract infections. Serum levels of immunoglobulins A and E characteristically are reduced; affected children also may show reduced levels of immunoglobulin G and elevated levels of immunoglobulin M.

335. The answer is B (1, 3). *(McRae, Acta Radiol 5:55, 1966.)* Lacunar skull results from abnormal membranous bone formation; it probably begins in utero and resolves by six months of age. The cause is not known but, contrary to popular belief, does not have any relation to increased intracranial pressure, even though it is associated frequently with encephalocele or meningomyelocele. Thinning of bone, which occurs in the thickest parts of the frontal, parietal, and upper portion of the occipital bones, creates the impression that there are holes in the skull.

Infectious Diseases and Immunology

Richard P. Lipman

DIRECTIONS: Each question below contains five suggested answers. Choose the **one best** response to each question.

336. The best single-drug treatment for individuals who have meningitis caused by *Hemophilus influenzae*, type b, is with intravenous

(A) ampicillin
(B) gentamicin
(C) cephalothin
(D) chloramphenicol
(E) erythromycin

337. An eight-year-old boy who has no history of sexual contact develops dysuria and a purulent urethral discharge. Culture on chocolate agar shows a few colonies of *Escherichia coli*. Forty-eight hours later, his left ankle becomes swollen, hot, and tender, coincident with the onset of chills, fever, and a stiff neck. A lumbar puncture shows cloudy cerebrospinal fluid. The cause of his disease is most likely to be

(A) *Neisseria gonorrhoeae*
(B) *Mycoplasma hominis*
(C) T-strain *Mycoplasma*
(D) *Chlamydia*
(E) herpesvirus hominis, type 2

338. All of the following diseases or infectious agents are characteristically associated with eruptions involving both the mouth and hands EXCEPT

(A) Kawasaki disease
(B) *Rickettsia rickettsii*
(C) group A coxsackievirus
(D) Herpesvirus hominis (type 1)
(E) syphilis

339. A two-year-old Pakistani child, staying with relatives in the United States, suddenly becomes lethargic and develops a fever of 40°C (104°F). Eruptions of clear, fragile vesicles begin to appear on the trunk. During the next four days, new eruptions involve the face and extremities, and the older vesicles become pustular; the fever is unabated, and the child remains severely ill. The most likely diagnosis of this child's condition is

(A) smallpox
(B) chickenpox
(C) shingles
(D) hand-foot-and-mouth disease
(E) cat scratch fever

340. Following a mild two-week upper respiratory tract infection, a six-month-old girl develops a severe cough that is not relieved by expectorants. The cough is paroxysmal and exhausting, and copious amounts of sticky, clear mucus issue from the nose and mouth. Treatment with ampicillin is ineffective, and hospitalization is required after a brief convulsion during a coughing spell on the tenth day following onset of the severe cough. A presumptive diagnosis of this child's disorder can be made by a

(A) throat culture
(B) white blood cell count
(C) chest x-ray
(D) Gram stain of the tracheal aspirate
(E) Gram stain of the nasal discharge

341. All of the following statements about acute osteomyelitis are true EXCEPT that

(A) it most commonly is caused by *Staphylococcus aureus*
(B) it often arises following development of deep cellulitis
(C) tenderness in the region of infection is diffuse, not localized
(D) bony changes are not visible radiographically for five to ten days after onset of infection
(E) antibiotic therapy usually is required for at least four weeks

342. A three-year-old boy develops a fever and tender swellings below the angles of the mandible. His tonsils are red, swollen, and covered with white exudate, which contains many bacteria but no polymorphonuclear leukocytes. Although the spleen is not palpable, the inguinal nodes are visibly enlarged. These findings are most consistent with infection caused by

(A) mumps virus
(B) group A β-hemolytic streptococci
(C) group A coxsackievirus
(D) Epstein-Barr virus
(E) *Streptococcus (Diplococcus) pneumoniae*

343. A 15-year-old boy develops fever and tachypnea following five days of sore throat, headache, and gradually worsening cough. Chest x-ray shows bilateral hilar infiltrates. White blood cell count is normal. Gram stain of a nasopharyngeal swab shows large numbers of lancet-shaped gram-positive diplococci. The causative organism most likely is

(A) *Streptococcus (Diplococcus) pneumoniae*
(B) *Mycoplasma pneumoniae*
(C) *Mycoplasma hominis*
(D) *Mycobacterium tuberculosis*
(E) *Legionella pneumophila*

344. A three-year-old boy has had a temperature of 39°C (102.2°F) and a stiff back for the last three days. Examination shows a red throat, large nontender anterior and posterior cervical nodes, and slight resistance of the neck to flexion. Immediate management should include a

(A) lumbar puncture
(B) heterophil test
(C) throat culture and oral penicillin for seven days
(D) throat culture and oral penicillin for ten days
(E) throat culture, white blood cell count, and re-examination in 24 hours

345. All of the following clinical observations are characteristic of staphylococcal pneumonia EXCEPT

(A) hilar adenopathy on chest x-ray
(B) rapid progression of dyspnea to respiratory failure
(C) pleural effusion
(D) air-filled pulmonary blebs
(E) distended abdomen with diminished bowel sounds

346. Which of the following infections typically has an incubation period of less than two weeks?

(A) Mumps
(B) Varicella
(C) Rubella
(D) Measles
(E) Rabies

347. Which of the following statements about measles encephalitis is true?

(A) It occurs relatively rarely (1 per 10,000 cases of measles)
(B) It occurs more frequently in association with severe rather than mild cases of measles
(C) An immunologic demyelinating reaction may play a role in development of the disease
(D) Direct viral invasion of the central nervous system is not a significant factor
(E) The prognosis usually depends on the degree of coma

348. A 14-year-old girl awakens with a mild sore throat, low-grade fever, and a diffuse maculopapular rash. During the next 24 hours she develops tender swelling of her wrists and redness of her eyes. In addition, her physician notes mild tenderness and marked swelling of her posterior cervical and occipital lymph nodes. Four days after the onset of her illness the rash has vanished.

The most likely diagnosis of this girl's condition is

(A) rubella
(B) rubeola
(C) roseola
(D) erythema infectiosum
(E) acute infectious lymphocytosis

349. A three-year-old child awakens at night with a fever of 39.6°C (103.3°F), a severe sore throat, and a barking cough. Physical examination of the child, who is drooling, shows a very red throat and inspiratory stridor. The hypopharynx is obscured by yellow mucus. The lungs are clear and there is no respiratory distress. Optimal management would include

(A) immediate hospitalization for possible intubation
(B) immediate inhalation therapy with racemic epinephrine
(C) treatment with oral ampicillin, 50 mg/kg/day
(D) suctioning of the pharynx and hourly examinations of the hypopharynx
(E) a throat culture and initiation of expectorant and mist therapy

350. The leading cause of bacterial meningitis in children between the ages of six months and three years is

(A) group A β-hemolytic *Streptococcus*
(B) group C *Neisseria meningitidis*
(C) type 5 *Streptococcus* (*Diplococcus*) *pneumoniae*
(D) type b *Hemophilus influenzae*
(E) untypable *Hemophilus influenzae*

351. The management of salmonellal gastroenteritis ordinarily includes the administration of

(A) ampicillin
(B) chloramphenicol
(C) tetracycline
(D) cephaloridine
(E) none of the above

352. A three-day-old infant develops *Escherichia coli* meningitis. Treatment with intravenous chloramphenicol, 40 mg/kg daily, produces prompt clinical improvement; beginning on the fifth day of therapy, however, she becomes progressively lethargic and refuses feedings. Because her temperature is subnormal, she is placed on a heated bed. No specific physical or hematologic abnormalities are found, and examination of cerebrospinal fluid shows improvement over results obtained five days earlier.

For the immediate management of this child, the physician involved should

(A) obtain an electroencephalogram
(B) obtain a CAT scan of the skull
(C) begin treatment with ampicillin
(D) increase the dose of chloramphenicol
(E) reduce the dose of chloramphenicol

353. A 14-month-old infant suddenly develops a fever of 40.2°C (104.4°F). Physical examination shows an alert, active infant who drinks milk eagerly. No physical abnormalities are noted. The white blood cell count is 22,000/mm^3 with 78% polymorphonuclear leukocytes, 18% of which are band forms. The most likely diagnosis is

(A) pneumococcal bacteremia
(B) roseola
(C) streptococcosis
(D) typhoid fever
(E) diphtheria

354. A five-year-old boy develops a mild sore throat, malaise, a low-grade fever, and a faint, generalized, rough, fine red papular rash most obvious on the trunk. His tongue is coated as shown in figure **A** below. After three days the rash has faded, and his tongue appears as in figure **B**. One week later there is a sudden, alarming loss of the superficial layers of skin from his fingers.

The most likely diagnosis of this child's condition is

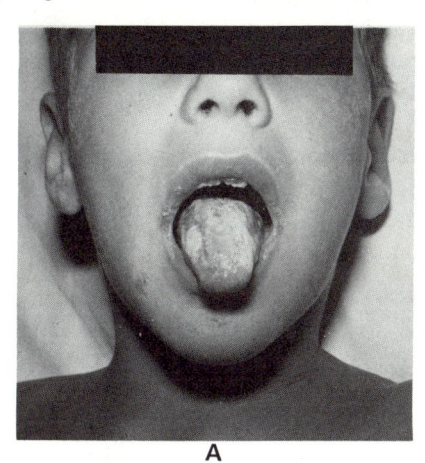

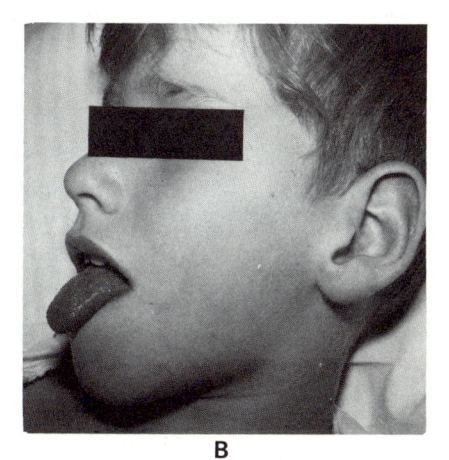

(A) rubella
(B) fifth disease
(C) roseola
(D) scarlet fever
(E) thrush

Pediatrics

Questions 355-356

A nine-year-old girl has a persistently high fever, constipation, and progressive abdominal pain, tenderness, and distension. Development of these symptoms follows three days of malaise, headache, and intermittent fever. Physical examination reveals a disoriented, somnolent child who has a temperature of 39.8°C (103.6°F), diffuse inspiratory rales, a moderately enlarged spleen, and a distended, tender abdomen. A faint maculopapular rash is present on the trunk.

355. The organism most likely to be responsible is

(A) *Rickettsia rickettsii*
(B) *Neisseria meningitidis*
(C) *Salmonella typhi*
(D) *Brucella melitensis*
(E) *Shigella dysenteriae*

356. During the first week of this girl's illness, laboratory identification of the etiologic pathogen can best be accomplished by

(A) stool culture
(B) blood culture
(C) urine culture
(D) duodenal fluid culture
(E) measurement of serum agglutinins

357. The rash and mucous-membrane lesions shown below develop in an infant five days after a nonspecific upper respiratory tract infection. Which of the following is LEAST likely to be responsible?

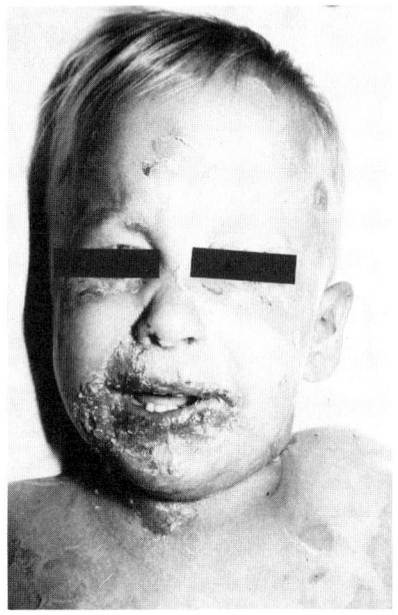

(A) *Mycoplasma pneumoniae*
(B) Herpesvirus hominis, type 1
(C) Rubella virus
(D) Phenobarbital ingestion
(E) Penicillin therapy

358. Which of the following statements about aplastic anemia caused by chloramphenicol therapy is correct?

(A) It occurs with an incidence of about 0.01 percent
(B) It is usually dose-related
(C) It disappears when treatment is discontinued
(D) It appears during therapy rather than after therapy
(E) None of the above

359. A stool culture from a four-year-old child who has mild diarrhea grows enteropathogenic *Escherichia coli*. All of the following statements about this organism are true EXCEPT that

(A) it may be invasive
(B) it may be noninvasive and toxigenic
(C) it is a rare cause of diarrhea in infants
(D) infections in young children respond to oral neomycin
(E) infections in older children do not require antibiotic therapy

360. Streptococcal pyoderma (impetigo) is best described as

(A) a vesicular or bullous infection in which the blisters rupture over a period of many hours
(B) a vesicular infection in which blisters rupture early and crusts develop
(C) a vesicular infection characterized by painful, brown, crusted lesions that spread out on the face
(D) a vesicular infection producing painful, indurated, thick-walled vesicles on a red fingertip
(E) a vesicular infection in which painful vesicles are arranged in a linear pattern

Pediatrics

DIRECTIONS: Each question below contains four suggested answers of which **one** or **more** is correct. Choose the answer:

A	if	1, 2, and 3	are correct
B	if	1 and 3	are correct
C	if	2 and 4	are correct
D	if	4	is correct
E	if	1, 2, 3, and 4	are correct

361. A 15-year-old boy returned to his pediatrician because of a persistent, but moderately improved, urethral discharge two weeks following treatment with intramuscular procaine penicillin G, 4.8 million units, and oral probenecid, 1 g. A Gram stain of the original discharge had shown many gram-negative diplococci within abundant leukocytes. When re-examined, no organisms could be identified either by stain or bacteriologic culture. Manifestations of disease in other individuals infected with the boy's persistent pathogen or with related serotypes would be likely to include

(1) persistent tachypnea, cough, and inspiratory rales in a two-month-old infant
(2) purulent conjunctival discharge in a three-day-old infant
(3) fever and tender swollen inguinal lymph nodes
(4) interstitial pneumonia in a sixteen-year-old girl who works in a pet store

362. Common features of infections with hepatitis A virus include which of the following?

(1) Prolonged presence of virus in stools
(2) Short incubation period (15 to 50 days)
(3) Frequent occurrence of extrahepatic manifestations
(4) Sudden onset of fever, nausea, and vomiting

363. Twelve hours after eating her Christmas dinner, a three-year-old girl develops vomiting, abdominal cramps, low-grade fever, and profuse watery diarrhea that fails to improve with a clear liquid diet. Stool cultures obtained on the fourth day because of persistent diarrhea show neither *Salmonella* nor *Shigella* species. However, additional studies might be expected to show

(1) *Yersinia enterocolitica*
(2) a rotavirus infection
(3) *Campylobacter fetus*
(4) *Clostridium difficile*

364. A newborn infant has an abnormally small head; skull x-ray is shown below. The radiographic findings are characteristic of infection with which of the following organisms?

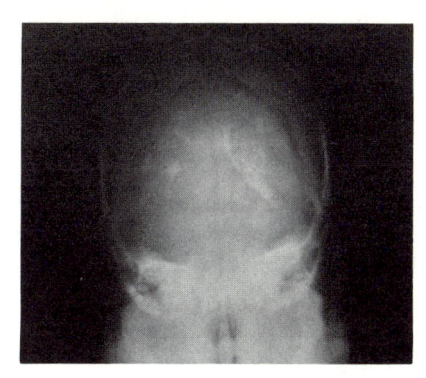

(1) *Toxoplasma gondii*
(2) *Treponema pallidum*
(3) Cytomegalovirus
(4) Rubella virus

365. Neurologic complications can develop from the administration of which of the following vaccines?

(1) Oral polio vaccine (Sabin)
(2) Diphtheria-pertussis-tetanus vaccine
(3) Smallpox vaccine
(4) Measles vaccine

366. A toxin that has a direct pathogenic effect on the heart can be produced by which of the following organisms?

(1) *Rickettsia rickettsii*
(2) *Corynebacterium diphtheriae*
(3) *Clostridium tetani*
(4) Group A β-hemolytic streptococci

367. A newborn infant becomes markedly jaundiced on the second day of life, and a faint petechial eruption first noted at birth is now a generalized purpuric rash. Hematologic studies for hemolytic diseases are negative. Appropriate measures at this time would include

(1) radiographic examination of the long bones
(2) isolation of the infant from pregnant hospital personnel
(3) a blood culture
(4) measurement of the level of serum immunoglobulin M

368. A lumbar puncture of a child who has signs of meningitis shows a white blood cell count of 600/mm^3 (62% polymorphonuclear leukocytes and 38% lymphocytes) and a glucose level of 40 mg/100 ml (blood glucose is 110 mg/100 ml). Gram staining is unproductive. Organisms likely to cause this clinical picture include

(1) *Mycobacterium tuberculosis*
(2) group A coxsackievirus
(3) *Cryptococcus neoformans*
(4) lymphocytic choriomeningitis virus

369. Examination of the stool from a patient who has fever and diarrhea shows red blood cells and many polymorphonuclear leukocytes. This clinical picture is consistent with intestinal disease caused by

(1) *Salmonella typhimurium*
(2) *Salmonella typhi*
(3) *Shigella sonnei*
(4) enteropathogenic *Escherichia coli*

SUMMARY OF DIRECTIONS

A	B	C	D	E
1, 2, 3 only	1, 3 only	2, 4 only	4 only	All are correct

370. Which of the following blood test results can provide evidence of a current case of infectious mononucleosis?

(1) An elevated titer of antibody to Epstein-Barr virus
(2) A white blood cell differential that includes at least 5 percent atypical, vacuolated lymphocytes
(3) Absorption of sheep red blood cell agglutinins by guinea pig kidney cells
(4) Absorption of sheep red blood cell agglutinins by beef red blood cells

371. Which of the following drug therapies can provide effective oral treatment of individuals who have group A β-hemolytic streptococcal pharyngitis?

(1) Penicillin G, 400,000 units three times daily for ten days
(2) Phenoxymethyl penicillin (penicillin V), 250 mg four times daily for seven days
(3) Erythromycin, 44 mg/kg daily for ten days
(4) Sulfadiazine, 100 mg/kg daily for fourteen days

372. A two-month-old infant has a temperature of 39.6°C (103.3°F); physical examination is completely normal. This child could have which of the following types of infection?

(1) Roseola infantum
(2) Bacterial meningitis
(3) Streptococcal pharyngitis
(4) Urinary tract infection

373. In addition to the familiar maculopapular rash, measles typically is characterized by which of the following symptoms?

(1) Cough
(2) Moderate or high fever
(3) Coryza
(4) Conjunctivitis

374. Correct statements about patients who have histoplasmosis include which of the following?

(1) Chest x-ray may show intrathoracic calcification similar to that of tuberculosis
(2) A positive skin test usually indicates active infection
(3) A diffuse pneumonia may occur
(4) Tetracycline is an effective treatment

375. A positive Mantoux test in a child is likely to

(1) develop within two to ten weeks after infection
(2) indicate infection with atypical mycobacteria
(3) indicate a need for antimicrobial therapy
(4) become negative for a brief period after immunization with live viruses

376. A three-year-old black male developed a painful tender swelling of his foot, accompanied by a temperature of 39°C (102.2°F). His white blood cell count was 10,600/mm^3 (72% polymorphonuclear leukocytes and 28% lymphocytes), and his erythrocyte sedimentation rate was 56 mm per hour. An x-ray of his foot is shown below. True statements about this child's illness include which of the following?

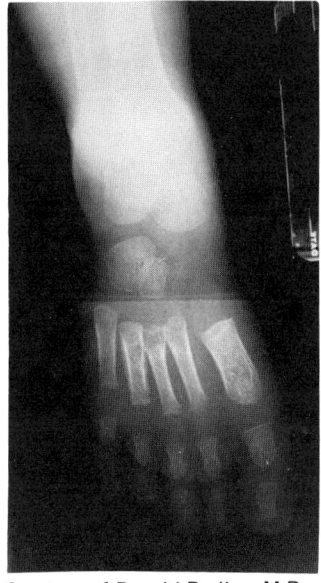

Courtesy of Donald Darling, M.D.

(1) *Salmonella* organisms may be found in his blood
(2) His sodium metabisulfite blood test is likely to be abnormal
(3) Polyvalent pneumococcal vaccine may significantly reduce his future morbidity
(4) Intravenous sodium oxacillin is the treatment of choice

377. Meningococcemia can lead to which of the following complications?

(1) Acute adrenal failure
(2) Arthritis
(3) Gastrointestinal hemorrhage
(4) Pericarditis

378. Disease is produced by which of the following parasites in the course of their migration through the parenchyma of body tissues?

(1) *Necator americanus*
(2) *Ascaris lumbricoides*
(3) *Toxocara canis*
(4) *Enterobius vermicularis*

379. A child who has croup can be expected to

(1) have a low-grade fever
(2) wheeze during inspiration
(3) be infected with parainfluenza virus
(4) show patchy lung infiltrates on chest x-ray

380. Two weeks ago, a five-year-old boy developed diarrhea, which has persisted to the present time in spite of dietary management. His stools have been watery, pale, and frothy. He has been afebrile. Microscopic examination of his stools might show

(1) *Trichuris trichiura*
(2) *Entamoeba histolytica*
(3) *Giardia lamblia*
(4) *Toxoplasma gondii*

SUMMARY OF DIRECTIONS

A	B	C	D	E
1, 2, 3 only	1, 3 only	2, 4 only	4 only	All are correct

381. True statements about poliomyelitis include which of the following?

(1) It can be asymptomatic or nonparalytic
(2) It is accompanied by fever, sore throat, and myalgia
(3) Aseptic meningitis can be a prominent feature
(4) Hypertension and urinary retention sometimes arise as complications

382. Three days after swellings first appeared at the angle of his mandible, a seven-year-old boy suddenly develops a severe headache, fever, and stiff neck. His cerebrospinal fluid contains 300 leukocytes/mm^3 (62% polymorphonuclear leukocytes and 38% lymphocytes), 40 mg/100 ml of protein, and 60 mg/100 ml of glucose. His blood glucose level is 120 mg/100 ml. His physician should

(1) repeat the lumbar puncture in four to six hours
(2) obtain a serum amylase level
(3) order a heterophil test
(4) begin antibiotic therapy immediately

383. A 12-day-old infant is brought to an emergency room because of lethargy and anorexia. White blood cell count is 4000/mm^3 with a normal differential. Except for lethargy, no specific findings are evident on physical examination. The examining physician should

(1) do an immediate lumbar puncture
(2) obtain a urine culture
(3) obtain a blood culture
(4) re-examine the infant in 24 hours

384. A newborn infant has the desquamating rash depicted in the figure below. The child might also be expected to develop which of the following conditions?

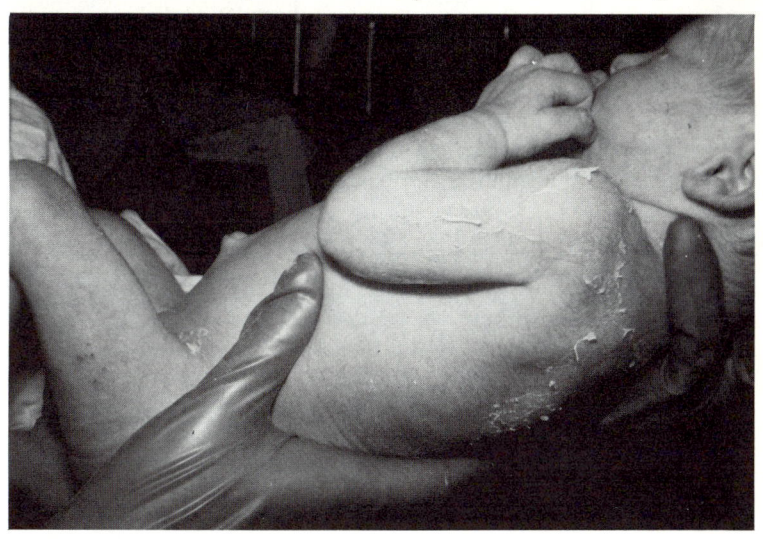

(1) Purulent umbilical drainage
(2) Pneumonia
(3) Progressive enlargement of one breast
(4) An asymmetric Moro reflex

Pediatrics

DIRECTIONS: The groups of questions below consist of lettered choices followed by several numbered items. For each numbered item select the **one** lettered choice with which it is **most** closely associated. Each lettered choice may be used once, more than once, or not at all.

Questions 385-388

For each of the immunologic abnormalities listed in the table below, select the syndrome or disease with which it is most closely associated.

(A) Bruton disease
(B) DiGeorge syndrome
(C) Wiskott-Aldrich syndrome
(D) Job-Buckley syndrome
(E) Swiss-type immunodeficiency disease

	Serum IgG	Serum IgA	Serum IgM	T-Cell Function	Parathyroid Function
385.	Normal	Normal	Normal	Decreased	Decreased
386.	Low	Low	Low	Normal	Normal
387.	Low	Low	Low	Decreased	Normal
388.	Normal	High	Low	Decreased	Normal

Questions 389-390

For each of the phagocytic disorders described below, select the syndrome or disease with which it is most closely associated.

(A) Lazy leukocyte syndrome
(B) Chediak-Higashi syndrome
(C) Chronic granulomatous disease
(D) Ataxia-telangiectasia
(E) None of the above conditions

389. Abscesses, pneumonia, and osteomyelitis accompany this sex-linked or autosomal recessive condition in which leukocytes manifest normal attachment and phagocytosis but are not microbicidal for catalase-positive organisms because of defective oxidative metabolism

390. Recurrent, severe bacterial and viral infections occur in this neutropenic disorder in which leukocytes demonstrate defective chemotaxis, delayed degranulation of giant lysosomes, and normal, but delayed, intracellular killing

# Infectious Diseases and Immunology

Answers

336. The answer is D. *(Feldman, Pediatrics 61:406-409, 1978. Katz, Pediatrics 55:6-8, 1975.)* Until the emergence of resistant strains of type b *Hemophilus influenzae*, intravenous ampicillin was the treatment of choice for patients who had meningitis caused by this organism. Now, however, single-agent use of intravenous chloramphenicol, which produces excellent spinal fluid levels compared with other antibiotic drugs, is recommended. To forestall the development of hematologic problems, ampicillin therapy can be instituted later if the causative strain is not resistant to the drug. Daily doses of ampicillin, 200-400 mg/kg, must be given to maintain adequate levels in the spinal fluid; antibiotic diffusion across the meninges diminishes as meningeal inflammation is reduced. Some authorities recommend initial therapy with both ampicillin and chloramphenicol because they are sometimes synergistic. Chloramphenicol may then be discontinued if the organism proves to be sensitive to ampicillin. Cephalosporins do not generally reach therapeutic levels in the spinal fluid.

337. The answer is A. *(Krugman, ed 7. pp 77-89. Taylor-Robinson, N Engl J Med 302:1003-1010, 1063-1067, 1980. Vaughan, ed 11. pp 761-763.)* If vaginal or urethral discharge is present, gonococcal infection must be suspected, regardless of the affected individual's age or sexual history. Laboratory demonstration of *Neisseria gonorrhoeae* is usually but not always possible using both a Gram stain of the exudate and a culture on Thayer-Martin medium, which is more selective than chocolate agar. Gonococci can spread either hematogenously or by direct extension; infection can cause inflammation or abscess formation in the epididymis, prostate gland, fallopian tubes, peritoneal cavity, liver, and joints. Gonococcal endocarditis or meningitis, though rare, occasionally can develop. Nongonococcal urethritis accompanied by dysuria and purulent discharge, once attributed to T-strain mycoplasmas, is now thought to be caused mainly by species of *Chlamydia*. However, although this infection may be complicated by arthritis and conjunctivitis (Reiter's syndrome), meningitis does not occur. Most authorities no longer acknowledge *Mycoplasma hominis* to be a cause of symptomatic urethritis. The genital strain (type 2) of herpesvirus hominis produces a painful vesiculating balanitis or vulvitis.

338. **The answer is B.** *(Hoekelman, pp 1178-1180. Kato, Pediatrics 63:175-179, 1979. Vaughan, ed 11. pp 673, 843-846, 869, 951, 953, 955-956.)* Individuals bitten by ticks which harbor *Rickettsia rickettsii* are at great risk to develop Rocky Mountain spotted fever, which is characterized by high fever, excruciating headache, a confused mental state, hepatosplenomegaly, hyponatremic edema, and a generalized macular or petechial rash, which typically begins on the extremities, including the palms and soles. Oral exanthems are unusual. The rickettsia-induced vasculitis is associated with such serious complications as cerebral arteritis, myocarditis, and disseminated intravascular coagulation. Treatment with chloramphenicol or tetracycline has reduced the fatality rate from 20 to 5 percent. **Kawasaki disease** (mucocutaneous lymph node syndrome), of unknown etiology, affects chiefly infants and toddlers and is potentially fatal in cases complicated by coronary arteritis and resultant aneurysm or occlusion. Initially, affected individuals commonly manifest redness of the conjunctivae, tongue, and lips (sometimes with peeling), a diffuse blotchy red rash, redness of the palms and soles, desquamation of the fingers or toes, cervical adenitis, and marked elevation of both the erythrocyte sedimentation rate and the white blood cell count, with a shift to the left. Its occurrence in clusters suggests the involvement of an infectious agent. Among the many clinical syndromes associated with the more than 20 members of the **group A coxsackieviruses** are the following: (1) nonspecific febrile summer illnesses, often with exanthems; (2) aseptic meningitis; (3) acute myocarditis or pericarditis; (4) herpangina, characterized by high fever, sore throat, and ulcerations of the anterior faucial pillars, tongue, posterior palate, and inner aspect of the lips; and (5) hand-foot-and-mouth disease, a common, easily identified syndrome characterized by fever, vesicles and ulcers in the mouth, thick-walled vesicles on the hands and feet, and variable degrees of maculopapular rash. Children with **herpetic stomatitis** who suck their fingers or thumb may develop an unusual painful herpetic infection of the fingertip (herpetic whitlow) with spreading vesicles, redness, and swelling. Among the many lesions associated with both congenital and acquired **syphilis** are a maculopapular rash, which involves the palms and soles, and oral mucous patches. In addition, mucocutaneous lesions about the mouth (rhagades) are seen in congenital syphilis.

339. **The answer is B.** *(Krugman, ed 7. pp 486-504. Vaughan, ed 11. pp 873-875, 921, 949.)* Chickenpox (varicella) is caused by varicella-zoster virus. Although often a mild disease, it may be associated with a high fever and severe clinical course more typical of smallpox. The vesicles of children who have chickenpox are superficial and sometimes umbilicated, spreading centrifugally from the trunk to the extremities. Because the vesicles continue to erupt for three or four days, the vesicles are in all stages of development, from macules to pustules or crusts. In smallpox, on the other hand, the vesicles are deep and umbilicated, spreading centrally from the extremities. The lesions are all in the same

stage of development and tend to cluster in areas where the skin is tight or traumatized, such as over the nasal bridge or belt line. Herpes zoster infection (shingles) represents a reactivation of the varicella-zoster virus in an immune individual. After a latent period of infection of the posterior nerve roots, the virus causes clusters of painful vesicles to appear along dermatomes. Hand-foot-and-mouth disease, caused by coxsackieviruses, is characterized by fever and a generalized macular rash that produces vesicles on the palms and soles as well as in the pharynx, where they ulcerate. Cat scratch fever, symptoms of which include malaise, headache, and low-grade fever, is identified by local suppurating lymphadenitis near the scratch.

340. The answer is B. *(Baraff, Pediatrics 61:224-230, 1978. Krugman, ed 7. pp 242-251. Vaughan, ed 11. pp 766-769.)* Pertussis (whooping cough) should be strongly suspected in a child who, after a two-week illness resembling a common cold, develops a paroxysmal, strangling cough accompanied by profuse, thick mucus that pours from the nose and mouth. The characteristic inspiratory whoop at the end of a paroxysm, which is diagnostic for pertussis, may be absent in affected children less than six months of age. Complications include atelectasis, pneumonia, otitis media, and convulsions. Marked leukocytosis, often as high as 45,000/mm^3, with an absolute lymphocytosis is a characteristic laboratory finding. Identification of the pathogen, *Bordetella pertussis (Hemophilus pertussis)*, cannot be made by microscopic examination of secretions, except by fluorescent antibody staining techniques. Unless nasopharyngeal cultures are obtained during the first two weeks of illness or very early in the paroxysmal phase, the organism is difficult to isolate. Erythromycin is useful as prophylaxis for exposed family members and to shorten the duration of infectivity for affected infants. It does not, however, alter the course of the disease.

341. The answer is C. *(Vaughan, ed 11. pp 713-716.)* Acute osteomyelitis tends to begin abruptly with fever and marked, localized bone tenderness that usually occurs at the metaphysis. Redness and swelling frequently follow. Although usually the result of hematogenous bacterial spread, particularly of *Staphylococcus aureus*, acute osteomyelitis may follow an episode of deep cellulitis and should be suspected whenever deep cellulitis occurs. Diagnosis must often be based on clinical grounds, because bone changes may not be visible on x-ray for up to 12 days after onset of the disease. However, bone scans with technetium radioisotopes may be extremely useful in the early diagnosis of osteomyelitis and in its differentiation from cellulitis and septic arthritis. Antibiotic treatment must be initiated immediately to avoid further extension of infection into bone, where adequate drug levels are difficult to achieve. Treatment is usually continued for at least four weeks. In addition to x-rays and white blood cell count, erythrocyte sedimentation rate is useful in monitoring a patient's recovery.

342. The answer is D. *(Vaughan, ed 11. pp 739, 869-870, 887, 891.)* Although infectious mononucleosis, which is caused by the Epstein-Barr virus, develops most often in older children and adolescents, it also occurs commonly in children between the ages of two and ten years. It is characterized by fever, pharyngitis, a generalized macular red rash, hepatitis, and enlargement of lymph nodes and spleen, which may not become palpable until the second week of the illness. The accompanying pharyngitis, which often produces a white exudate containing a multitude of heterogeneous bacteria but few leukocytes, may be hard to distinguish clinically from streptococcal pharyngitis, the exudate of which is more yellow in color and contains many leukocytes but relatively few bacteria. Mumps produces no significant redness or exudate; and group A or group B coxsackievirus infection causes discrete ulcerations in the pharynx.

343. The answer is B. *(Denny, J Infect Dis 123:74-92, 1971. Sanford, N Engl J Med 300:654, 656, 1979. Vaughan, ed 11. pp 1214-1215.)* Bilateral hilar or interstitial pneumonia, especially when accompanied by a normal white blood cell count, is typical of nonbacterial disease. The picture may be confused if the patient is a coincidental carrier of pneumococci in the nasopharynx; lancet-shaped, gram-positive, α-hemolytic streptococci also may be abundantly present in pairs and resemble pneumococci. In such cases, cultures and Gram stain of tracheal aspirates are significant. Prodromal symptoms of sore throat, headache, a gradually worsening cough, and subsequent development of interstitial or hilar pneumonia are characteristic of both viral disease and *Mycoplasma pneumoniae* pneumonia, a condition highly prevalent in adolescents. Pneumonia caused by the latter agent can often be identified by specific serologic tests for *M. pneumoniae* or suggested by a significant rise in the serum cold agglutinin titer, which occurs in at least 50 percent of affected individuals.

Legionnaires' disease, caused by the gram-negative bacillus *Legionella pneumophila* is characterized by a severe bilateral interstitial pneumonia, with myalgia, headache, high fever, gastrointestinal symptoms, central nervous system dysfunction, and moderate leukocytosis and neutrophilia. Tuberculosis must be suspected if hilar adenopathy or pulmonary calcifications are present. *Mycoplasma hominis* is a genitourinary pathogen sometimes associated with postpartum fever and pelvic inflammatory disease.

344. The answer is A. *(Dodge, N Engl J Med 272:954-960, 1003-1010, 1965. Vaughan, ed 11. pp 722-723.)* A fever accompanied by inability to flex rather than rotate the neck immediately suggests meningitis. An indolent clinical course does not rule out bacterial meningitis: *Hemophilus influenzae* may produce meningeal symptoms (fever, headache, and stiff neck or back) that are so mild that several days can elapse before medical advice is sought. The large cervical nodes characteristic of streptococcal pharyngitis may limit rotational or lateral neck movement if their tenderness is exacerbated by contraction of the sternocleidomastoid muscles. Initial symptoms of infectious mononucleosis with associated aseptic meningitis usually are pharyngitis, adenopathy (often nontender), and meningeal signs. A lumbar puncture is of prime diagnostic importance in determining the presence of bacterial meningitis, which requires immediate antibiotic therapy. A delay in treatment of even one hour may lead to such complications as cerebrovascular thrombosis, obstructive hydrocephalus, cerebritis with seizures or acute increased intracranial pressure, coma, or death.

345. The answer is A. *(Vaughan, ed 11. pp 1210-1212.)* Staphylococcal pneumonia, which usually occurs in children younger than one year of age, also may follow viral respiratory infections such as influenza in older children and adolescents. The sudden onset of fever, cough, and tachypnea tends to be followed by very rapid development of severe dyspnea, cyanosis, shock, and, occasionally, abdominal ileus. Extensive destruction of lung tissue is common and can lead to pneumatoceles, empyema, and pyopneumothorax. Long-term follow-up studies of survivors, however, tend to show a normal chest x-ray and pulmonary function. Hilar adenopathy that is accompanied by either pleural fluid or air-filled cavities suggests tuberculosis rather than an acute pyogenic infection.

346. The answer is D. *(Yow, ed 18. pp 132-133, 150, 211, 243, 305.)* The usual incubation periods of several important diseases are as follows: measles, 10 to 12 days; varicella, 10 to 21 days; rubella, 14 to 21 days; mumps, 14 to 21 days; and rabies, 14 to 56 days. The durations of infectivity are as follows: measles, from the onset of the catarrhal stage through the fifth day of the rash; varicella, from one day before the eruption until the last vesicle has dried (approximately seven days); rubella, from seven days before the onset of the rash to up to eight days after its disappearance; mumps, from one day before parotid swelling through the third day after it subsides; and rabies (dogs), from five days before the onset of signs through the course of the disease.

347. The answer is C. *(Vaughan, ed 11. p 860.)* Encephalitis is a serious complication of measles; it occurs relatively commonly (1 per 750 cases of measles). It may develop during any stage of measles infection, even during the pre-eruptive period; in this stage, direct viral invasion of the central nervous system can cause encephalitis. More commonly, encephalitis is noted first between two and five days after the exanthem appears; it is characterized at this time by a demyelinating process. Measles encephalitis is associated with a high mortality rate and a high incidence of permanent neurologic impairment. No relationship, however, exists either between the initial severity of encephalitis and its eventual outcome or between the severity of measles and the severity of the accompanying encephalitis.

348. The answer is A. *(Vaughan, ed 11. pp 857-867, 950.)* Symptoms of rubella, usually a mild disease, include a diffuse maculopapular rash that lasts for three days, marked enlargement of the posterior cervical and occipital lymph nodes, low-grade fever, mild sore throat, and, occasionally, conjunctivitis, arthralgia, or arthritis. Individuals who have rubeola develop a severe cough, coryza, photophobia, conjunctivitis, and a high fever that reaches its peak at the height of the generalized macular rash, which typically lasts for five days; Koplik's spots on the buccal mucosa are diagnostic. Roseola is a viral exanthem of infants in which the high fever abruptly abates as a rash appears. Erythema infectiosum (fifth disease) begins with bright erythema on the cheeks ("slapped cheek" sign), followed by a red maculopapular rash on the trunk and extremities. A high white blood cell count (above 20,000/mm^3 with 60% to 95% lymphocytes), mild sore throat, morbilliform rash, and gastrointestinal symptoms can appear in individuals who have acute infectious lymphocytosis.

349. The answer is A. *(Vaughan, ed 11. pp 765, 1193-1197.)* Children who have acute epiglottitis, a life-threatening infection of the hypopharynx and epiglottis caused by *Hemophilus influenzae*, typically present with high fever, extremely sore throat, and a croupy cough. Physical examination characteristically shows a very red throat and a red, swollen epiglottis that may be obscured by exudate or so distorted that its identity is misinterpreted. Affected children often are unable to swallow saliva; and because the swollen epiglottis can unpredictably and suddenly cause total and fatal airway obstruction, immediate hospitalization is mandatory. Most authorities recommend prompt tracheotomy or endotracheal intubation, even in the absence of severe respiratory distress. If a diagnosis of acute epiglottitis is uncertain, a lateral x-ray of the neck will differentiate epiglottic from subglottic swelling, the latter of which is associated with a less serious disease, croup.

350. The answer is D. *(Vaughan, ed 11. pp 764-766.)* *Hemophilus influenzae*, in a nonencapsulated, untypable form, can cause chronic lung disease and acute otitis media. Encapsulated strains are typed a through f, with type b being responsible for almost all of the serious infections—including meningitis, pneumonia, bacteremia, and epiglottitis—caused by this organism. The incidence of these infections increases at about the age of six months, when levels of passively transferred maternal antibody and opsonins decline, and decreases at about five years of age, presumably following repeated infections with this organism.

351. The answer is E. *(Vaughan, ed 11. p 777.)* Salmonellal gastroenteritis is usually a self-limited disease with a course rarely altered by treatment with antibiotics. Rather than eliminating the pathogen, such treatment tends to prolong the carrier state. Recommended treatment includes the administration of a diet low in roughage and fats and sufficient oral fluids to maintain blood volume and replace fecal fluid losses. Intravenous fluid hydration and maintenance, coupled with temporary discontinuation of oral intake, may be necessary in severe cases. The value of oral kaolin or pectin remains unproven.

352. The answer is E. *(Meissner, Pediatrics 64:348-356, 1979.)* The maximum daily dose of chloramphenicol for premature infants and for all infants during the first week of life is only 25 mg/kg. However, even this low dose can produce blood levels that exceed the therapeutic range (10 to 20 μg/ml) and suppress protein synthesis, leading to progressive lethargy, loss of sucking, a gray skin color, hypothermia, bradycardia, hypotension, and death ("gray syndrome"). Blood levels of chloramphenicol in newborn infants must be measured, regardless of the dosage, if symptoms of the gray syndrome appear.

353. The answer is A. *(Feder, Clin Pediatr 19:457-462, 1980. Vaughan, ed 11. pp 737, 746-752.)* In an infant who appears otherwise normal, the sudden onset of high fever together with a marked elevation and shift to the left of the white blood cell count suggests pneumococcal bacteremia. Viral infections such as roseola seldom cause such profound shifts in the blood leukocyte count. Streptococcosis refers to prolonged, low-grade, insidious nasopharyngitis that sometimes occurs in infants infected with group A β-hemolytic streptococci. Neither typhoid fever nor diphtheria produces markedly high white blood cell counts; both are characterized by headache, malaise, and other systemic signs.

354. The answer is D. *(Vaughan, ed 11. p 739.)* Scarlet fever results when group A β-hemolytic streptococci infecting the throat or other sites produce an erythrogenic toxin that acutely inflames the skin, kidneys, joints, or heart. The disease is easily identified by the following features: a primary site of bacterial infection, usually in the throat; a generalized, fine, papular rash that has a "sandpaper" texture, is worse in the skin creases, and often involves the tongue, on which red papillae project above a thick white coat (strawberry tongue); and, following the rash, desquamation of branlike scales especially from the fingers and the tongue, causing the latter to appear red and denuded (raspberry tongue). The streptococcal infection of scarlet fever can vary in severity from very mild to fatal.

355. The answer is C. *(Klein, Pediatr Clin North Am 21:450, 1974. Vaughan, ed 11. pp 777-781, 794, 796.)* The symptom complex of progressive elevation of temperature, mental obtundation, abdominal distension and tenderness, splenomegaly, pneumonia, and a faint, pink maculopapular rash on the trunk is highly characteristic of typhoid fever. Constipation or diarrhea also may occur. Brucellosis, although also characterized by splenomegaly and fever (not usually undulant in children), is associated with prominent cervical and axillary lymphadenopathy; a rash, changes in mentation, and acute abdominal findings are not ordinarily part of the syndrome. The generalized rash of Rocky Mountain spotted fever, which is caused by *Rickettsia rickettsii*, is usually purpuric or petechial and can involve the palms and soles. Chloramphenicol is the antibiotic of choice in the treatment of individuals who have typhoid fever. Ampicillin, although also effective, is characterized by more treatment failures and a slower response than chloramphenicol; its only advantage, other than avoiding bone marrow suppression associated with chloramphenicol therapy, is a lower rate of both relapse and development of a chronic carrier state. For strains of *Salmonella typhi* that are resistant to both chloramphenicol and ampicillin, administration of trimethoprim together with sulfamethoxazole may be effective.

356. The answer is B. *(Vaughan, ed 11. p 779.)* During the first few days of typhoid fever, invasion of the bloodstream by *Salmonella typhi* occurs through infection sites in the proximal small intestine. Following the clearance of bacteria by the reticuloendothelial system, secondary local infections develop in the spleen, liver, and lymph nodes; septicemia then recurs, causing bacterial seeding of many organs. As a result, *S. typhi* appears in stool and urine later than in the bloodstream. Serum agglutinins do not rise significantly until the second week of infection.

357. The answer is C. *(Vaughan, ed 11. pp 678-679.)* The combination of erythema multiforme and vesicular, ulcerated lesions of the mucous membranes of the eyes, mouth, anus, and urethra defines the Stevens-Johnson syndrome (erythema multiforme exudativum). Fever is common and pulmonary involvement occasionally is noted; the mortality rate can approach 10 percent. Common complications include corneal ulceration, dehydration due to severe stomatitis and subsequently poor fluid intake, and urinary retention caused by dysuria. Among the known causes of the Stevens-Johnson syndrome are allergy to various drugs (including barbiturates, sulfonamides, and penicillin) and infection with *Mycoplasma pneumoniae*. Some authorities believe that herpesvirus hominis, type 1, also can cause Stevens-Johnson syndrome.

358. The answer is E. *(Meissner, Pediatrics 64:348-356, 1979.)* Aplastic anemia induced by chloramphenicol is relatively uncommon (1 case in every 60,000 to 100,000 individuals receiving the drug). Not usually dose-related, it is an idiosyncratic reaction that can occur either during therapy or up to many months after; it usually has a fatal outcome. In contrast, chloramphenicol-induced bone marrow suppression is extremely common, is dose-related, occurs during therapy, and responds satisfactorily to a reduction in dose or cessation of treatment.

359. The answer is C. *(Gangarosa, N Engl J Med 296:1210-1213, 1977. Ulshen, N Engl J Med 302:99-101, 1980. Vaughan, ed 11. pp 769-773.)* Enteropathogenic *Escherichia coli* includes a large number of arbitrarily selected serotypes, including some which either, (1) are invasive; (2) produce a heat-labile or heat-stable enterotoxin; (3) disrupt the small bowel microvilli by direct adhesion; or (4) are nonpathogenic. Pathogenicity can be determined with certainty only by laboratory demonstration of invasiveness or of toxicity for epithelial tissue. An important cause of diarrhea in children under 18 months of age, especially in diarrhea epidemics, enteropathogenic *E. coli* infections usually are treated effectively with oral neomycin. In older children who have diarrhea, the presence of another pathogen should be suspected when enteropathogenic *E. coli* is reported, particularly if the diarrhea is mild. In such cases, the diarrhea can be expected to subside without antibiotic treatment.

360. The answer is B. *(Dillon, Am J Dis Child 115:530-541, 1968. Vaughan, ed 11. pp 739-740, 867-871, 875-876.)* Streptococcal impetigo is a superficial pyoderma in which thin-walled vesicles rupture very rapidly, creating oozing or crusted honey-colored sores; these sores may be the first lesions noted by an affected individual. The vesicles of staphylococcal impetigo are more durable and may not rupture as the lesions spread. Impetigo is usually painless; painful, crusted, spreading lesions on the face are ordinarily caused by herpesvirus hominis, type 1, which also can cause a distinctive painful, red swelling of a fingertip with clusters of thick-walled vesicles. Herpes zoster infection features painful vesicles in a linear arrangement along dermatomes.

361. The answer is B (1, 3). *(Lumicao, Pediatr Clin North Am 26:269-282, 1979. Tipple, Pediatrics 63:192-197, 1979.)* Chlamydial species include *Chlamydia psittaci* and *Chlamydia trachomatis*, both of which are pathogenic for man. *C. psittaci* causes ornithosis, an infection ordinarily contracted from birds, principally parrots, parakeets, turkeys, and ducks. Ornithosis is characterized by interstitial pneumonia, fever, headache, and myalgias. Much more prevalent are infections with various serotypes of *C. trachomatis*, which cause trachoma, chlamydial conjunctivitis of the newborn, chlamydial pneumonia of infancy, nongonococcal and postgonococcal urethritis, and lymphogranuloma venereum. Chlamydial conjunctivitis of the newborn (inclusion blenorrhea) can be differentiated from other causes of neonatal conjunctivitis by the time of onset and by culture and staining techniques. In contrast to the chemical conjunctivitis produced by silver nitrate eye drops, which occurs within the first two days of life, and to bacterial conjunctivitis, which often develops within the first week of life and which can be identified with routine bacteriologic cultures and Gram stain, inclusion blenorrhea typically appears at approximately 10 to 14 days of life. The characteristic inclusion bodies may be seen within the cytoplasm of epithelial cells obtained by conjunctival swabbing and Giemsa staining. Chlamydial pneumonia of infancy usually occurs between one and three months of age and develops gradually. Characterized clinically by a frequent and persistent cough, tachypnea, inspiratory rales, normal temperature, and a chest x-ray pattern of interstitial infiltrates and hyperinflation, the illness tends to continue for several weeks. Lymphogranuloma venereum (LGV) is a sexually transmitted disease caused by three relatively invasive serotypes of *C. trachomatis*. Following the production of a primary lesion on the genitals or urethra, a second stage occurs, with tender enlargement of the regional lymph nodes, often accompanied by fever. A third stage, with tissue destruction leading to rectal strictures, may occur.

362. The answer is C (2, 4). *(Hoekelman, pp 777-781. Seto, Pediatr Clin North Am 26:305-314, 1979.)* Hepatitis A (infectious hepatitis) is characterized by a relatively short incubation period (15 to 50 days) following transmission of the virus, primarily by the fecal-oral route. Its onset is abrupt, with sudden fever, nausea, vomiting, anorexia, and liver tenderness, soon followed by jaundice. Elevated serum levels of bilirubin and aspartate aminotransferase (glutamic-oxaloacetic transaminase, SGOT) are transient, usually not persisting more than three weeks. Viremia is brief and the period of maximum infectivity of stools usually occurs during the two-week period prior to the onset of jaundice. Hepatitis B (serum hepatitis), usually transmitted parenterally via blood or blood products, may also be transmitted nonparenterally via body fluids such as saliva or semen. Following a long incubation period (40 to 180 days), there is gradual onset of low fever, anorexia, and jaundice, often preceded or accompanied by extrahepatic manifestations such as macular rashes, arthralgias, or urticaria, which may mimic serum sickness. Serum levels of SGOT and bilirubin may be elevated for months, the latter sometimes rising to levels greater than 20 mg/100 ml when associated with the fulminant hepatitis more often seen with hepatitis B infection. Viremia usually persists throughout the clinical course of hepatitis B infections and may progress to a chronic carrier state in 10 percent of individuals, most of whom are asymptomatic. These may be identified by the persistence of the viral surface antigen HB_sAg in their blood. A large number of patients with viral hepatitis do not develop antibodies to either the hepatitis A or B virus, suggesting the existence of at least one additional type (non-A/non-B viral hepatitis).

363. The answer is A (1, 2, 3). *(Kohl, Pediatr Clin North Am 26:433-443, 1979. Prince, Pediatr Clin North Am 26:261-268, 1979. Steinhoff, J Pediatr 96: 611-622, 1980. Torphy, Pediatrics 64:898-903, 1979.)* Yersinia enterocolitica is a gram-negative, invasive member of the Enterobacteriaceae family. As the etiologic agent of one form of prolonged diarrhea, with vomiting, fever, and abdominal pain that may resemble acute appendicitis, it is rarely identified by routine bacteriologic cultures. Because it can be isolated easily with special bacteriologic techniques, some authorities predict that *Y. enterocolitica* will prove to be an important cause of common-source outbreaks of gastroenteritis. Human rotavirus infection is characterized by winter outbreaks of sudden vomiting, fever, and diarrhea, often accompanied by upper respiratory tract symptoms. It may affect both adults and children within families and appears to be the single most important etiologic agent in childhood gastroenteritis. *Campylobacter fetus* (formerly *Vibrio fetus*) is emerging as an important cause of both common-source and sporadic diarrhea. The enteritis commonly is associated with severe abdominal cramps and diarrheal stools, which may contain blood or mucus. In addition to enteritis, at least two other patterns of human disease occur with infection with this pathogen: bacteremia and focal infections in older, debilitated men, and perinatal infections of mothers or infants. Special bacteriologic techniques are required to isolate this organism. During either oral or parenteral therapy with antibiotics, particularly ampicillin, penicillin, and clindamycin, the normal bowel flora are markedly reduced in number, allowing proliferation of *Clostridium difficile*. This bacteria elaborates a toxin which then produces profuse watery diarrhea, fever, vomiting, and abdominal distension, with typical pseudomembranous plaques visible by proctoscopy. This syndrome, known as antibiotic-associated pseudomembranous colitis, usually remits when the antibiotic is stopped but may in some cases progress to toxic megacolon, peritonitis, and shock. In such cases, intravenous fluid replacement and eradication of the clostridia with vancomycin may be lifesaving.

364. The answer is B (1, 3). *(Krugman, ed 7. pp 4-8, 417-425.)* Microcephaly accompanied by intracranial calcification, particularly in the ventricular ependyma, is highly characteristic of congenital toxoplasmosis or infection with cytomegalovirus. Definitive diagnosis of either disease may be made by demonstration of a rising antibody titer to either pathogen; in addition, cytomegalovirus can be cultured from the urine of affected individuals. It is important to note that maternal immunoglobulin G antibodies may passively cross the placenta and initially produce positive serologic titers in the newborn for *Toxoplasma*, *Treponema*, cytomegalovirus, or rubella. Therefore, to document that an antibody is of fetal origin, a stable or rising antibody titer must be demonstrated or the nondiffusable immunoglobulin M antibody fraction must be tested.

365. The answer is E (all). *(Hopkins, JAMA 210:694-700, 1969. Krugman, ed 7. pp 556-559. Vaughan, ed 11. pp 769, 861, 882.)* Encephalitis is a rare but serious complication of immunization with smallpox, pertussis, and measles vaccines. It occurs most commonly following smallpox vaccination (1 case per

100,000 in the United States, up to 1 case per 4000 in Europe, with a mortality rate of 50 percent). The incidence of encephalitis following live measles vaccination may approach 3 cases for every 1 million children vaccinated. Pertussis antigen must not be given to a child who has a history of convulsions following previous exposure to pertussis vaccine. Simple febrile convulsions following administration of these three vaccines are not rare in susceptible children less than three years of age. Development of poliomyelitis following trivalent oral polio vaccination occurs less often than 1 child per 10 million apparently normal children. A greater risk, however, occurs for adults, both those in contact with vaccinated children and those being vaccinated themselves; it is advised, therefore, that adults should not be vaccinated routinely. Live-virus vaccines should not be used in immunosuppressed individuals.

366. The answer is C (2, 4). *(Krugman, ed 7. pp 13-16. Vaughan, ed 11. pp 739, 746-752.)* The erythrogenic toxin of scarlet fever, caused by group A β-hemolytic streptococci, can produce myocarditis. *Corynebacterium diphtheriae*, in association with a specific bacteriophage, also produces a potent toxin, which causes extensive destruction of tissue at the site of infection and, as a result, promotes local growth of the pathogen. This destruction stimulates formation of the characteristic adherent necrotic membrane in the pharynx or, rarely, on the nasal septum. Laryngeal stridor and respiratory obstruction commonly ensue as the infection spreads downward. The toxin can disseminate systemically, binding to cells of the heart, kidneys, liver, adrenal glands, and central or peripheral nervous system. The subsequent toxic complications may occur as late as two to seven weeks after the original infection and are a major cause of death from diphtheria.

367. The answer is E (all). *(Krugman, ed 7. pp 7-8, 322-326, 395-399, 421-423. Vaughan, ed 11. pp 482-485, 842-847, 1010.)* Sepsis of the newborn may first manifest as jaundice and thrombocytopenic purpura. Among the important causes of neonatal sepsis are prenatal infections, including congenital syphilis, toxoplasmosis, cytomegalic inclusion disease, and rubella. Useful diagnostic studies, in addition to cultures for bacteria, include specific serologic tests for pathogens, viral cultures for cytomegalovirus, lumbar puncture, x-rays of the chest and long bones, and measurement of the cord-blood immunoglobulin M level, which often is increased in prenatal infections. Longitudinal striations in the metaphyses are characteristic of congenital rubella, while osteochondritis or periostitis usually indicates congenital syphilis. Congenital syphilis, cytomegalovirus disease, and rubella may be highly contagious. Urine may contain rubella virus for more than six months and is therefore a special hazard to nonimmune pregnant women.

368. The answer is B (1, 3). *(Krugman, ed 7. pp 162-167, 462. Vaughan, ed 11. pp 727-728.)* The aseptic meningitis syndrome refers to a variety of disorders characterized by meningitis associated with a conspicuous number of lymphocytes but no organisms visible on Gram stain. Causes include infections with viruses, rickettsiae, spirochetes, fungi, protozoa, and mycobacteria. Among noninfectious causes are tumors, leukemia, poisons such as lead, and meningeal irritation from intrathecally injected material, contiguous lesions, or allergy. In contrast to the typically low cerebrospinal fluid (CSF) glucose levels (less than half the blood glucose level) in bacterial meningitis, the CSF glucose level in aseptic meningitis ordinarily is normal. Important exceptions include infections with *Mycobacterium tuberculosis* and fungi, which usually produce low CSF glucose levels; virus infections very rarely depress the CSF glucose level. Once suspected, tubercle bacilli can be visualized by an acid-fast stain, and the yeast *Cryptococcus neoformans* (torula) by an india-ink preparation. The presence of minute amounts of alcohol in the CSF results from the fermentation of glucose and indicates the presence of fungi.

369. The answer is B (1, 3). *(Vaughan, ed 11. pp 771-776, 779, 784.)* The stools of patients infected with invasive gastroenteric organisms, such as *Salmonella typhimurium* and *Shigella sonnei*, usually contain many polymorphonuclear leukocytes and red blood cells. In individuals who have typhoid fever, leukocytes also are abundant in the stool, but most of these cells are mononuclear. Infection with noninvasive enteropathogenic *Escherichia coli* causes green, foul-smelling stools with mucus but few, if any, red or white blood cells.

370. The answer is D (4). *(Vaughan, ed 11. p 888.)* The Paul-Bunnell-Davidsohn heterophil agglutinin test, in which sheep red blood cell agglutinins are titrated, is a nonspecific antigen-antibody reaction that is very useful in diagnosing infectious mononucleosis. Differential absorption of serum antibodies by beef red blood cells or guinea pig kidney cells can distinguish the agglutinins associated with infectious mononucleosis both from other naturally occurring sheep red blood cell agglutinins and from those associated with serum sickness. In infectious mononucleosis, the heterophil agglutinins can be absorbed only by beef red blood cells and not by guinea pig kidney cells. Naturally occurring sheep red blood cell agglutinins, on the other hand, can be absorbed by guinea pig but not beef cells; and in serum sickness, both beef and guinea pig cells can absorb the sheep red blood cell agglutinins. A rise in the titer of antibody to Epstein-Barr virus indicates a current infection; a stable but elevated titer, however, may indicate a past infection. Large, vacuolated, atypical lymphocytes are characteristic of infectious mononucleosis when they comprise more than 10 percent of peripheral leukocytes. A smaller percentage can be associated with certain nonbacterial infections.

371. The answer is B (1, 3). *(Peter, N Engl J Med 297:365-370, 1977. Vaughan, ed 11. p 690. Yow, ed 18. p 270.)* In order to eradicate group A β-hemolytic streptococci in individuals who have pharyngitis, ten days of antibiotic treatment must be given. Penicillins G and V are the oral drugs of choice, in a daily dose of at least 800,000 units or the equivalent administered in at least three divided doses. In patients allergic to penicillin, erythromycin may be used; this drug, however, is associated with a higher relapse rate. Sulfonamides, although satisfactory in the prophylaxis of streptococcal pharyngitis, are not effective therapy for patients who have acute streptococcal infections.

372. The answer is C (2, 4). *(Vaughan, ed 11. pp 468-473.)* The prodromal features of bacterial meningitis during the first six months of life may be very subtle; symptoms may include lethargy and anorexia. High fever may not occur, but when present during this period, it is an extremely important sign of sepsis; urine and blood cultures and a lumbar puncture should be performed. The classic indications of meningitis—fever, stiff neck, bulging fontanelle, high-pitched cry, vomiting, and convulsions—may be absent in small infants who have the disease. In the differential diagnosis of fever in children less than six months of age, streptococcal pharyngitis and roseola infantum are extremely unusual; urinary tract infections, however, must be considered carefully and are often associated with congenital anomalies involving the urinary tract.

373. The answer is E (all). *(Vaughan, ed 11. pp 857-862.)* Measles is a generalized viral infection that can affect many organ systems. The disease characteristically is heralded by a severe respiratory infection that produces a harsh cough, profuse clear nasal discharge, red conjunctivae, photophobia, and high fever. A widespread, blotchy, red rash appears on the fourth or fifth day, and the symptoms worsen as the rash spreads. The rash and other symptoms abate in approximately five days. Koplik's spots on the buccal mucosa are pathognomonic. Complications of measles that are often encountered include encephalitis, primary viral or secondary bacterial pneumonia, viral myocarditis, group A β-hemolytic streptococcal pharyngitis or otitis media, and thrombocytopenic purpura with hemorrhages into the skin ("black measles").

374. The answer is B (1, 3). *(Vaughan, ed 11. pp 967-970.)* The symptoms and manifestations of histoplasmosis, which can range from subclinical to severe, resemble those of tuberculosis. The primary infection usually produces single or multiple miliary calcifications that arise in the lungs and mediastinum. Complications developing after the primary infection may be intrathoracic or extrathoracic and include pneumonia, cavitation, mediastinal lymphadenopathy, and localized lesions in any body tissue, including skin, lymph node, meninges, heart, adrenal gland, and bone. *Histoplasma capsulatum* can be identified by culture or stained smears of blood or biopsy tissue. A positive skin test also is extremely useful, because it indicates sensitization; it does not, however, necessarily imply active infection. Sulfonamides and amphotericin B are effective therapeutic agents.

375. The answer is E (all). *(Vaughan, ed 11. pp 823-824, 835. Yow, ed 18. pp 285-299.)* Allergic response to tubercle bacilli is the basis for the intracutaneous Mantoux test for tuberculosis; the test becomes positive within two to ten weeks after infection. Cross-reactions to atypical mycobacteria sometimes occur and can be differentiated from positive reactions for tuberculosis by the relatively larger intradermal reaction to the specific atypical antigen. The Mantoux test may become negative either during advanced stages of tuberculosis or briefly after immunization with live-virus vaccines (such as measles, rubella, and smallpox), administration of corticosteroids or immunosuppressive drugs, or development of a febrile illness or dehydration. Except in regions where atypical mycobacterial disease is endemic, a positive skin test in a child warrants antimicrobial therapy for at least one year.

376. The answer is A (1, 2, 3). *(Hoekelman, pp 1012, 1014.)* In a black child with the typical features of acute osteomyelitis depicted in the x-ray that accompanies the question (periosteal new bone formation and cortical destruction involving the fourth metatarsal bone), underlying sickle cell disease should be strongly suspected. Because of the strikingly high frequency of osteomyelitis due to *Salmonella* in patients with sickle cell disease, initial therapy should include an antibiotic with known effectiveness against that organism. Many patients with sickle cell disease eventually develop functional hyposplenism and thus have a high incidence of pneumococcal bacteremia. Accordingly, prophylactic administration of polyvalent pneumococcal vaccine is recommended.

377. The answer is E (all). *(Vaughan, ed 11. pp 724, 758-761.)* Meningococcemia may be complicated by a variety of septic disorders, including meningitis, purulent pericarditis, endocarditis, pneumonia, otitis media, and arthritis. (Arthritis associated with meningococcemia may occasionally be toxic rather than purulent.) The potent endotoxin of the causative organism, *Neisseria meningitidis*, can induce shock, disseminated intravascular coagulation with associated hemorrhaging, and acute adrenal failure caused by localized intra-adrenal bleeding; these reactions can be collectively referred to as the Waterhouse-Friderichsen syndrome. Vaccines against *N. meningitidis* group A and C are now available, but they fail to protect young infants, who comprise a majority of the civilian population at risk. Prophylaxis with rifampin or minocycline for persons in close contact with affected individuals is recommended by many authorities.

378. The answer is A (1, 2, 3). *(Vaughan, ed 11. pp 972-980.)* *Ascaris lumbricoides* larvae travel through the intestinal wall and end up, by way of the liver, in the lungs, where they commonly produce pneumonia and peripheral eosinophilia (Löffler's syndrome); worms mature in the small intestine, where they sometimes cause obstruction. The larvae of *Toxocara canis* migrate from the intestine to all parts of the body, where granulomatous reactions may occur (visceral larva migrans). Hookworms (*Necator americanus*) can cause intestinal blood loss from mucosal laceration; cutaneous larva migrans occurs when hookworm larvae fail to enter cutaneous blood vessels after penetrating the skin. Pinworms (*Enterobius vermicularis*) develop only in the colon, producing no internal disease other than a rare case of appendicitis. However, gravid worms crawl out of the anus at night, disturbing sleep and causing severe pruritus. Vaginitis and salpingitis may occur if the worms then enter the vagina.

379. The answer is B (1, 3). *(Vaughan, ed 11. pp 1193-1197.)* Croup, an infection of early childhood, involves the larynx and trachea; it usually is caused by parainfluenza or respiratory syncytial viruses. Symptoms include a low-grade fever, barking cough, and hoarse inspiratory stridor without wheezing. The pharynx may be normal or slightly red, and the lungs usually are clear. In children in severe respiratory distress, prolonged dyspnea can progress to physical exhaustion and fatal respiratory failure. Because agitation may be a sign of hypoxia, sedation should not be ordered.

380. The answer is A (1, 2, 3). *(Vaughan, ed 11. pp 977, 1010-1017.)* Persistent, nonsuppurative diarrhea can be caused by amebas, whipworms (trichuriasis), or *Giardia lamblia*. Amebas produce an ulcerating colitis that may be very mild or extremely destructive. Amebic liver abscess should be suspected when fever, chills, leukocytosis, and right upper quadrant pain or tenderness follow diarrhea. Whipworm infection can lead to chronic irritation of the bowel wall and thus to diarrhea and rectal prolapse. Diarrhea associated with giardiasis probably occurs because of malabsorption resulting from extensive coating of intestinal mucosa by the parasite. Infestation often results from contaminated municipal or well water and is accompanied by intermittent abdominal cramps and flatulence, as well as by prolonged diarrhea. Acquired *Toxoplasma gondii* can infest any body tissue, resulting in fever, myalgia, lymphadenopathy, maculopapular rash, hepatomegaly, pneumonia, encephalitis, chorioretinitis, and myocarditis. This intracellular parasite does not ordinarily cause diarrhea and is not found in stools. Congenital toxoplasmosis may occur if a mother first acquires the parasite during pregnancy. Her infected newborn infant may demonstrate jaundice, hepatosplenomegaly, hydrocephalus or microcephaly, intracranial calcification, or chorioretinitis.

Infectious Diseases and Immunology

381. The answer is E (all). *(Vaughan, ed 11. pp 924-931.)* Poliomyelitis infection, though familiarly paralytic, also can be asymptomatic, producing only a brief viremia after the virus has multiplied in the intestinal tract. In both the nonparalytic and paralytic varieties, fever, sore throat, muscle pains, and aseptic meningitis with nuchal rigidity are prominent features. Complications include gastric ulcers, hypertension, bladder paralysis, and respiratory paralysis. Polio will continue to occur sporadically as long as lax immunization practices persist.

382. The answer is A (1, 2, 3). *(Vaughan, ed 11. pp 719-726.)* In individuals who have meningitis, a glucose level in the cerebrospinal fluid that is less than 50 percent of the blood glucose level suggests a bacterial, fungal, or, occasionally, viral infection. Early in the course of bacterial meningitis, the white blood cell count in cerebrospinal fluid may be difficult to interpret; within hours, however, the characteristically high percentage (90%) of polymorphonuclear leukocytes appears. In mild, equivocal cases (leukocyte count less than 1000/mm^3), antibiotic treatment might well be delayed pending a second lumbar puncture four to six hours after the initial tap. Nonbacterial meningitis that has developed in association with an illness causing submandibular or cervical swelling suggests mumps or infectious mononucleosis; abnormal serum amylase concentration or heterophil agglutination test results, respectively, are diagnostic.

383. The answer is A (1, 2, 3). *(Patterson, Bacteriol Rev 40:774-792, 1976. Philip, Pediatrics 65:1036-1041, 1980. Wilson, Pediatr Clin North Am 21:571-581, 1974.)* The sudden onset in a newborn infant of lethargy, poor feeding, or other symptoms indicating a rapid, nonspecific change in behavior should suggest sepsis with possible meningitis, especially if leukopenia also is present. At present, the most common cause of bacterial meningitis in the neonate is group B β-streptococci; this disease is almost always contracted from the mother, who may be an asymptomatic carrier, or from the newborn nursery. Various gram-negative bacilli, such as *Pseudomonas* and *Proteus*, are also common pathogens in newborns. Following a lumbar puncture, which should be performed immediately in affected infants, cultures from other sources, including blood, urine, and stool, should be taken. Continuous close observation is essential.

384. The answer is E (all). *(Krugman, ed 7. pp 366-367, 370, 372-373. Vaughan, ed 11. p 481.)* Colonization of a newborn infant with *Staphylococcus aureus* commonly occurs either through the skin or by way of the umbilicus, the latter leading to a purulent drainage that progresses to local redness and swelling. Although the resulting dermatitis is usually pustular, it occasionally may appear as pemphigus neonatorum, which is characterized by bulla formation, or as the "scalded skin syndrome," which features generalized erythema, tenderness, and exfoliation, especially after stroking (Nikolsky's sign). Staphylococcal neonatal mastitis is associated with a progressive enlargement of one or both breasts beyond the normal hypertrophy often noted at birth. In a newborn infant, osteomyelitis, which usually is staphylococcal, causes pseudoparalysis or point tenderness over a long bone; staphylococcal pneumonia and meningitis also can develop. Fever and other clinical signs of systemic sepsis may not be present in infants who have staphylococcal infections.

385-388. The answers are: 385-B, 386-A, 387-E, 388-C. *(Hoekleman, pp 1065-1068. Vaughan, ed 11. pp 590-597, 609.)* Many primary immunologic deficiencies may be classified as defects of T-lymphocyte function (containment of fungi, protozoa, acid-fast bacteria, and certain viruses) and B-lymphocyte function (synthesis and secretion of immunoglobulins). Among the T-cell diseases is the **DiGeorge syndrome** in which defective embryologic development of the third and fourth pharyngeal pouches results in hypoplasia of both thymus and parathyroid glands. Primary B-cell diseases include panhypogammaglobulinemia **(Bruton disease)**, an X-linked deficiency of all three major classes of immunoglobulins, as well as other selective deficiencies of the immunoglobulins or their subgroups. Combined T- and B-cell diseases include the X-linked **Wiskott-Aldrich syndrome** of mild T-cell dysfunction, diminished serum IgM, marked elevation of IgA and IgE, eczema, recurrent middle ear infections, and thrombocytopenia. Patients with the catastrophic combined T- and B-cell disease known as combined immunodeficiency disease **(Swiss-type lymphopenic agammaglobulinemia)** lack functioning T and B cells. Consequently, there are both marked lymphopenia and agammaglobulinemia, as well as hypoplasia of the thymus. Chronic diarrhea, rashes, recurrent serious bacterial, fungal, or viral infections, wasting, and early death are characteristic. Other T- and B-cell deficiencies include ataxia-telangiectasia and chronic mucocutaneous candidiasis. **Job-Buckley syndrome** is a disorder of phagocyte cell chemotaxis associated with hypergammaglobulin E, eczema, and recurrent severe staphylococcal infections.

389-390. The answers are: 389-C, 390-B. *(Hoekleman, pp 1068-1069. Vaughan, ed 11. pp 606-610.)* Disorders of leukocytes include (1) defective locomotion out of the bone marrow, (2) depressed chemotaxis involving cellular defects, chemotactic inhibitors, or deficiencies of chemotactic factors, and (3) inability to ingest or kill microorganisms. Sometimes several disorders are present concurrently. **Defective locomotion** results in the neutropenia characteristic of the lazy leukocyte syndrome, in which abnormal chemotaxis, otitis media, and stomatitis are also part of the clinical picture. **Depressed cellular chemotaxis** is associated with the Job-Buckley syndrome (hyperimmunoglobulin E, eczema, and recurrent staphylococcal infections), Down's syndrome, and the Chediak-

Higashi syndrome (see below), among others. Inhibition of chemotaxis is seen in association with excesses of certain plasma proteins, including IgA. These excesses sometimes occur with rheumatoid arthritis, the Wiskott-Aldrich syndrome, and Hodgkin's disease. Deficiency of chemotactic factors, most of which are components of the complement system, may in association with deficient levels of complement produce recurrent, severe infections caused by encapsulated bacteria. Among the diseases associated with the **inability of leukocytes to kill** ingested microorganisms is chronic granulomatous disease, sex linked in 80 percent of cases. In individuals so affected, severe recurrent pneumonia and abscesses of lymph nodes and of the liver are caused by a variety of catalase-positive bacteria. These can survive ingestion by the defective leukocytes which lack normal oxidative metabolism and cannot produce microbicidal superoxide and hydrogen peroxide. These leukocytes can be identified in the laboratory by their failure to reduce nitroblue tetrazolium (**NBT** test). Chediak-Higashi syndrome, caused by another leukocyte defect, is characterized by abnormally large intracytoplasmic lysosomes, visible as giant granules (Dohl bodies), which degranulate in a delayed manner after phagocytosis of pathogens. Thus, oxidative metabolism and consequent microbial killing are delayed. Neutropenia, depressed chemotaxis, and recurrent pyogenic infections are accompanying abnormalities.

Hematologic and Neoplastic Diseases

Uma S. Rai

DIRECTIONS: Each question below contains five suggested answers. Choose the **one best** response to each question.

391. The spleen indisputably shortens red blood cell survival in which of the following conditions?

(A) Pyruvate kinase deficiency
(B) Hexokinase deficiency
(C) Glucose-6-phosphate dehydrogenase deficiency
(D) Hereditary spherocytosis
(E) Acquired idiopathic hemolytic anemia

392. In a group of children with symptomatic thrombocytopenia, the measurement of platelet-associated immunoglobulin G (PAIgG) will give a positive clue to the diagnosis of

(A) Wiscott-Aldrich syndrome
(B) disseminated intravascular coagulation
(C) idiopathic thrombocytopenic purpura
(D) hypoplastic anemia
(E) hypersplenism

393. Which of the following laboratory tests would be LEAST helpful in evaluating the role of hemolysis in neonatal hyperbilirubinemia?

(A) Serum haptoglobin concentration
(B) Serum bilirubin concentration
(C) Reticulocyte count
(D) Hemoglobin percentage
(E) Blood carbon monoxide concentration

394. At 12 hours of age, a polycythemic infant looks anxious, sweaty, and jittery. The most important part of the definitive treatment of this child's hematologic disorder should be

(A) phlebotomy
(B) phlebotomy followed by replacement with normal saline
(C) infusion of normal saline
(D) a partial plasma exchange transfusion
(E) institution of intravenous glucose therapy

395. A six-year-old black girl is hospitalized because of pallor and fatigue of a few weeks duration. When she was 18 months of age, she had iron-deficiency anemia that responded to oral iron and blood transfusion therapy; at that time a stool guaiac of 3+ was attributed to excessive milk intake. When she was four years of age, her anemia recurred; treatment with intramuscular iron was effective. Except for her pallor, physical examination is unremarkable. Laboratory results are hemoglobin, 5 g/100 ml; reticulocytes, 3%; and microcytic, hypochromic erythrocytes in the peripheral blood smear. Neither the child nor her parents has been aware of her having gastrointestinal symptoms or blood in the stools.

The cause of this child's anemia would best be established by

(A) screening for sickle cell hemoglobin
(B) testing for serum iron and total iron-binding capacity
(C) a hemolytic workup
(D) a barium study of the gastrointestinal tract
(E) a red blood cell survival test (^{51}chromium labeling)

396. In children who have sickle cell disease, which of the following conditions most frequently has its onset during the first and second years of life?

(A) Aplastic crisis
(B) Hemolytic crisis
(C) Intrasplenic sequestration crisis
(D) Septic complications
(E) Cerebrovascular accident

397. The most common cause of death in children who have homozygous β-thalassemia is

(A) hepatic insufficiency
(B) diabetes mellitus
(C) cardiac arrhythmias and congestive heart failure
(D) overwhelming bacterial sepsis
(E) hypoadrenalism

398. In the long-term treatment of iron overload in children with homozygous thalassemia, the most effective iron chelation is accomplished when deferoxamine (Desferol) is given by

(A) mouth
(B) intramuscular injection
(C) intravenous infusion
(D) subcutaneous infusion
(E) subcutaneous infusion with vitamin C supplementation

399. A 10-year-old boy who has moderately severe hemophilia A and is on a home treatment program has just suffered a mild spontaneous hemorrhage into his right knee joint. Knowing that infusion of 1 unit of factor VIII per kg body weight raises the plasma factor VIII level by 2 percent with a subsequent half-life of 12 hours, what level should be attained for adequate initial control?

(A) 5 to 10 percent of normal
(B) 10 to 20 percent of normal
(C) 20 to 30 percent of normal
(D) 30 to 40 percent of normal
(E) 40 to 50 percent of normal

400. Different varieties of hemoglobin (Hb) vary markedly in their capacities to interact and participate in sickling with sickle hemoglobin (Hb S). Which of the following heterozygous hemoglobinopathies is associated with the LEAST amount of sickling?

Hemoglobinopathy	Percent Hb S	Percent Non-Hb S
(A) Hb S and Hb A (sickle cell trait)	40	60 (Hb A)
(B) Hb S and Hb C	50	50 (Hb C)
(C) Hb S and Hb D	45	55 (Hb D)
(D) Hb S and hereditary persistence of Hb F	70	30 (Hb F)
(E) Hb S and β-thalassemia	60-90	10-40 (Hb A + Hb F)

401. A six-month-old infant presents with failure to thrive, psychomotor deterioration, and hepatosplenomegaly. Wright-Giemsa staining of a bone marrow aspirate shows large numbers of cells, as illustrated below. These findings are associated most closely with

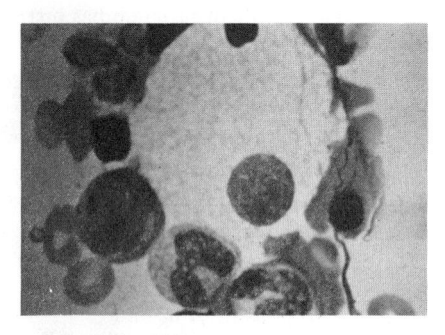

(A) histiocytosis X
(B) Gaucher's disease
(C) Niemann-Pick disease
(D) Hurler's syndrome
(E) myelogenous leukemia

402. Until the mid-1960s, the therapy of acute lymphoblastic leukemia (ALL) in childhood was comprised of induction remission with vincristine and prednisone and maintenance with methotrexate and 6-mercaptopurine. However, since then, a patient's chances for five to seven years of continuous and complete remission have improved from 20 to 50 percent. This progress is most likely associated with

(A) availability of platelets and granulocyte transfusion for supportive care
(B) addition of L-asparaginase or daunorubicin in induction remission treatment
(C) addition of cyclophosphamide and arabinosylcytosine in maintenance therapy
(D) central nervous system prophylaxis with cranial irradiation and intrathecal methotrexate
(E) more aggressive early chemotherapy for patients with poor prognostic indicators

403. The value of free erythrocyte porphyrin:hemoglobin ratio (FEP:Hg) is usually abnormal in all of the following conditions EXCEPT

(A) early, mild iron deficiency anemia
(B) severe iron deficiency anemia
(C) α- or β-thalassemia trait
(D) lead poisoning
(E) erythropoietic protoporphyria

404. Granulocyte transfusions are most likely to be effective in which of the following patients with acute leukemia?

(A) A neutropenic patient in remission with documented septicemia
(B) A neutropenic patient in remission with *Pneumocystis carinii* infection
(C) A neutropenic patient in relapse with undocumented infection
(D) A patient with refractory acute leukemia with infection and pancytopenia
(E) A patient in remission following bone marrow transplantation

405. Premature infants three to six months of age and older are more prone to develop significant anemia than are comparably aged full-term infants. This late anemia of prematurity is most likely to be the consequence of

(A) a lack of erythropoietin synthesis
(B) a decreased oxygen requirement and an increased oxygen unloading capacity
(C) decreased red blood cell survival
(D) rapid growth and diminished iron reserves
(E) poor utilization of available iron in food

406. During the last 30 years, the two-year disease-free survival rate of children who have Wilms' tumor has improved from 30 to 90 percent. Which of the following therapeutic factors have contributed most to this increased survival rate?

(A) Improved surgical techniques
(B) A megavoltage apparatus during radiation therapy
(C) Actinomycin D
(D) Vincristine
(E) Actinomycin D and vincristine in combination

407. Neuroblastoma can be associated with all of the following statements EXCEPT

(A) tumor-specific antigens are present on neuroblastoma cells
(B) two-thirds of patients, when first seen, have metastases
(C) three-fourths of all tumors secrete catecholamines
(D) prognosis strongly depends on disease stage and therapy
(E) there is a high rate of spontaneous regression

Questions 408-410

An eight-year-old boy is admitted to a hospital because of malaise, a mild cough, and a small mass in the left cervical area; symptoms first appeared two weeks ago. Examination of the boy, who looks well nourished, reveals two enlarged, rubbery, nontender, left posterior cervical lymph nodes; the rest of the examination is normal. Chest x-ray reveals enlarged left perihilar nodes associated with questionable infiltration in an area (1 to 2 cm) of the neighboring lung field. Biopsy of the cervical nodes confirms the diagnosis of Hodgkin's disease of the nodular sclerosing type. Staging laparotomy and splenectomy do not reveal the presence of disease in the abdomen.

408. This patient's disease falls into which of the following staging classifications?

(A) Stage I-B
(B) Stage II-B
(C) Stage II$_E$-A
(D) Stage III-A
(E) Stage III$_E$-A

409. Which of the following treatments would be recommended for the child described?

(A) Chemotherapy
(B) Chemotherapy followed by nodal irradiation
(C) Radiotherapy with mantle covering the involved area
(D) Radiotherapy followed by chemotherapy
(E) Extended-field radiotherapy

410. Early and long-term complications that could develop in the child described above after the completion of recommended therapy include all of the following EXCEPT

(A) overwhelming sepsis
(B) pneumonitis
(C) growth retardation
(D) occurrence of another malignancy
(E) portal hypertension

411. Which of the following regimens of combination chemotherapy is associated with the fewest side effects in maintaining long-lasting remission in children who have acute lymphoblastic leukemia?

(A) 6-Mercaptopurine, methotrexate, and cyclophosphamide
(B) 6-Mercaptopurine, methotrexate, cyclophosphamide, and cytosine arabinoside
(C) A half-dosage combination of 6-mercaptopurine and methotrexate
(D) A full-dosage combination of 6-mercaptopurine and methotrexate
(E) A two-week course of oral prednisone and intravenous vincristine once every ten weeks

412. The polymorphonuclear neutrophil shown in the illustration below is most likely to be associated with

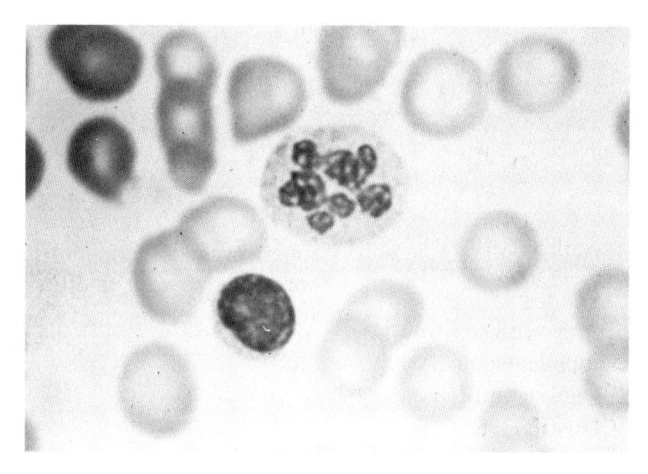

(A) malignancy
(B) iron deficiency
(C) folic acid deficiency
(D) Döhle's inclusion bodies
(E) the Pelger-Hüet nuclear anomaly

413. All of the following therapies would constitute a suitable treatment of choice for at least one of the following anemias — **acquired aplastic anemia, Fanconi's anemia, congenital hypoplastic anemia,** or **transient erythroblastopenia of childhood** — EXCEPT

(A) doing nothing
(B) performing bone marrow transplantation from HLA-matched donor
(C) administering prednisone
(D) administering androgens (oxymetholone)
(E) administering glutathione

DIRECTIONS: Each question below contains four suggested answers of which **one** or **more** is correct. Choose the answer:

A	if	1, 2, and 3	are correct
B	if	1 and 3	are correct
C	if	2 and 4	are correct
D	if	4	is correct
E	if	1, 2, 3, and 4	are correct

414. Von Willebrand's disease can be associated with which of the following pathologic states?

(1) Concordant decrease in the levels of antihemophilic factor (factor VIII AHF) and factor VIII antigen (factor VIII AGN)
(2) Abnormal platelet aggregation by collagen, adenosine diphosphate, and epinephrine in most patients
(3) Abnormal ristocetin-induced platelet aggregation in most patients
(4) Frequency of hemarthrosis equal to that in classical hemophilia A

415. Incidental factors affecting hemoglobin concentration and hematocrit values in a normal newborn infant include

(1) the site of blood sampling
(2) previous fetomaternal blood exchange
(3) the length of time between birth and blood sampling
(4) the manner in which the umbilical cord is clamped at the time of delivery

416. Assay of serum ferritin is a new tool in evaluating iron nutrition. Its advantages over the traditional measurements of hemoglobin, hematocrit, and serum transferrin saturation include which of the following?

(1) It allows evaluation of iron status within the normal range as well as in deficiency and excess
(2) Return of serum ferritin to normal levels reflects the effect of iron supplementation more reliably than do such returns of hematocrit and transferrin saturation
(3) In anemia caused by infection or chronic disease, consistently elevated values of serum ferritin are a more reliable indicator of iron status than are values of transferrin saturation
(4) Serum ferritin is a better estimate of a mobile pool of iron than transferrin saturation

417. Correct statements about osteosarcoma include which of the following?

(1) Epiphyses of the long bones are the common primary sites
(2) Lungs are the most common site of metastasis
(3) Amputation with no subsequent chemotherapy is the treatment of choice
(4) Preoperative chemotherapy has significantly prolonged the disease-free survival period

418. The overall prevalence of iron-deficiency anemia in American children between the ages of six months and two years has remained stable during the last three decades despite the increasing availability of iron-fortified foods. True statements regarding preventive measures against iron-deficiency anemia include which of the following?

(1) Breast milk is a better source of iron than cow's milk
(2) Cow's milk is a better source of iron than commercial formulas
(3) Iron supplementation for premature infants should begin at two months of age
(4) The best commercial cereals are those containing sodium iron pyrophosphate

419. A 22-year-old Rh-negative primigravid woman (at 12 weeks gestation) went to a prenatal clinic after a two-day episode of spotting of blood. Indirect antiglobulin screening, which was negative at four weeks gestation, again was negative, and the woman returned home. The rest of the pregnancy was uneventful (indirect antiglobulin screening at 28 weeks was negative). Delivery was spontaneous with slight antepartum hemorrhage, and she gave birth to a healthy Rh-positive ABO-compatible infant who had no evidence of hemolytic disease. The woman received a single 300 μg prophylactic dose of Rh-immune globulin within 72 hours of delivery. Six months postpartum, however, she showed evidence of Rh sensitization, and her next pregnancy ended in the delivery of an infant who had moderately severe erythroblastosis fetalis.

Which of the following factors could have contributed to the apparent failure of Rh-immune globulin protection in this case?

(1) The woman was not monitored adequately during pregnancy
(2) The woman suffered a threatened abortion at 12 weeks and should have received a dose of Rh-immune globulin then
(3) Rh isoimmunization could have occurred between the 28th gestational week and the time of delivery
(4) Massive transplacental fetomaternal hemorrhage warranting more than a single prophylactic dose of Rh-immune globulin could have occurred

SUMMARY OF DIRECTIONS

A	B	C	D	E
1, 2, 3 only	1, 3 only	2, 4 only	4 only	All are correct

420. Because of fetal distress, labor is induced at 41 weeks gestation in a 40-year-old diabetic mother who has had moderate toxemia of pregnancy. Induction of labor leads to the spontaneous delivery of an infant who on examination is small for gestational age, looks plethoric, and is in mild respiratory distress. Signs of Down's syndrome also are present. Laboratory data include a venous hemoglobin concentration of 26 g/100 ml and a venous hematocrit of 75%.

The polycythemia in this newborn may be attributable to

(1) maternal diabetes
(2) placental insufficiency
(3) maternal-fetal transfusion
(4) Down's syndrome

421. Poor prognostic signs in children who have acute lymphocytic leukemia include which of the following?

(1) Age below two years or above ten years
(2) Median white blood cell count at diagnosis of 50,000/mm³ or more
(3) Presence of a mediastinal mass
(4) Early central nervous system leukemia

422. The splenectomy of a two-year-old child has been recommended. In regard to the child's chances of developing an overwhelming infection after surgery it is true that

(1) institution of high-dose penicillin therapy for febrile illnesses can reduce the chances
(2) the salvaging of at least part of the spleen, if possible, can reduce the chances
(3) immunization with pneumococcal polysaccharide (PPS) vaccine can reduce the chances
(4) the chances are higher in this child than in a splenectomized four-year-old child

423. A young primigravid woman gives birth to a male infant after an uneventful full-term pregnancy and a prolonged vertex delivery. Except for ecchymoses of the occipital area and a few purpuric spots over the shoulder and chest, the infant appears to be well. His platelet count is 30,000/mm³; all other tests are normal. The mother's platelet count is normal and serologic examination is negative for antiplatelet antibodies. On the third day after birth, the child appears mildly jaundiced, lethargic, and jittery, and he refuses his feedings.

At this point, ideal management of the child's thrombocytopenia would include

(1) partial excision of the spleen
(2) exchange transfusion using fresh whole blood
(3) administration of corticosteroids
(4) transfusion of washed maternal platelets

424. A two-year-old child in shock has fulminant meningococcemia; petechiae are noted and oozing from puncture sites has been observed. The child's peripheral blood smear, presented below, shows fragmented red blood cells and few platelets. Clotting studies are likely to show

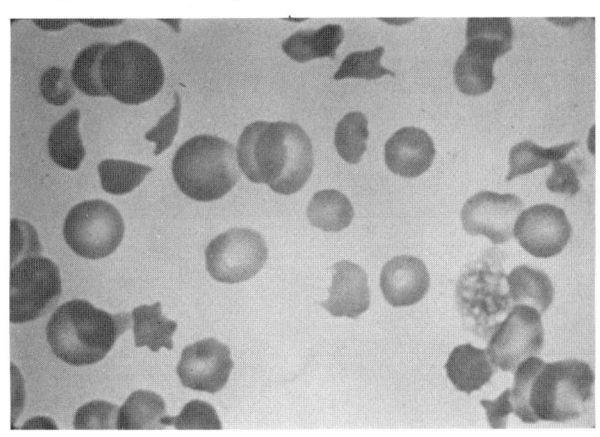

(1) decreased levels of factors V and VIII
(2) a decreased prothrombin level
(3) a decreased fibrinogen level
(4) the presence of fibrin split products

425. Factors within the spleen that may adversely affect red blood cell metabolism include

(1) glucose deprivation
(2) acidic pH
(3) hypoxia
(4) high microsomal heme oxygenase activity

426. Hypochromic anemia is likely to be associated with which of the following disorders?

(1) Iron deficiency
(2) Anemia due to lead intoxication
(3) Thalassemia
(4) Pyridoxine-responsive anemia

427. Intramuscular iron preparations as a treatment for children who have iron-deficiency anemia can be associated with which of the following statements?

(1) Their therapeutic response is significantly more rapid than oral iron preparations
(2) They are useful in children who also have a malabsorption syndrome
(3) They are chemically less complex than oral iron preparations
(4) They have significant side effects

DIRECTIONS: The groups of questions below consist of lettered choices followed by several numbered items. For each numbered item select the **one** lettered choice with which it is most closely associated. Each lettered choice may be used once, more than once, or not at all.

Questions 428-432

For each description or disorder listed, select the peripheral blood smear below with which it is most likely to be associated.

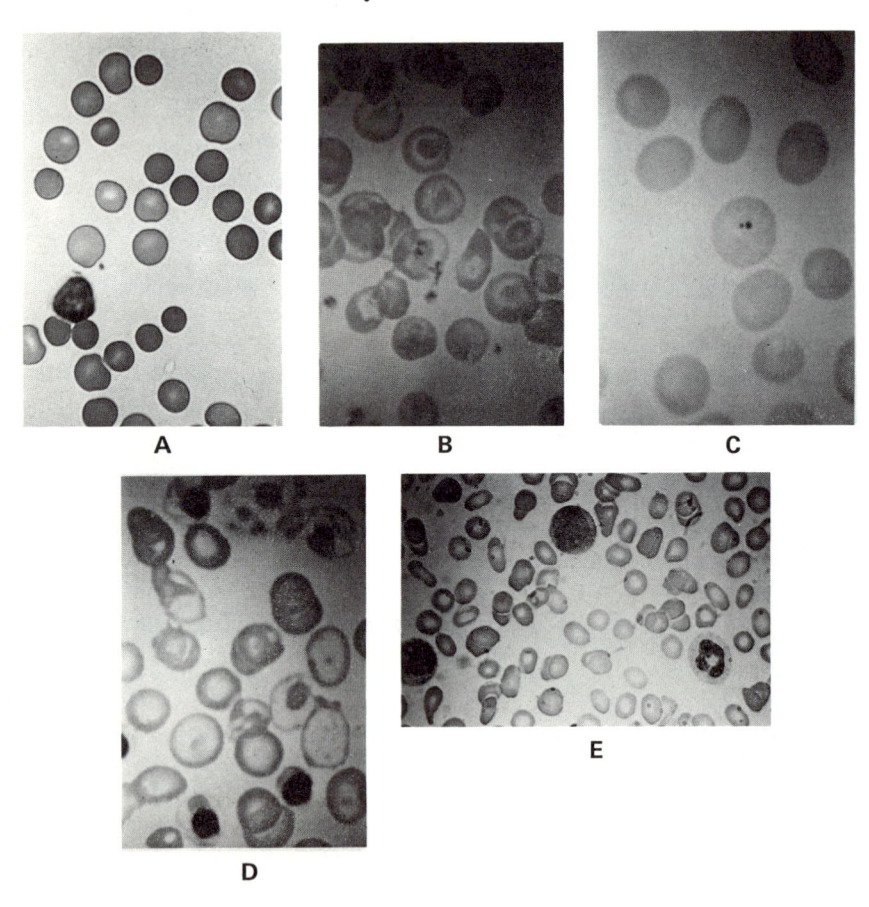

A

B

C

D

E

428. Howell-Jolly bodies in a splenectomized child
429. Basophilic stippling in a child who has lead intoxication
430. Thalassemia major
431. Hereditary spherocytosis
432. Hemoglobin C disease

Hematologic and Neoplastic Diseases 199

Questions 433-435

For each type of childhood leukemia listed, choose the bone marrow photomicrograph below with which it is most likely to be associated.

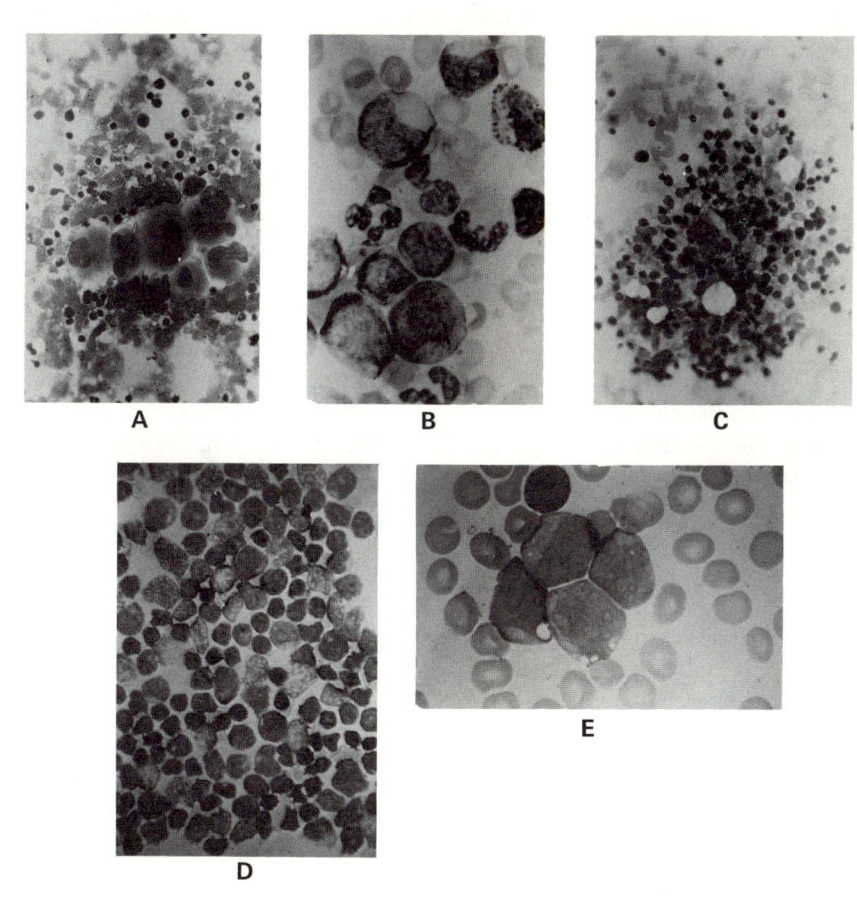

A

B

C

D

E

433. Acute lymphoblastic leukemia (ALL)
434. Acute myeloblastic leukemia (AML)
435. Chronic granulocytic leukemia (CGL)

Questions 436-440

Circulating hemoglobin mass reflects the balance between red blood cell production and destruction. For each of the following types of nutritional anemia, select the hematologic disorder with which it is most likely to be associated.

(A) Primarily a failure of red blood cell production often associated with increased plasma volume
(B) Primarily a failure of red blood cell production often complicated by mild to moderate red blood cell destruction
(C) Primarily red blood cell destruction that is incompletely compensated by red blood cell production
(D) Primarily red blood cell destruction accompanied by complete failure of red blood cell production (erythroid aplasia)
(E) None of the above

436. Iron-deficiency anemia

437. Folate-deficiency anemia

438. Vitamin B_{12}-deficiency anemia

439. Vitamin E-deficiency anemia

440. Anemia of uncomplicated protein-calorie malnutrition

Questions 441-445

Match the following chemotherapeutic agents with their corresponding mechanisms of action (as supported by cell kinetic studies).

(A) Impairs DNA synthesis by competitive inhibition of DNA polymerase
(B) Damages the microtubules in the mitotic spindle
(C) Alkylates purine bases in the DNA chain, leading to inhibition of DNA synthesis
(D) Binds to dehydrofolate reductase to prevent pyrimidine synthesis
(E) Blocks purine synthesis by inhibiting key enzymatic reactions

441. Cyclophosphamide

442. 6-Mercaptopurine

443. Methotrexate

444. Cytosine arabinoside

445. Vincristine

Hematologic and Neoplastic Diseases

Answers

391. The answer is D. *(Lux, Pediatr Clin North Am 27:463-486, 1980. Sullivan, Pediatr Ann 9:38-42, 1980.)* During its usual life span of 120 days, the red cell not only must maintain an adequate energy supply through utilization of glucose, but it also must keep a structural integrity and deformability to be able to negotiate its passage through small capillaries (2 to 3 μ) and the mechanically and metabolically stressful environment of the spleen. In the last few years, new data about red cell structural proteins and membrane skeleton (spectrin, actin, and ankyrin) suggest the existence of a qualitative defect that renders hereditary spherocytic red cells unstable and easily fragmented. The sequence of changes which ends with red cell death begins with loss of membrane fragments, which causes a decreased surface area/volume ratio (spherocytosis), with decreased cellular deformability. This leads to splenic entrapment and red cell death. The congested, acidic, hypoglycemic environment of the splenic cords accelerates spherocyte formation in hereditary spherocytosis (HS) more than in other conditions. Because it abolishes the hemolytic process, splenectomy is almost curative in HS. The red cells take on a more uniform morphology after splenectomy. Although splenectomy may be of marginal benefit in pyruvate kinase deficiency and hexokinase deficiency, it is of no benefit in glucose-6-phosphate dehydrogenase deficiency and acquired idiopathic hemolytic anemia.

392. The answer is C. *(Hymes, Blood 56:84-87, 1980. Lightsey, J Pediatr 94: 201-204, 1979.)* Idiopathic thrombocytopenic purpura (ITP) is a common disorder which accounts for the majority of cases of childhood thrombocytopenia. Almost 90 percent of affected children have spontaneous and permanent recovery within six months of onset. Because of the role of the humoral immune system in producing platelet antibodies in ITP, this disease has been categorized as an immune thrombocytopenia. A reliable in vitro test has been developed to assist in the diagnosis, follow-up, and differentiation of acute and chronic disease. It is based on a study of 20 children with ITP in whom the mean platelet-associated immunoglobulin G (PAIgG) levels were 1446, 12,552, and 3956 ng IgG/10^9 platelets in normal children and those with acute and chronic ITP, respectively. In age-matched children with thrombocytopenia due to other causes, values were in the normal range. The PAIgG has been further classified as the heavy chain subclass of antibodies bound to the platelets. In Wiscott-Aldrich syndrome, there are ultrastructural abnormalities in both megakaryocytes and platelets. The platelet abnormality in disseminated intravascular coagulation is one of excessive consumption. In hypersplenism of any cause, there is increased pooling of platelets in the enlarged spleen with a productive marrow.

393. The answer is A. *(Necheles, Acta Pediatr 65:361-367, 1976. Piomelli, vol 1. pp 151-192.)* Determining the concentration of serum haptoglobin, which binds free hemoglobin, is of little value in assessing hemolysis in newborn infants who have hyperbilirubinemia, because only 10 percent of neonates have detectable levels in the serum. The normal adult range (30 to 100 mg/100 ml) is not reached until the first month of life. Furthermore, in most neonates who have hemolytic disease, the spleen is the site of red blood cell destruction; thus, only in very severe intravascular hemolysis is free hemoglobin present in the plasma. In the digestion of heme by heme oxygenase, a splenic microsomal enzyme, carbon monoxide is released. In a recent study, levels of carbon monoxide consistently were increased in infants who had significant hyperbilirubinemia and reticulocytosis, which indicate hemolysis. The measurement of carbon monoxide in the whole blood by gas chromatography has become a common laboratory procedure. It is probably the most sensitive test to reflect increased red blood cell hemolysis, but its accuracy depends upon measurement of ambient air carbon monoxide.

394. The answer is D. *(Nathan, ed 2. pp 219-222.)* After reaching a critical point (venous hematocrit 60% to 65%), hyperviscosity increases exponentially, resulting in a decreased peripheral flow. The lungs, heart, and central nervous system are most affected; common symptoms and signs include respiratory distress, cyanosis, congestive heart failure, convulsions, and jaundice due to increased hemolysis. Although polycythemic patients should be monitored for evidence of hypoglycemia, hypocalcemia, and hyperbilirubinemia, in a symptomatic infant timely partial exchange transfusion using fresh frozen plasma to bring the postexchange hematocrit to 60% or below not only dramatically relieves most of the symptoms but also lessens the likelihood of future complications. The goal is to reduce the hematocrit (Hct) while maintaining the blood volume. The formula commonly employed to approximate the volume of exchange is:

$$\text{Volume of Exchange (ml)} = \frac{\text{Blood Volume} \times (\text{Observed Hct} - \text{Desired Hct})}{\text{Observed Hct}}$$

Usually one exchange transfusion is adequate to allay the effects of a hyperviscosity problem.

395. The answer is D. *(Shumway, Pediatr Clin North Am 19:855, 1972. Woodruff, Am J Dis Child 124:26, 1972.)* Intestinal blood loss is frequently a contributing factor in the pathogenesis of iron-deficiency anemia. This blood loss almost always ceases once iron replacement treatment is started and intake of cow's milk is reduced. Blood loss also can occur due to anatomic lesions, such as Meckel's diverticula, intestinal duplications, hemorrhagic telangiectasia, or bleeding ulcers; unfortunately, these are easily overlooked in a child because of their uncommon occurrence and paucity of symptoms. Blood loss caused by these lesions must be suspected in anemic children older than two years of age or whose intestinal blood loss or anemia persists or recurs after iron treatment.

Two errors were made in the management of the patient presented in the question. First, the presence of occult blood in the stool should have been tested after the initiation of iron treatment at 18 months of age. Second and more significant, when the child was four years of age and iron-deficiency anemia recurred, an immediate search for occult blood loss should have begun. A hemolytic anemia is not suggested by the data presented, and it certainly would not have responded to iron therapy.

396. The answer is D. *(Oski, 1975. pp 107-120. Schwartz, vol 3. pp 192-213.)* During the first or second years of life of children who have sickle cell disease, septic complications and vaso-occlusive phenomena constitute the gravest threat and cause the most serious symptoms. Autosplenectomy and poor tissue defense due to vaso-occlusion are two factors that increase susceptibility to infection; the most common pathogenic offender is *Streptococcus (Diplococcus) pneumoniae*. The most frequent complication of homozygous sickle cell anemia in all age groups is acute pulmonary involvement. In addition, bacterial meningitis may be 600 times more common in these patients than in normal children. In one study, bacterial septicemia and infection were the cause of death in 63 percent of sickle cell children during their first decade of life. The overall mortality in the first year of life is 16 percent. Parents should be alerted that fever and chills may reflect a serious infection (e.g., sepsis, pneumonia, meningitis, or osteomyelitis). Likewise, appropriate cultures should be done, and parenteral antibiotic coverage should be started, based on clinical grounds, while awaiting culture results. It is common practice now to give prophylactic pneumococcal vaccine at two years of age. Although intrasplenic sequestration crises can also occur early in life, they are not as common as septic complications. Aplastic crises due to temporary suppression of bone marrow activity by intercurrent infection may be followed by a recovery phase of marked reticulocytosis, which is sometimes referred to as a hemolytic crisis. These complications, in addition to acute vaso-occlusion in the brain, may occur at any age, but are less common then septic complications in the first two years of life.

397. The answer is C. *(Schwartz, vol 3. pp 317-334.)* Homozygous β-thalassemia, or Cooley's anemia, is a severe inherited anemia due to decreased synthesis of beta globin chains. Almost every patient requires frequent transfusion therapy. Each 250 ml unit of packed red blood cells contains approximately 250 mg of iron; the usual requirement of 2 units every three or four weeks will result in an excess accumulation of 50 g of iron in ten years. (The total body iron in a normal adult is 4 to 5 g.) These patients also have increased iron absorption due to excess erythropoiesis and some hypoxia due to anemia. This excess iron can damage liver, spleen, pancreas, and almost any other organ, but the worst effect is on the heart. Acute pericarditis (19 of 46 patients in one series) is a rather benign complication that has its onset at about 11 years of age. However, cardiac arrhythmias and congestive heart failure were the leading causes of death in this series (24 of 25 patients). The average age of onset was 16 years; 14 died within 3 months of onset of this complication, and only 7 lived more than 1 year after the onset of heart failure. Autopsy findings showed severe myocardial hemosiderosis. More effective chelation therapy may postpone this inevitable complication.

398. The answer is E. *(Schwartz, vol 3. pp 335-355.)* Deferoxamine (Desferol) is the only clinically useful iron-chelating drug in widespread usage. Theoretically, about 100 mg of deferoxamine can bind 9.35 mg of iron to the water-soluble complex in the urine. The major source of chelatable iron appears to be ferritin and hemosiderin in the storage pool of reticuloendothelial and parenchymal cells. The problem has been to accomplish effective chelation from these sites to achieve negative iron balance. Although the intramuscular route has been conventionally used for the last several years, poor solubility, painful injections, and rapid drug excretion (four to six hours) have been drawbacks. A 24-hour intravenous infusion of an equivalent dose can increase urinary iron excretion by 300 percent, but this requires hospitalization. A small lightweight infusion pump has been devised by which a 12-hour subcutaneous infusion of deferoxamine, 750 mg, can be given, increasing iron excretion by slightly over 100 percent in comparison with the same dose administered intramuscularly. This excretion is further increased by 20 to 250 percent when supplemental vitamin C is given orally to maintain a normal leukocyte vitamin C concentration. A dose of 200 mg daily is adequate. Other chelating agents still under investigation are rhodotorulic acid and 2,3-dihydrobenzoic acid.

399. The answer is A. *(Levine, N Engl J Med 291:1381-1384, 1974. Stirling, Lancet 1:813-814, 1979.)* In recent years, with the development of concentrated plasma fractions, the management of hemophilia has shifted dramatically from physician's office, emergency room, or inpatient setting to successful home treatment programs. Prompt therapy has reduced costs, decreased morbidity, slowed the progression of hemophilic arthropathy and considerably normalized the life-style of the patient as well as of the family. Several recent studies have shown that if treatment is given as soon as the symptoms of a limp, failure to move an extremity, or a peculiar sensation in a joint are recognized, plasma levels of 5 to 10 percent factor VIII are adequate to control the simple spontaneous joint hemorrhages in severe hemophiliacs. With a delay in diagnosis or treatment the physical signs of a full-blown hemarthrosis often develop, with an immobile, red, warm, swollen, and tender joint. In such cases, much higher doses of factor VIII are required.

400. The answer is D. *(Nathan, ed 2. pp 693-697. Schwartz, vol 3. pp 215-248.)* Whenever sickle cell disease is doubly heterozygous, the affected individuals have varying degrees of hemolytic anemia and clinical manifestations, ranging from no symptoms to a disease state indistinguishable from severe sickle cell disease (Hb SS). The mechanisms for the interaction and protection of the hemoglobin molecules in these heterozygous combinations and for the expression of sickle cell disease are not completely understood. In addition to the interaction of abnormal hemoglobins, the intracellular hemoglobin concentration and distribution of fetal hemoglobin in the red cell modify the sickling, the former directly and the latter inversely. Of all the hemoglobinopathies listed in the question, the disorder characterized by hemoglobin S (Hb S) and hereditary persistence of fetal hemoglobin (Hb F) is associated with the least sickling, even though the percent of Hb S is almost twice that of sickle cell trait (70 percent versus 40 percent). In this condition Hb F, which participates poorly (if at all) in sickling, is distributed uniformly in all cells. In sickle cell disease (Hb SS), on the other hand, it is distributed randomly and heterogeneously in red blood cells; this is why patients with sickle cell disease show no correlation between their clinical course and percentage of Hb F. The other sickle syndromes listed in the question produce less sickling than sickle cell disease.

401. The answer is C. *(Williams, ed 2. pp 1151-1152.)* The clinical history and the presence of foam cells in the bone marrow of the infant described in the question are typical of Niemann-Pick disease (sphingomyelin lipidosis). A deficiency of the lysosomal enzyme sphingomyelinase in several tissues causes the accumulation of sphingomyelin, which is ingested by reticuloendothelial cells. The resulting rounded or oval cells (foam cells) have an eccentric nucleus with prominent nucleoli; however, the distinguishing characteristic is the appearance of small, glittering droplets in the cytoplasm. These abnormal cells can be found in the bone marrow, liver, spleen, lymph nodes, thymus, brain, and many other organs. The foam cells of Gaucher's disease typically look different; the cytoplasm of these Gaucher cells appears to be stuffed with many long, wavy fibrils of variable length, giving the appearance of wrinkled tissue paper.

402. The answer is D. *(Mauer, Blood 56:1-10, 1980. Simone, Br J Haematol 45:1-4, 1980.)* The arachnoid meninges act as a sanctuary for proliferation of leukemic blast cells because of relatively poor diffusion of antileukemic drugs into the cerebrospinal fluid. More than 50 percent of patients experience their first relapse in that site before the advent of central nervous system (CNS) prophylaxis treatment. St. Jude's Children's Hospital (Memphis) has been instrumental in introducing, soon after induction remission, 2400 rads of cranial radiation and five doses of intrathecal methotrexate. It has been shown that only 15 percent of children not given CNS prophylaxis had complete remission for five years, whereas 47 percent of children who received the St. Jude treatment had continuous and complete remission for five to seven years. The availability of supportive measures and other chemotherapeutic agents has contributed to therapeutic refinement and some improvement. Lately, because of continuous long-term survival of several children with acute lymphoblastic leukemia, it has become apparent that CNS prophylaxis carries some risk of CNS damage (e.g., altered neuropsychological function, leukoencephalopathy, or mineralizing vasculopathy). Different regimens are still under trial to replace CNS radiation (e.g., combined intrathecal and intravenous use of methotrexate).

403. The answer is C. *(Oski, Pediatr Clin North Am 27:237-252, 1980. Piomelli, Pediatrics 57:136-141, 1976.)* The last step of heme synthesis is the incorporation of iron into the protoporphyrin ring catalyzed by the enzyme heme synthetase. In iron deficiency, due to paucity of available iron, and likewise in the presence of lead, which inhibits the action of the heme synthetase, there is accumulation of protoporphyrin within the erythrocytes. Recently, a rapid, simple, inexpensive micromethod for the measurement of the erythrocyte porphyrin: hemoglobin ratio (FEP:Hg) has become well established. By fingerprick, blood samples are spotted on a filter paper which can be left on the shelf for up to three months at room temperature. An inexpensive filter fluorometer is used for reading. The cost is a few cents per test, and one technician can run 200 tests each day, making the test applicable for field studies. Its major usefulness is in differentiating the three common causes of microcytic anemia: iron deficiency, β-thalassemia trait, and lead poisoning. The test results are normal in β-thalassemia trait because there is plenty of available iron and the defect is in decreased globin chain synthesis. Further, if a child with iron deficiency anemia has an intercurrent upper respiratory infection, or has already been started on iron therapy, the parameters of seum iron and transfusion saturation and ferritin may not reflect iron deficiency, whereas the FEP:Hg ratio remains high during iron therapy following the sequential senescence of microcytic red cells. The values return to normal in approximately 15 weeks. The values of FEP:Hg ratio are: less than 2.8 $\mu g/g$ = normal; 3.5 to 17.0 $\mu g/g$ = iron deficiency, lead poisoning, or both; and greater than 17.5 $\mu g/g$ = lead poisoning or erythropoietic protoporphyria.

404. The answer is A. *(Higby, Blood 55:2-8, 1980.)* In the selection of patients with acute leukemia for granulocyte transfusions, only with neutropenia patients (absolute neutrophil count of 500/mm^3 or less) and documented septicemia have granulocyte transfusions definitely improved the survival. With infections not accompanied by septicemia and infections caused by nonbacterial organisms (*Pneumocystis carinii* and fungi), the contribution of granulocyte transfusions to survival is not as well documented. In addition to the severity and the type of infection, the overall chances of recovery from neutropenia and of subsequent survival must also be taken into account in deciding whether to initiate granulocyte transfusion. About 3 to 5 percent of leukemic children are refractory to therapy, and they almost always die during induction therapy. The effective treatment involves administration of at least 10^{10} functional granulocytes per day (four transfusions per day) for seven days. In a post-transplant patient, the HLA match may be difficult due to the greater chances of immunologic reactions. Granulocyte transfusions are costly and not without the hazards of alloimmunization and the transmission of viruses.

405. The answer is D. *(Committee on Nutrition, Pediatrics 58:765, 1976. Oski, 1975. pp 3-8.)* It is generally accepted that late anemia of prematurity stems from nutritional deficiencies (largely iron deficiency) caused by rapid growth and early depletion of already poor reserves. Full-term and premature newborns begin life with standard iron reserves of approximately 70 mg/kg body weight. In contrast to full-term infants whose birth weights double by five months of age and triple by one year of age, premature infants may triple their birth weights by six months of age. Early physiologic anemia of newborn infants, which is most evident between six and twelve weeks after birth, results from decreased red blood cell survival, decreased oxygen requirements, increased oxygen unloading capacity, and an absence of erythropoietin synthesis. These factors are all common in newborns but are somewhat more pronounced in premature infants. This is why iron supplementation is recommended for premature infants at two months of age.

406. The answer is E. *(D'Angio, Cancer 45:1791-1798, 1980.)* The primary role of surgery (nephrectomy) is indisputable in the broad therapeutic approach to Wilms' tumor; it can confirm the diagnosis as well as contribute to clinicopathologic staging. The most significant major advance in the last decade in treating Wilms' tumor, however, has been the initiation of maintenance combination chemotherapy with actinomycin D and vincristine. The National Wilms' Tumor Study has shown that when actinomycin D or vincristine is used alone, the two-year disease-free rate is 55 percent; with combination therapy it rises to 90 percent. Similar results have been reported from Toronto and the Medical Research Council in the United Kingdom. This maintenance chemotherapy has eliminated the use of routine postoperative radiation therapy in group I disease where tumor is limited to the kidney and is completely excised. This minimizes the late consequences of radiation therapy. The results of trial of a third combination drug, adriamycin, are still inconclusive.

407. The answer is D. *(Evans, Cancer 45:833-839, 1980. Evans, Pediatr Clin North Am 23:161-170, 1076. Vaughan, ed 11. p 1445.)* The natural course of neuroblastoma remains an enigma. On the one hand, it has the highest rate of spontaneous regression of any human cancer; on the other, the two-year overall survival rate is the same today (32 percent) as it was before the advent of chemotherapy. Prognosis is influenced most strongly by age: the younger the child, the better the prognosis, regardless of the stage of the tumor or type of therapy. Chemotherapy with vincristine, cyclophosphamide, and adriamycin, either singly or in combination, has been reported to prolong the median survival time by a few months. A cell-mediated immune response may explain the spontaneous regression of neuroblastoma in situ. One study investigated 17 cases of stage IV-S disease (a category comprising very young children—most under six months—with small primary tumors but disseminated disease with distant foci in the liver, skin, or bone marrow) in a total series of 207 neuroblastoma patients. Six of eleven survivors had spontaneous regression of all or part of their disease. This high rate of regression suggests that the prognosis in neuroblastoma is not strongly dependent on the disease stage and therapy.

408. The answer is C. *(Kaplan, Cancer 45:2439-2474, 1980. Nathan, ed 2. pp 1030-1033.)* The stages (I through IV) of Hodgkin's disease define the location and dissemination of the disease process; each stage can be further classified as being associated with systemic symptoms ("B") or not ("A") or with extension to a contiguous extralymphatic site (subscript "E"). The boy described in the question has stage II_E disease: involvement of two or more lymph nodes on the same side of the diaphragm with spread to an extralymphatic site (in this case, a lung). Malaise, fatigue, and generalized weakness are deemed to be too nonspecific and difficult to document to be considered in staging. Presence of fever, night sweats, and unexplained loss of 10 percent or more of body weight in the six months preceding the time of diagnosis are indicative of systemic involvement; the presence of these signs is noted by the suffix "B." The absence of significant fever, night sweats, and weight loss further delineates the boy's Hodgkin's disease as stage II_E-A (the child's mild cough could be due to a local lung reaction). Clinical staging and histopathologic diagnosis are essential in planning therapy.

409. The answer is C. *(Kaplan, Cancer 45:2439-2474, 1980. Nathan, ed 2. pp 1033-1036.)* The development of megavoltage equipment has made radiotherapy an extremely effective treatment for Hodgkin's disease. It now is possible to give high-dose focused radiotherapy and spare the adjacent normal tissues. Recent trials using this treatment modality in children who have stage I or stage II disease have produced five-year survival rates in excess of 80 percent. Mantle covers the cervical and mediastinal nodes in addition to the involved lung field. Extended field radiotherapy has many more side effects than a mantle covering the involved area. Chemotherapy is primarily for stage III and IV disease with systemic involvement (B). However, in one clinical trial, stage I-A and II-A patients were randomized to receive high-dose involved-field radiotherapy plus six cycles of MOPP (nitrogen mustard, oncovin, prednisone, and procarbazine) as opposed to irradiation alone. The relapse-free four-year survival rate was 95.8 percent in the combined-therapy group as against 86.7 percent in the radiotherapy-alone group. More such trials in the pediatric age group are necessary. The late occurrence of a second malignancy is more common in patients initially treated with both radiation therapy and chemotherapy than with either alone.

410. The answer is E. *(Kaplan, Cancer 45:2439-2474, 1980. Nathan, ed 2. pp 1036-1037. Rutherford, Br J Haematol 44:347-358, 1980.)* Many individuals who have Hodgkin's disease have deficient cell-mediated immunity, which becomes aggravated by the early effects of therapy. Children in particular are prone to viral diseases such as herpes zoster, overwhelming pneumococcal sepsis, and a variety of infections after splenectomy, and in addition, radiation-induced pneumonitis could make them very prone to infection with opportunistic organisms *(Pneumocystis carinii)*. Later, the long-term sequelae of radiation and chemotherapy, such as pulmonary fibrosis, pericarditis, retardation of bone growth, thyroid dysfunction, and testicular or ovarian failure may become evident. Recently, the risks of staging laparotomy, such as sepsis or intestinal obstruction, (including splenectomy) in symptomatic Hodgkin's disease have been thought to outweigh the benefits conferred by accurate knowledge of stage. The rate of morbidity with laparotomy (from a data base of 900 cases) is 6.4 percent, with a mortality rate of 3 percent. The rate of late death from overwhelming infection is 2.52 percent. In any case, use of pneumococcal vaccine and prophylactic penicillin is recommended for splenectomized children. On long-term, 10-year follow-up of Hodgkin's disease patients who had combined modality treatment (radiation therapy and chemotherapy), the cumulative risk of developing acute leukemia is 5 percent and a second non-Hodgkin's lymphoma, 10 to 15 percent.

411. The answer is D. *(Pinkel, Pediatr Clin North Am 23:117-130, 1976. Simone, Br J Haematol 45:1-4, 1980.)* Studies by St. Jude's Children's Hospital (Memphis) on the effectiveness of different combination chemotherapeutic regimens for children who have acute lymphocytic leukemia have shown the following results:

Regimen	No. Children in Complete Remission for Five Years	No. Deaths
6-Mercaptopurine and methotrexate	54 of 64	0
6-Mercaptopurine, methotrexate, and cyclophosphamide	44 of 62	2
6-Mercaptopurine, methotrexate, cyclophosphamide, and cytosine arabinoside	50 of 62	4

The latter two regimens were associated with a marked increase of immunosuppression and thus an increased incidence of deaths due to *Pneumocystis carinii* pneumonia. Half-dose combination of 6-mercaptopurine and methotrexate reduced median remission time by about 50 percent compared to full-dose combination. The prednisone-vincristine regimen described in the question is not effective remission therapy unless administered with other drugs.

One of the most urgent needs of the 1980s is a method for detecting minimal residual disease in the bone marrow as well as elsewhere in the body. Is it possible to detect one leukemic cell in a million? What is the biologic basis of resistance? It is because of such uncertainties that, 30 years since its introduction, we are still seeking the optimal schedule and dosage for methotrexate.

412. The answer is C. *(Lindenbaum, Br J Haematol 44:511-513, 1980. Nathan, ed 2. pp 349-352.)* The finding of hypersegmented neutrophils (average count: > 3 lobes per cell) in the peripheral blood is one of the most useful laboratory aids in making an early diagnosis of folate deficiency. In adults put on a folate-deficient diet, serum folate levels become low in three weeks, and hypersegmented neutrophils appear in the bone marrow in five weeks and in the peripheral blood in seven weeks. It is only after 17 to 19 weeks that megaloblastic anemia develops. In a recent retrospective study of 357 patients with megaloblastic anemia, in 351 (98.3 percent) patients, the peripheral blood smear was found to have at least one hypersegmented neutrophil with six or more lobes per 100 cells. In contrast, only 1 of the 50 controls had a single six-lobed neutrophil. The Pelger-Hüet anomaly is an inherited disorder in which neutrophils have no more than two lobes. Neutrophils in severe bacterial infections have toxic granulation, Döhle's inclusion bodies, and cytoplasmic vacuoles.

413. The answer is E. *(Lipton, Pediatr Clin North Am 27:217-235, 1980.)* Although uncommon, aplastic anemia is a serious childhood disease. It is strictly defined as acquired or constitutional bone marrow failure, which involves erythrocytes, granulocytes, and platelets, with peripheral pancytopenia; evidence of reduced or absent production of blood cells in the bone marrow; and replacement of normal cellular elements by fat. In a recent review of 205 pediatric patients with aplastic anemia ranging in age from newborn to 20 years of age, 30 percent had congenital or inherited types. The peak age incidence for acquired aplastic anemia was three to five years, with a poorer prognosis in the severe forms, in which the median survival was less than six months. Although there may be rare cases of spontaneous recovery or improvement, bone marrow transplantation should be performed without delay in those patients with histocompatible donors. The three-year survival rate with this procedure is approximately 50 to 70 percent, which is considerably higher than with any other therapeutic modality. Chronic graft-versus-host disease remains a morbid problem. Prior to the effective use of androgens, almost all patients with Fanconi's anemia died of complications of pancytopenia. With androgen therapy, 50 percent survive for more than seven years, but there are reports of malignant disease appearing in long-term survivors. Congenital hypoplastic anemia (Diamond-Blackfan syndrome) is a rare pure red blood cell aplasia which usually presents at birth. One-third of the patients may show short webbed neck and thumb abnormalities. Oral prednisone therapy induces a response within four weeks in 80 to 85 percent of children. The long-term prognosis is excellent. Transient erythroblastopenia of childhood is, as the name implies, a transient suppression of erythropoiesis following a viral infection. Spontaneous total recovery occurs without sequelae, and no treatment is required.

414. The answer is B (1, 3). *(Williams, ed 2. pp 1434-1440, 1977.)* Von Willebrand's disease (VWD) usually presents as epistaxis and easy bruising in early childhood. In contrast to classical hemophilia A, hemarthrosis and fatal bleeding are unusual. Although factor VIII procoagulant activity (factor VIII AHF) is decreased in both disorders, hemophiliac plasma contains an antigen that is precipitated by a rabbit antibody to factor VIII (factor VIII AGN), whereas patients with severe VWD lack this antigen. The prolonged bleeding time in VWD is due to a defect in platelet adhesiveness as documented by significant impairment of ristocetin-induced platelet aggregation in the majority of patients. This factor, which is missing in plasma in VWD, is called von Willebrand's factor (factor VIII VWF). Platelet aggregation by collagen, adenosine diphosphate, and epinephrine is normal in most patients with VWD. These tests are used to confirm the diagnosis of VWD and to differentiate it from classical hemophilia A.

415. The answer is E (all). *(Nathan, ed 2. pp 27-31.)* Capillary blood samples from a heel prick have hemoglobin values 10 percent higher than venous samples. This error can be minimized by warming the area, eliciting a brisk blood flow, and discarding the initial drops. Within the first few hours after birth, plasma volume decreases and hemoglobin concentration increases (from 15 to 25 percent). The placental vessels at birth contain 75 to 125 ml of blood, about a quarter of which normally gets into a newborn infant within 15 seconds of birth. Cord-related factors can make a difference of 40 percent in neonatal blood volume; for example, because the umbilical arteries constrict shortly after birth, whereas the vein remains dilated, delayed cord clamping was associated in one study with an average red blood cell mass of 49 ml/kg at 72 hours as compared to 31 ml/kg in infants with immediate cord clamping. Fetomaternal transfusion in the last phases of pregnancy and labor can lead to anemia in the newborn; conversely, maternal-fetal transfusion can result in plethora.

416. The answer is A (1, 2, 3). *(Burks, J Pediatr 88:224-226, 1976. Saarinen, Acta Paediatr Scand 67:745, 1978.)* Serum ferritin concentration is a very sensitive reflection of iron stores from birth to adult life. Its assay requires less than 0.1 ml of serum, and because samples can be stored for several months, it is a useful tool in nutritional surveys. The normal value in children between the ages of 6 months and 15 years is 30 ng/ml; the level in children who have iron deficiency anemia is 10.0 ng/ml. In iron overload (sickle cell disease) levels may be over 500 ng/ml. In the natural sequence of stages in iron deficiency, depletion of **iron stores**, as manifested by a fall in serum ferritin concentration, is the first readily detectable event. This is then followed by a fall in serum transferrin saturation (which represents the **mobile iron pool**). Only when transferrin saturation drops below 15 percent does the marrow feel the pinch of iron deficiency. Anemia is a late and nonspecific manifestation of iron deficiency; in fact, iron deficiency, as reflected first by decreased ferritin levels and then by transferrin saturation, may exist for several weeks before there are clinical manifestations of anemia. Infection and chronic disease may cause transferrin synthesis but not serum ferritin concentration to drop, thus making transferrin saturation a less reliable laboratory index than serum ferritin under these conditions.

Some investigators reported measuring serum ferritin in assessment of iron nutrition in 238 infants on seven occasions in the first year of life. The values of iron-supplemented infants remained consistently higher.

417. The answer is C (2, 4). *(Jaffe, vol 2. pp 109-121.)* Among cancers in children under 14 years of age, malignant bone tumors are relatively rare, being only the sixth most common malignancy. However, osteosarcoma comprises 60 percent of all malignant bone tumors in this age group. The peak incidence is in the 10 to 20-year-old age group, coinciding with the pubertal growth spurt. The metaphysis of long bones, particularly the lower end of the femur, is the most common site of the primary tumor, with lungs being the primary site of hematogenous metastasis. Using massive doses of methotrexate (MTX 7.5 to 12 g/m^2/ six hour infusions) followed by folinic acid (citrovorum factor rescue; CF 10 mg every six hours x 10) was the first major effective advance in the treatment of children with metastatic disease. This was followed by the introduction by different study groups of high-dose MTX-CF in combination with vincristine, adriamycin, and cyclophosphamide, given eight to ten weeks prior to surgery for primary tumor. The four-year disease-free survival rate in over 100 patients treated with this regimen is 74 percent compared with 20 percent in 300 historical controls who received no preoperative chemotherapy. A trial of *cis*-dichlorodiamine platinum II (DPP) is still inconclusive.

418. The answer is B (1, 3). *(American Academy of Pediatrics, Pediatrics 58: 765-768, 1976. Dallman, p 6.)* The Committee on Nutrition of the American Academy of Pediatrics states that iron supplementation from one or two sources, such as the newer iron-fortified cereals (that do not contain the poorly absorbed iron pyrophosphate) or iron-containing drops, should begin at four months of age for term infants and two months for premature infants. Breast-feeding is preferred, and iron-fortified formulas and other heat-treated milk products are better than cow's milk as substitutes for human breast milk during the first six to twelve months of an infant's life. After the age of six months, infants receiving cow's milk should have their daily milk intake limited to 750 ml and should begin eating iron-rich solid foods. Excessive milk ingestion increases occult blood loss in the gastrointestinal tract and thus contributes to iron-deficiency anemia. Unless milk drinking is discouraged and better methods of iron supplementation for infants are adopted, iron deficiency will remain all too common. It has recently been shown by using an external tagging method (^{59}FeSO$_4$) that breast-fed infants absorb 49 percent of the iron in the breast milk in contrast to infants fed cow's milk or unfortified cow's milk formula who absorbed only 10 to 12 percent of the available iron. Assessment of iron nutrition by serum ferritin measurements indicates that routine iron supplementation may not be necessary in term infants who continue to be breast-fed.

419. The answer is E (all). *(Bowman, pp 40-47.)* The incidence of Rh immunization can be reduced from 15 percent to 2 percent by postdelivery injections of Rh-immune globulin. The case history presented illustrates several problems in reducing the failure rate of Rh prevention. Proper monitoring of this woman should have included a Kleihauer acid elution test (to demonstrate fetal cells in her circulation) at the time of the threatened abortion and also, because of antepartum hemorrhage, after delivery. Furthermore, if initial sensitization produced minimal antibody levels, more sensitive screening techniques should have been used, even after 28 weeks gestation; the usual indirect antiglobulin antibody screen alone may be negative. Thus, she should have received one dose of Rh-immune globulin at 12 weeks and more than one dose after delivery, if there was significant fetomaternal bleeding.

420. The answer is E (all). *(Nathan, ed 2. pp 1509-1510.)* Polycythemia (hemoglobin, >22 g/100 ml; hematocrit, $>65\%$) in an infant during the first week of life can lead to several undesirable complications. Although the etiology may be obscure, placental insufficiency leading to intrauterine hypoxia seems to play a central role in the majority of the conditions associated with plethora. Maternal diabetes, another common cause, may be related to placental dysfunction. In infants who have Down's syndrome, evidence of a myeloproliferative disorder is not uncommon; it can affect in the neonatal period any of the formed blood elements and very often is associated with myeloid hyperplasia that can be confused with congenital leukemia.

421. The answer is E (all). *(Mauer, Blood 56:1-10, 1980. Pinkel, Pediatr Clin North Am 23:117-130, 1976.)* Age less than two years or more than ten years, the presence at diagnosis of central nervous system leukemia or a white blood cell count of 50,000/mm^3 or higher, and the appearance of a mediastinal mass all indicate a poor prognosis for children who have acute lymphocytic leukemia. Most of the children having these poor prognostic signs have the thymic (T cell) variety of the disease. These children, usually older boys, possess surface antigens specific for thymocytes. In addition to the conventionally employed regimen of prednisone and vincristine, other chemotherapeutic agents, such as daunorubicin or L-asparaginase, should be administered. Children with T-cell acute lymphocytic leukemia run a greater risk of bleeding and infection during the first four weeks of remission induction therapy. Only 20 percent of these patients with poor prognostic features can be expected to achieve long-term disease-free survival, and once they relapse, which is very often in the first few months, virtually none of them go into remission despite aggressive chemotherapy.

Hematologic and Neoplastic Diseases

422. The answer is E (all). *(Gellis, pp 115-116.)* The immune functions of the spleen, other than the filtration and phagocytosis of bacteria in the reticuloendothelial system, are not completely known. After splenectomy, the serum level of immunoglobulin M falls and opsonization of encapsulated organisms like *Streptococcus (Diplococcus) pneumoniae* becomes defective. These factors may contribute to the development of overwhelming pneumococcal infections in splenectomized children, especially those who are less than four years of age, who have a severe hematologic disease, or who require chemotherapy for a lymphoma. A recent follow-up evaluation of 71 splenectomized or autosplenectomized patients who were immunized with pneumococcal polysaccharide (PPS) vaccine revealed that this vaccine is effective in preventing pneumococcal sepsis. Although the use of prophylactic penicillin in splenectomized children has, on occasion, been recommended, it is not known for how many years prophylaxis should be continued or whether it can prevent sepsis caused by gram-negative organisms. An aggressive approach to febrile illnesses in these children should be undertaken, including institution of high-dose penicillin therapy before blood culture results are available.

423. The answer is C (2, 4). *(Gellis, pp 270-271.)* Isoimmune neonatal purpura is the most common cause of neonatal thrombocytopenia; it is associated with significant morbidity and mortality, particularly due to bleeding in the central nervous system. The pathogenesis is very similar to that of isoimmune Rh-immunization. The techniques for the determination of platelet antigens and the antibodies directed against them are, unfortunately, limited; the diagnosis is made largely by the exclusion of idiopathic thrombocytopenic purpura in the mother and intrauterine infection and sepsis in the neonate. Platelet transfusion may be of both therapeutic and diagnostic value. Because platelets from an affected infant's mother may be associated with a significant dose of plasma antibodies, they should be washed before transfusion into the child. Exchange transfusion with fresh whole blood also removes the circulating antibodies as well as partially damaged platelets. Isoimmune neonatal purpura is likely to recur in subsequent pregnancies; cesarean section therefore should be done in the case of cephalopelvic disproportion to avoid birth trauma to the fetal head.

424. The answer is E (all). *(Nathan, ed 2. pp 1223-1228.)* The clinical history and blood-smear findings presented in the question are typical of disseminated intravascular coagulation. The disorder, which can be triggered by endotoxin shock, results ultimately in the initiation of the intrinsic clotting mechanism and the generation of thrombin. Fibrin deposited in the microcirculatory system can lead to tissue ischemia and necrosis, further capillary damage, release of thromboplastic substances, and increased thrombin generation. Simultaneous activation of the fibrinolytic system produces increased amounts of fibrin split products, which inhibit thrombin activity. Of utmost importance in the treatment of children who have disseminated intravascular coagulation is the management of the condition that precipitated the disorder.

425. The answer is A (1, 2, 3). *(Nathan, ed 2. pp 269-271.)* Stasis and slow circulation through the congested red pulp of the spleen bring about hypoxia, a fall in glucose content, and a fall in pH due to lactic acid formation. These factors together affect the metabolism and deformability of every red blood cell, especially those that are aged or abnormal. For example, a fall in pH can lower 2,3-diphosphoglycerate activity in red blood cells, and a decrease in glucose concentration can affect the red blood cell glycolytic pathway. The effect of these environmental factors is a decrease in the deformability of red blood cells. Microsomal heme oxygenase is a heme-splitting enzyme that acts only when hemoglobin is released from a hemolyzed red blood cell; thus, it does not affect red blood cell metabolism or membrane function.

426. The answer is E (all). *(Nathan, ed 2. pp 329-332.)* Red blood cells emerging from the bone marrow with decreased amounts of hemoglobin first become smaller (microcytic) in order to sustain an adequate mean corpuscular hemoglobin concentration and only later become hypochromic and show increased central pallor on peripheral-smear examination. The impairment could be in the synthesis of globin or heme. In thalassemia, there is a quantitative decrease in globin-chain synthesis due to a genetic disorder. In iron deficiency, synthesis of heme is impaired due to a lack of iron; and lead can block incompletely many enzymatic steps in heme manufacture. In pyridoxine-responsive anemia, the exact mechanism causing hypochromicity is unknown, but the impairments resemble those of lead poisoning and result in poor utilization of adequate iron stores situated in the normoblasts.

427. The answer is C (2, 4). *(Nathan, ed 2. pp 321-322.)* Administration of intramuscular iron seldom is required. The injections are quite painful and often accompanied by skin discoloration. Severe anaphylactic reactions have occurred, and deaths, though rare, have been reported in association with the use of intramuscular iron. Children who have iron-deficiency anemia do not respond significantly differently to oral versus intramuscular iron therapy. Indications for the use of intramuscular iron can include an apparent lack of response to oral therapy, malabsorption syndromes, and major surgery in severely iron-deficient children. Oral iron preparations are simple iron salts, whereas intramuscular iron preparations are iron-carbohydrate complexes.

Hematologic and Neoplastic Diseases 217

428-432. The answers are: 428-C, 429-E, 430-D, 431-A, 432-B. *(Nathan, ed 2. pp 277, 296, 396-404, 492-502, 731-734.)* Howell-Jolly bodies (slide C) are small, spherical nuclear remnants seen in the reticulocytes and, rarely, erythrocytes of individuals who have no spleen—either due to congenital asplenia or splenectomy—or who have a poorly functioning spleen (e.g., hyposplenism associated with sickle cell disease). Ultrafiltration of blood is a unique function of the spleen that cannot be assumed by other reticuloendothelial organs.

Basophilic stippling (slide E) represents abnormal aggregates of ribosomes within reticulocytes. This condition occurs whenever the utilization of iron for hemoglobin synthesis is impeded, as in lead intoxication and thalassemia. The presented peripheral blood smear of a child who has lead poisoning also provides evidence (microcytic, hypochromic red blood cells) of associated iron deficiency.

A target cell is an erythrocyte with a membrane that is too large for its hemoglobin content; a thin rim of hemoglobin at the cell's periphery and a small disc in the center give the cell a target-like appearance. Target cells, which are more resistant to osmotic fragility than other erythrocytes, are seen in children who have β-thalassemia, hemoglobin C disease, or liver disease (e.g., obstructive jaundice or cirrhosis). Thalassemia major (slide D) can be diagnosed by the presence of poorly hemoglobinized normoblasts in addition to target cells in the peripheral blood.

Uniformly small microspherocytes (less than 6 μm in diameter) are typical of hereditary spherocytosis (slide A). Because of a decreased surface-to-volume ratio, these osmotically fragile red blood cells have an increased density of hemoglobin. Although spherical red blood cells also may appear in other hemolytic states, such as immune hemolytic anemia, microangiopathy, ABO incompatibility, and hypersplenism, their cellular volume is only irregularly augmented.

Although hemoglobin C disease (slide B) is a mild disorder, target cells comprise a far greater percentage of total red blood cells than in thalassemia major. Target cells are the only manifestations of hemoglobin C disease; targeting is so striking because hemoglobin C has a greater tendency than normal hemoglobin to aggregate and precipitate during the drying of cells on a glass slide.

433-435. The answers are: 433-D, 434-E, 435-B. *(Nathan, ed 2. pp 979-984.)* The differentiation of the types of leukemia is based mainly on morphologic characteristics as revealed by Wright's-stained smears of peripheral blood and bone marrow. Only occasionally are special cytochemical stains helpful in confirming the diagnosis.

Acute lymphoblastic leukemia is the most common type of childhood leukemia and is associated with the best prognosis. The marrow is filled with one kind of cell; most of the volume of this cell is occupied by an immature nucleus, which includes chromatin clumped around a few nucleoli. There may be folding of the nucleus. The scanty cytoplasm is blue and nongranular. Periodic acid-Schiff stain may be positive.

Acute myeloblastic leukemia is less common and has a poorer prognosis. The myeloblasts are mostly in one phase of maturity and show thin, spongy nuclear chromatin and several distinct punched-out nucleoli. The blue-gray cytoplasm is more abundant than in lymphoblasts and often contains typical Auer rods, which are abnormal lysosomes never seen in lymphoblasts. Myeloperoxidase stain may be positive.

Chronic granulocytic leukemia progresses through two stages: chronic and blastic. Bone marrow examination during the chronic phase reveals a proliferation of granulocytic cells of intermediate maturity; increased platelets also may be noted. The blastic phase, which is much harder to treat, is characterized by an increased number of less differentiated blast cells.

436-440. The answers are: 436-B, 437-B, 438-B, 439-C, 440-A. *(Nathan, ed 2. pp 289-298.)* One of the best clinical approaches in the evaluation of anemia is the determination of the status of red blood cell production and destruction. Destruction reflects a decrease in the life span of red blood cells, as evidenced by hemolysis or blood loss. The bone marrow's response to anemia is reflected by the reticulocyte count or by the presence of polychromasia in the peripheral smear. In deficiencies of iron, folate, or vitamin B_{12}, the marrow responds with increased cellularity of erythroid precursors; due to a lack of substrate, however, not enough mature red blood cells are released, and the reticulocyte count decreases. All three of these deficiencies, particularly in the advanced stages, further are complicated by red blood cell destruction both in the marrow and the peripheral blood.

In the anemia of protein-calorie malnutrition, which is due to a lack of essential amino-acid substrates, the bone marrow shows a decreased erythroid-to-myeloid ratio and a reduced population of reticulocytes. Red blood cell survival is normal. If uncomplicated (i.e., if there is no significant iron or folate deficiency due to regional environmental factors), the anemia is moderate; however, plasma volume is increased disproportionately due to hypoalbuminemia.

In premature infants, vitamin E deficiency can lead to hemolytic anemia. Because one of the metabolic roles of vitamin E compounds is to protect lipids in biologic membranes from oxidative damage, injury to red blood cell membranes can occur in vitamin E-deficient infants. Red blood cell survival is moderately decreased; and although red blood cell production is increased (reticulocyte counts usually are 10 percent), it fails to compensate completely.

441-445. The answers are: **441-C, 442-E, 443-D, 444-A, 445-B.** *(Lampkin, Semin Hematol 9:211-223, 1972. Vietti, Pediatr Clin North Am 23:67-92, 1976.)* Because experimental data concerning the use of chemotherapeutic agents are incomplete and at times, perhaps, inaccurate, much of cancer chemotherapy still is given on an empirical basis. However, since the introduction of tritiated thymidine, accurate studies of DNA synthetic activities and of the proliferative characteristics of normal and leukemic cells now are possible, and a reasonably good correlation between in vivo and in vitro studies of leukemic cells has emerged. Several treatment advances, such as multimodal therapy using cytosine arabinoside in the treatment of children who have acute myelogenous leukemia, have resulted from these more sophisticated scientific studies.

The five anti-neoplastic drugs listed in the question all have different mechanisms of action. **Methotrexate** is a folic acid analog that binds in a "pseudoreversible" reaction with the enzyme dehydrofolate reductase, which is essential for the synthesis of pyrimidines. **Cytosine arabinoside** (cytarabine, ara-C) is a pyrimidine analog that impairs DNA synthesis by competitive inhibition of DNA polymerase. Both of these agents exert their antimetabolic effects during the S phase of the mitotic cycle.

Cyclophosphamide is a nitrogen mustard alkylating agent that inhibits DNA synthesis by the alkylation of purine bases. It blocks the mitotic cycle at the premitotic (G_2) stage. **Vincristine** is a vinca alkaloid, derived from the periwinkle plant; by damaging the microtubules necessary for the formation of mitotic spindles, this chemotherapeutic agent arrests mitosis during metaphase. The purine analog **6-mercaptopurine** is an effective antineoplastic drug because it blocks purine synthesis by inhibiting two enzymatic reactions: the conversion of 5-phosphoribosyl-1-pyrophosphate to 5-phosphoribosyl-1-amine and the conversion of inosinic acid to xanthylic acid.

Endocrine, Metabolic, and Genetic Disorders

Abdollah Sadeghi-Nejad

DIRECTIONS: Each question below contains five suggested answers. Choose the **one best** response to each question.

446. In the evaluation of thyroid function, the tests most frequently used are total serum thyroxine and T_3 resin uptake. The test T_3 uptake indirectly measures the concentration of

(A) total T_3
(B) free T_3
(C) reverse T_3
(D) free T_4
(E) thyroxine-binding globulin

447. The earliest sign of puberty in boys is usually

(A) enlargement of the penis
(B) enlargement of the testes
(C) growth acceleration
(D) pubic hair growth
(E) axillary hair growth

448. A ten-year-old obese boy is diagnosed as having Cushing's syndrome on the basis of his fat distribution, his arrested growth, and the presence of hypertension, plethora, purple striae, and osteoporosis. Which of the following disorders is most likely to be responsible for the clinical picture that this boy presents?

(A) Bilateral adrenal hyperplasia
(B) Adrenal adenoma
(C) Adrenal carcinoma
(D) Craniopharyngioma
(E) Ectopic adrenocorticotropin-producing tumor

449. A 12-year-old girl has a mass in her neck. Physical examination reveals a thyroid nodule, but the rest of the gland is not palpable. A technetium scan reveals a "cold" nodule. The child appears to be euthyroid. Which of the following diagnoses is the LEAST likely?

(A) Simple adenoma
(B) Follicular carcinoma
(C) Papillary carcinoma
(D) Medullary carcinoma
(E) Dysgenetic thyroid gland

450. According to Greek mythology, Hermaphroditus was the son of Hermes and Aphrodite. As a youth, he rejected the love of Salmacis, a river nymph. The gods granted both her wish to remain with him always and his wish to die rather than submit to her love by fusing them into one ambisexual being as they drowned in a river. All of the following statements about true hermaphrodites are true EXCEPT that

(A) most are chromatin-positive
(B) most have parents with sex-chromosome aberrations
(C) their sex-chromosome patterns may be XX, XY, or a mosaic
(D) their internal genitalia reflect the composition of their gonads
(E) they may have both a testis and an ovary

451. A 16-year-old girl presenting with short stature, primary amenorrhea, and advanced bone age is most likely to have which of the following conditions?

(A) Cushing's syndrome
(B) Turner's syndrome
(C) Adrenogenital syndrome
(D) Anorexia nervosa
(E) An isolated deficiency of growth hormone

452. Individuals who have a 48,XXXY karyotype are tall, mentally retarded phenotypic males having a small phallus and small, abnormal testes. Cells obtained by buccal smear would be expected to contain how many Barr bodies?

(A) One
(B) Two
(C) Three
(D) Four
(E) None

453. True sexual precocity in girls is most likely to be caused by

(A) a feminizing ovarian tumor
(B) a gonadotropin-producing tumor
(C) a lesion of the central nervous system
(D) exogenous estrogens
(E) early onset of puberty

454. Examination of a 14-year-old boy with gynecomastia reveals that he is midpubertal; his breasts are moderately enlarged but there is no development of the areolae or nipples. In most cases the best therapy for gynecomastia would be

(A) administration of androgens
(B) administration of antiestrogens (e.g., clomiphene)
(C) administration of bromocriptine
(D) reassurance
(E) surgery

455. All of the following disorders are associated with neonatal hypoglycemia EXCEPT

(A) von Gierke's disease (glucose-6-phosphatase deficiency)
(B) Pompe's disease (acid maltase deficiency)
(C) panhypopituitarism
(D) prematurity
(E) nesidioblastosis

456. A four-month-old infant is brought to a physician because of hypoglycemia. Except for the finding of hepatomegaly, physical examination is within normal limits. Laboratory studies reveal lipemia, fasting hypoglycemia, and an increased anion gap. The most likely diagnosis is

(A) "leucine-sensitive" hypoglycemia
(B) neonatal hepatitis
(C) lipid storage disease (Gaucher's disease)
(D) von Gierke's disease (glucose-6-phosphatase deficiency)
(E) galactokinase deficiency

457. A full-term infant is born to a woman who has poorly controlled, insulin-dependent diabetes. All of the following laboratory findings are likely to be associated with this infant EXCEPT

(A) hypoglycemia
(B) hypocalcemia
(C) hyperketonemia
(D) hyperinsulinemia
(E) hyperbilirubinemia

458. A ten-day-old infant is admitted to a hospital for evaluation of the following symptoms: poor feeding, irritability, vomiting, and jaundice. Physical examination reveals a markedly enlarged liver. The blood glucose level is low, and the infant has aminoaciduria. The most likely diagnosis is

(A) transferase-deficiency galactosemia
(B) galactokinase deficiency
(C) cytomegalic inclusion disease
(D) rubella syndrome
(E) erythroblastosis fetalis and hypoglycemia

459. A six-year-old girl has been referred to an endocrinologist because a reducing substance was found in her urine during a routine examination. Physical examination and glucose tolerance test results are normal; her urine reacts with Clinitest tablets but not with Clinistix. The most likely diagnosis is

(A) diabetes mellitus
(B) renal glycosuria
(C) hereditary fructose intolerance
(D) essential fructosuria
(E) deficiency of fructose-1,6-diphosphatase activity

460. A one-day-old infant develops tetany and convulsions. Serum calcium is 6.2 mg/100 ml. Which of the following diagnoses is the LEAST likely in this infant?

(A) Perinatal asphyxia
(B) High phosphorus intake
(C) Maternal diabetes mellitus
(D) Maternal hyperparathyroidism
(E) Prematurity

461. Maple syrup urine disease (classical branched-chain ketoaciduria) is a hereditary disorder transmitted as an autosomal recessive trait. If the gene frequency for heterozygosity is 1 in 250, the expected incidence of the disease would be

(A) 1 in 1000
(B) 1 in 25,000
(C) 1 in 62,500
(D) 1 in 250,000
(E) 1 in 625,000

462. Hereditary disorders transmitted as an X-linked recessive trait would be best described by which of the following statements?

(A) Females are not affected
(B) Heterozygous females are less severely affected than hemizygous males
(C) Hemizygous males are not affected
(D) Hemizygous males are less severely affected than heterozygous females
(E) Hemizygous males and heterozygous females are affected with equal frequency

463. Which of the following laboratory findings is unusual in patients with simple (nutritional) rickets?

(A) Aminoaciduria
(B) Hyperphosphaturia
(C) Elevated serum alkaline phosphatase levels
(D) Hypercalciuria
(E) Hypophosphatemia

464. Hypertension is associated with all of the following tumors EXCEPT

(A) aldosteronoma
(B) adrenocortical carcinoma
(C) thyroid carcinoma
(D) neuroblastoma
(E) pheochromocytoma

465. A ten-year-old boy is suspected of having angina pectoris. Physical examination shows multiple xanthomas and a corneal arcus. Which of the following types of hyperlipoproteinemia is most likely to be present?

(A) Type I (hyperchylomicronemia)
(B) Type II (hypercholesterolemia)
(C) Type III ("broad beta" disease)
(D) Type IV (hyperprebetalipoproteinemia)
(E) Type V (mixed hyperprebetalipoproteinemia and hyperchylomicronemia)

466. An infant is brought to a hospital because her wet diapers turn black when they are exposed to air. Physical examination is normal. Urine is positive both for reducing substance and when tested with ferric chloride. This disorder is caused by a deficiency of

(A) homogentisic acid oxidase
(B) phenylalanine hydroxylase
(C) L-histidine ammonia-lyase
(D) ketoacid decarboxylase
(E) isovaleryl-CoA dehydrogenase

467. Neonatal hypoglycemia is common in premature and small-for-gestational-age infants. The most common cause of hypoglycemia in these infants is

(A) inadequate stores of nutrients
(B) adrenal immaturity
(C) pituitary immaturity
(D) insulin excess
(E) glucagon deficiency

468. All of the following statements about anorexia nervosa are true EXCEPT that

(A) males are rarely affected
(B) the heart rate is usually slow
(C) endocrine gland function may be abnormal
(D) mental retardation is common
(E) a history of obesity is common

469. A seven-day-old boy is admitted to a hospital for evaluation of vomiting and dehydration. Physical examination is normal except for minimal hyperpigmentation of the nipples. Serum sodium and potassium concentrations are 120 mEq/L and 9 mEq/L, respectively. The most likely diagnosis is

(A) pyloric stenosis
(B) congenital adrenal hyperplasia
(C) secondary hypothyroidism
(D) panhypopituitarism
(E) hyperaldosteronism

DIRECTIONS: Each question below contains four suggested answers of which **one** or **more** is correct. Choose the answer:

A	if	1, 2, and 3	are correct
B	if	1 and 3	are correct
C	if	2 and 4	are correct
D	if	4	is correct
E	if	1, 2, 3, and 4	are correct

470. Hirsutism in females may be caused by

(1) increased ovarian androgens
(2) genetic predisposition
(3) increased adrenal androgens
(4) increased testicular (ectopic) androgens

471. Known complications of diabetes mellitus include which of the following?

(1) Cataracts
(2) Glomerulosclerosis
(3) Microangiopathy
(4) Blood vessel calcification

472. The best screening tests for growth hormone deficiency are fasting concentrations of growth hormone after exercise and after treatment with estrogens. The "definitive" tests usually used include the response of growth hormone to

(1) insulin-induced hypoglycemia
(2) L-dopa
(3) arginine infusion
(4) medroxyprogesterone acetate

473. Children who have the syndrome of inappropriate antidiuretic hormone secretion exhibit which of the following symptoms?

(1) Hyponatremia
(2) Overhydration
(3) Relatively concentrated urine
(4) Inappropriately low concentrations of antidiuretic hormone

474. An infant girl who has a 46,XX karyotype is hospitalized to determine the cause of her ambiguous genitalia. This child's virilization is likely to be caused by

(1) maternal exposure to progestins
(2) maternal androgen intake
(3) congenital adrenal hyperplasia
(4) neonatal Cushing's syndrome

475. Patients with the syndrome of testicular feminization are correctly described by which of the following statements?

(1) They are genotypic females
(2) Their breasts develop at puberty
(3) Their menses can be normal
(4) They exhibit end-organ resistance to testosterone

SUMMARY OF DIRECTIONS				
A	B	C	D	E
1, 2, 3 only	1, 3 only	2, 4 only	4 only	All are correct

476. A six-year-old boy with a two-week history of polyuria, polydipsia, and anorexia is admitted to a hospital. Which of the following diagnoses are likely?

(1) Insulin-dependent diabetes mellitus
(2) Nephrogenic diabetes insipidus
(3) Central diabetes insipidus
(4) Phosphate diabetes

477. Physical examination of a three-week-old infant suspected of having hypothyroidism is entirely normal. Routine newborn screening of the cord blood showed a low level of thyroxine and normal concentration of thyroid-stimulating hormone. These results were confirmed two weeks later on a venous blood sample. The differential diagnosis should include

(1) thyroid-binding globulin deficiency
(2) tertiary (hypothalamic) hypothyroidism
(3) secondary (pituitary) hypothyroidism
(4) primary hypothyroidism

478. Tall stature can be a feature of which of the following conditions?

(1) Klinefelter's syndrome
(2) A karyotype 47,XYY
(3) Marfan's syndrome
(4) Homocystinuria

479. Goitrous hypothyroidism can be present in a newborn infant as the result of which of the following factors?

(1) Peroxidase deficiency
(2) Maternal ingestion of thyroid hormone
(3) Maternal ingestion of iodide
(4) Thyroid-stimulating hormone deficiency

480. Cholecalciferol (vitamin D_3) is absorbed by the gut. In its enzymatic conversion to the active form of the vitamin, it must undergo

(1) hydroxylation at carbon 25
(2) hydroxylation at carbon 24
(3) hydroxylation at carbon 1
(4) hydroxylation at carbon 3

481. Ketonuria usually accompanies fasting in normal children. Other true statements regarding fasting in children include which of the following?

(1) Lipolysis is enhanced
(2) Blood glucose concentration frequently decreases during 24 hours of fasting
(3) Serum fatty acid levels are high
(4) Hyperinsulinemia is present

482. Depending on the individual patient, which of the following can be considered appropriate treatment for Cushing's disease?

(1) Trans-sphenoidal adenectomy
(2) Total adrenalectomy
(3) Pituitary irradiation
(4) Partial adrenalectomy

Pediatrics

DIRECTIONS: The groups of questions below consist of lettered choices followed by several numbered items. For each numbered item select the **one** lettered choice with which it is **most** closely associated. Each lettered choice may be used once, more than once, or not at all.

Questions 483-487

For each of the disorders listed below, select the serum concentration of calcium (Ca) and phosphate (PO_4) with which it is most likely to be associated.

(A) Low PO_4, normal Ca
(B) Low PO_4, high Ca
(C) Normal PO_4, low Ca
(D) Normal PO_4, normal Ca
(E) High PO_4, low Ca

483. Vitamin D-resistant rickets

484. Pseudohypoparathyroidism

485. Osteogenesis imperfecta

486. Hyperparathyroidism

487. Medullary thyroid carcinoma (primary hypercalcitoninemia)

Questions 488-493

All of the syndromes listed below are associated with obesity in children. For each of the other clinical findings that follow, select the syndrome with which it is most likely to be associated.

(A) Prader-Willi syndrome
(B) Laurence-Moon-Biedl syndrome
(C) Cushing's syndrome
(D) Frohlich's syndrome
(E) Pseudohypoparathyroidism

488. Cataracts

489. Hypotonia

490. Polydactyly

491. Brachydactyly

492. Basal ganglia calcification

493. Retinitis pigmentosa

Questions 494-500

For each of the following disorders, select the serum concentrations (mEq/L) of sodium (Na^+) and potassium (K^+) with which it is most likely to be associated.

(A) Na^+ 118, K^+ 7.5
(B) Na^+ 120, K^+ 3.0
(C) Na^+ 134, K^+ 6.0
(D) Na^+ 150, K^+ 2.9
(E) Na^+ 155, K^+ 5.5

494. Salt-losing 21-hydroxylase deficiency (adrenogenital syndrome)

495. Central diabetes insipidus

496. Nephrogenic diabetes insipidus

497. Hyperaldosteronism

498. Syndrome of inappropriate antidiuretic hormone (ADH) secretion

499. Addison's disease (in crisis)

500. Glucose-6-phosphatase deficiency (von Gierke's disease)

Endocrine, Metabolic, and Genetic Disorders

Answers

446. The answer is E. *(Gardner, ed 2. p 330. Williams, ed 5. p 136.)* The concentration of total serum thyroxine (T_4) is influenced by an individual's metabolic state and concentration of thyroxine-binding globulin (TBG). Thus, T_4 levels are high if TBG levels are high, as for example, in the newborn state, during pregnancy, or while taking oral contraceptives; conversely, T_4 levels are low in association with TBG deficiency. Because the measurement of TBG is tedious, triiodothyronine (T_3) uptake is used as an indirect measurement of TBG; uptake of T_3 and levels of TBG are inversely related. The product of T_3 uptake and total serum T_4, the free T_4 index, is used as an indicator of free (unbound) hormone which is metabolically active.

447. The answer is B. *(Gardner, ed 2. pp 20-21.)* While the onset of puberty is subject to marked individual variation, the sequence of pubertal development is relatively constant. The earliest sign of pubertal development in boys is the enlargement of the testes and the elongation and thinning of the scrotum. This is followed by growth of pubic hair and an increase in the size of the penis. Growth acceleration and axillary hair growth occur later.

448. The answer is A. *(Williams, ed 5. pp 255-263.)* Although the administration of exogenous adrenocorticotropic hormone or of glucocorticoids is the most common cause of Cushing's syndrome, it may also be caused by bilateral adrenal hyperplasia. In the latter case the concentration of adrenocorticotropic hormone is usually normal. The basic abnormality, however, is thought to be in the hypothalamic-pituitary axis, not the adrenal gland, because a distinct pituitary adenoma is found in some patients. Furthermore, many patients who have undergone bilateral adrenalectomy develop Nelson's syndrome (invasive pituitary adenoma) despite receiving adequate cortisol replacement.

449. The answer is E. *(DeGroot, ed 4. p 737.)* A "cold" thyroid nodule may be a benign or malignant lesion; and with the exception of anaplastic carcinomas, most thyroid malignancies are slow-growing. The management of individuals who have a "cold" nodule is controversial. A common approach is to attempt to suppress the nodule with a short course of thyroid hormone administration. If the nodule persists after three to six months, surgical excision is performed. A dysgenetic thyroid gland may appear as a neck mass; as a rule, however, it is functional and thus does not appear as a "cold" nodule on thyroid scan.

450. The answer is B. *(Federman, p 58. Williams, ed 5. pp 471-474, 1019.)* True hermaphrodites by definition have both ovarian and testicular tissue. Although the majority are XX (chromatin-positive), chromosomal mosaicism has been assumed to be present in all. Although their external genitalia are ambiguous, the majority of reported hermaphroditic children have been raised as males. Ductal differentiation (development of the epididymis and vas deferens or of the fallopian tubes) is dependent on the ipsilateral presence or absence of testicular tissue, which is capable of producing androgens and müllerian inhibiting factor. Uteri are usually present. Although a familial, autosomal recessive form of true hermaphroditism has been reported, the disorder usually appears sporadically; parental sex-chromosome aberrations have no known role in its pathogenesis.

451. The answer is C. *(Gardner, ed 2. p 476. Williams, ed 5. p 277.)* Girls who have adrenogenital syndrome (21-hydroxylase deficiency) show evidence of virilization and have amenorrhea and an advanced bone age; if untreated, they are tall during childhood but, because of early epiphyseal closure, short as adolescents and adults. A deficiency of 21-hydroxylase results in diminished ability to synthesize cortisol. Levels of adrenocorticotropin are elevated, and synthesis of adrenal androgens is increased. Excess amounts of androgens in turn suppress the hypothalamic-pituitary-gonadal axis. Although girls who have anorexia nervosa, Turner's syndrome, Cushing's syndrome, or isolated growth hormone deficiency may present with short stature and amenorrhea, they do not have an advanced bone age.

452. The answer is B. *(Williams, ed 5. p 430.)* A Barr (chromatin) body represents a partially inactivated X chromosome. The number of Barr bodies in each cell nucleus is equal to the number of X chromosomes **minus one**. Thus, normal males (XY) and females who have Turner's syndrome (XO) have no Barr bodies; normal females (XX) and males with Klinefelter's syndrome (XXY) have one Barr body in each cell.

453. The answer is E. *(Gardner, ed 2. p 619.)* The term "true sexual precocity" implies that the gonads have matured in response to the secretion of pituitary gonadotropins and have begun secreting sex steroids, causing the development of secondary sexual characteristics. Thus, ovarian tumors and exogenous estrogens, which suppress the function of the pituitary gland, do not cause true precocious puberty. In girls, the most common form of true precocious puberty is idiopathic and is thought to be caused by early maturation of an otherwise normal hypothalamic-pituitary-gonadal feedback system. In boys, true precocious puberty is relatively rare and is usually caused by lesions of the central nervous system. Gonadotropin-producing tumors, which are very rare, may cause true precocious puberty in both sexes.

454. The answer is D. *(DeGroot, pp 1583-1585.)* Gynecomastia is common in pubertal boys and as a rule is a self-limited problem lasting several months or years; nevertheless, it may result from underlying disease and should be carefully evaluated. The cause of pubertal gynecomastia is not known but is thought to be related to an imbalance in the estrogen:androgen ratio. This condition appears to be more severe in obese boys, usually due to a more marked accumulation of fat rather than an increase in breast tissue. When gynecomastia is accompanied by several psychosocial problems, plastic surgery may be necessary if weight reduction fails. However, reassurance is usually the only treatment required.

455. The answer is B. *(Senior, Clin Perinatology 3:79, 1976. Stanbury, ed 4. pp 146-148.)* Alpha-1,4-glucosidase (acid maltase) is a lysosomal enzyme that hydrolyzes glycogen fragments into glucose. Deficiency of this enzyme (Pompe's disease) leads to glycogen accumulation within lysosomes and, eventually, to cellular damage. This disorder affects heart and skeletal muscle and causes hypotonia, irritability, failure to thrive, and heart failure. Affected individuals have normal carbohydrate metabolism.

456. The answer is D. *(Senior, Clin Perinatology 3:79, 1976. Stanbury, ed 4. pp 143-146.)* Type I glycogen storage disease (glucose-6-phosphatase deficiency; von Gierke's disease) is an autosomal recessive disorder. Hepatomegaly, hypoglycemia, hyperlacticacidemia, hyperuricemia, and hypertriglyceridemia are the characteristic findings. Children who have "leucine-sensitive" hypoglycemia are hyperinsulinemic; hepatomegaly and hyperlipemia are not present. Hypoglycemia is usually not seen in conjunction with neonatal hepatitis or Gaucher's disease. Children with a deficiency of galactokinase may present with cataracts; they are not hypoglycemic.

457. The answer is C. *(Cornblath, ed 2. p 124.)* A high maternal glucose concentration stimulates beta cells in the fetal pancreas. At birth, the maternal delivery of glucose is interrupted; hyperinsulinemia persists, however, and hypoglycemia ensues. Hypocalcemia, too, often occurs, perhaps due to transient hypoparathyroidism or as a result of hypoglycemia-induced elevation of glucagon levels and subsequent stimulation of calcitonin secretion. Infants of diabetic mothers also have a high incidence of hyperbilirubinemia, but the cause of this condition is not known. Because high levels of circulating insulin inhibit lipolysis and ketone formation, hyperketonemia is not present in these infants.

458. The answer is A. *(Senior, Clin Perinatology 3:79, 1976. Stanbury, ed 4. p 164.)* Classic galactosemia is caused by a deficiency of the enzyme galactose-1-phosphate uridyltransferase. An autosomal recessive disorder, transferase-deficiency galactosemia results in the accumulation of galactose-1-phosphate, which leads to tissue damage in, for example, the liver and kidneys. It is also associated with mental retardation. Vomiting, jaundice, failure to thrive, and cataracts, usually appear within the first two weeks of life. A presumptive diagnosis is made on the basis of clinical findings and the presence of a reducing substance in the urine (note that results of glucose-specific urine tests—e.g., Labstix—will be negative). The diagnosis of transferase-deficiency galactosemia is confirmed by the absence of transferase activity in red blood cells. Total avoidance of galactose is the only treatment and will lead to the disappearance of abnormalities except those stemming from damage to the brain.

459. The answer is D. *(Senior, Clin Perinatology 3:79, 1976. Stanbury, ed 4. p 125.)* Clinitest tablets react with all reducing substances whereas Clinistix (glucose oxidase) is specific for glucose. A positive reaction with the former and a negative reaction with the latter suggest the presence of a reducing substance other than glucose in the urine. Children who have hereditary fructose intolerance as well as those who have essential fructosuria have reducing substances in their urine. Fructose intolerance, which presents during infancy, causes vomiting, hypoglycemia, and jaundice. Essential (benign) fructosuria (absence of fructokinase) is a rare autosomal recessive disorder that causes no symptoms and requires no therapy.

460. The answer is B. *(Gardner, ed 2. p 377. Root, J Pediatr 88:1, 177, 1976.)* Hypocalcemia of newborn infants may be divided into two groups: early (during the first 72 hours of life) and late (after 72 hours). The most common type of early neonatal hypocalcemia is the so-called idiopathic hypocalcemia. Current data suggest that in this heterogeneous group transient hypoparathyroidism may be present; maternal hyperparathyroidism is a rare cause of transient neonatal hypoparathyroidism. Maternal complications, including diabetes mellitus and toxemia, and neonatal disorders, such as hypoxia, prematurity, sepsis, and neonatal parathyroid disease, also may cause early hypocalcemia. Hypomagnesemia and high phosphate intake are the most common factors associated with late hypocalcemia.

461. The answer is D. *(Scriver, p 267.)* Maple syrup urine disease (classical branched-chain ketoaciduria) is an autosomal recessive disorder of amino acid metabolism in which the oxidative decarboxylation of branched-chain ketoacids is blocked. Because urine odor and body odor of affected individuals resemble the smell of maple syrup, the diagnosis may be suspected. The gene frequency of this disorder is approximately 1 in 250; thus, the likelihood of a union between two heterozygotes is 1 in 62,500. Because this disorder is inherited as a recessive trait, there is a 1 in 4 chance of heterozygous parents producing a homozygous offspring. Thus, the expected incidence of the disease is 1 in 250,000.

462. The answer is B. *(Williams, ed 5. p 1006.)* Because males have only one X chromosome (and are therefore hemizygous), they are affected by recessive traits linked to that chromosome. In each cell of heterozygous females, on the other hand, one X chromosome, either the normal X or the one carrying the abnormal allele, undergoes random inactivation (Lyon hypothesis); an X-linked recessive trait thus would be only partially expressed. For example, the X-linked recessive disorder nephrogenic diabetes insipidus produces a full-blown syndrome in males but only mild polyuria and polydipsia in heterozygous females.

463. The answer is D. *(Gardner, ed 2. p 854.)* Nutritional rickets is caused by a dietary deficiency of vitamin D and lack of exposure to sunlight. Intestinal absorption of calcium and phosphorus is diminished in vitamin D deficiency. Transient hypocalcemia stimulates the secretion of parathormone and the mobilization of calcium and phosphorus from bone; enhanced parathormone activity leads to phosphaturia and diminished excretion of calcium. In children with nutritional rickets, serum calcium concentration usually is normal and the phosphate level low. Aminoaciduria and increased serum alkaline phosphatase activity are common findings. The excretion of calcium in the urine is increased shortly after therapy with vitamin D has been instituted.

464. The answer is C. *(DeGroot, ed 4. p 666.)* Aldosteronoma, adrenocortical carcinoma, and pheochromocytoma are hormone-producing tumors that are often accompanied by hypertension. Neuroblastoma may produce excess catecholamines and cause an elevation of blood pressure. Thyroid carcinoma, on the other hand, is usually a nonfunctioning tumor; affected individuals are euthyroid and usually present with a neck lump that appears as a "cold" area on a thyroid scan.

465. The answer is B. *(Gardner, ed 2. p 115. Stanbury, ed 4. pp 617-633.)* Hypercholesterolemia (type II hyperlipoproteinemia) is the most common form of primary hyperlipoproteinemia in children. It is a familial disorder transmitted as an autosomal dominant trait. Evidence of coronary heart disease and xanthomas may appear in the first decade of life. Prognosis for homozygous children is grave, and heterozygotes usually die of coronary insufficiency in early adulthood.

466. The answer is A. *(Scriver, pp 352-353.)* The infant described in the question has alcaptonuria, an autosomal recessive disorder caused by a deficiency of homogentisic acid oxidase. The diagnosis is made in infants when their urine turns black on exposure to air due to the oxidation of homogentisic acid. Affected individuals are asymptomatic in childhood. In adults, ochronosis—the deposition of a bluish pigment in cartilage and fibrous tissue—develops; symptoms of arthritis may appear later. No specific treatment is available for individuals who have alcaptonuria. The other deficiencies listed in the question are found in phenylketonuria, histidinemia, maple syrup urine disease, and isovaleric acidemia, respectively.

467. The answer is A. *(Cornblath, ed 2. p 191.)* Glycogen and fat stores are diminished in premature and small-for-gestational-age infants. Energy stores are inadequate to meet the energy demands after the maternal supply of glucose is interrupted at birth, and hypoglycemia ensues. Deficiency of cortisol or growth hormone is a rare cause of neonatal hypoglycemia. Insulin excess, common in infants of diabetic mothers, is unusual in other infants. Hypoglycemia associated with a deficiency of glucagon has not been well documented.

468. The answer is D. *(Gardner, ed 2. p 1177.)* Anorexia nervosa usually is encountered in pubertal girls and young women. The underlying abnormality remains obscure. Many affected individuals have a history of voluntary dieting for obesity, and their body image may be distorted. Although most individuals with anorexia nervosa are intelligent, psychiatric disorders are common. Activity of the hypothalamic-pituitary axis may be suppressed; anorectic girls frequently come to the attention of endocrinologists because of primary or secondary amenorrhea. In some individuals, anorexia nervosa is a self-limiting disorder; for those requiring treatment, a combined psychiatric-medical approach is probably the best method of therapy.

469. The answer is B. *(Gardner, ed 2. p 482.)* Salt-losing congenital adrenal hyperplasia (adrenogenital syndrome; 21-hydroxylase deficiency) usually manifests during the first seven to ten days of life as anorexia, vomiting, diarrhea, and dehydration. Hypoglycemia also may occur. Affected infants may have increased pigmentation, and female infants show evidence of virilization—that is, ambiguous external genitalia. Hyponatremia, hyperkalemia, and urinary sodium wasting are the usual laboratory findings. Death may occur if the diagnosis is missed and appropriate treatment therefore is not instituted. Although adrenal aplasia, an extremely rare disorder, presents a similar clinical picture, it has an earlier onset than adrenal hyperplasia, and virilization does not occur.

470. The answer is A (1, 2, 3). *(DeGroot, pp 1451-1454.)* Most hirsute women have no demonstrable endocrine disorder. A genetic or constitutional cause is usually the basis for hairiness in women; for instance, Orientals and American Indians have scant body hair, whereas dark-haired individuals from Middle Eastern and Mediterranean countries tend to be hirsute. Development of sexual hair in females is dependent on the low concentration of androgens from the adrenal glands and ovaries. Excess androgen production by these organs is responsible for hirsutism in a minority of cases. Testicular tissue is not present in women. If it is present, the individual is, by definition, a hermaphrodite and usually presents with ambiguous genitalia.

471. The answer is E (all). *(Gardner, ed 2. p 960.)* The incidence and severity of complications in diabetes mellitus vary considerably. The extent to which good biochemical control affects the incidence is still a matter of controversy. Complications include retinopathy, neuropathy, nephropathy, vessel calcifications, and cataracts. As a rule, degenerative lesions are not clinically detectable until 10 to 20 years after the onset of disease. The basic abnormality in these lesions is not known.

472. The answer is A (1, 2, 3). *(DeGroot, p 1826. Williams, ed 5. p 53.)* The concentration of human growth hormone in blood varies markedly but with no regular periodicity in the course of 24 hours. There is a surge of growth hormone secretion during deep sleep (stage IV); lower values are associated with the rapid eye movement stage of sleep. Growth hormone concentrations can be increased by various stimuli including hypoglycemia, stress, and exercise. Certain amino acids (primarily arginine), vasopressin, pyrogen, and L-dopa can also increase growth hormone levels. Although their mode of action is unknown, these stimuli can be used to distinguish normal children from those who are growth-hormone-deficient because the latter will not exhibit increases in growth hormone levels. Medroxyprogesterone acetate has not been used as a stimulus for growth hormone secretion.

473. The answer is A (1, 2, 3). *(Vaughan, ed 11. p 1620.)* The syndrome of inappropriate antidiuretic hormone (ADH) secretion originally was described in adults who had bronchogenic carcinoma of the lung; the tumor in these patients secreted a peptide that had ADH-like properties. In children, the syndrome usually develops when administration of hypotonic intravenous fluids accompanies general anesthesia, central nervous system infection or trauma, or any other condition in which the secretion of endogenous ADH is enhanced. Because affected individuals are unable to excrete dilute urine, overhydration and hyponatremia result. The appropriate treatment is fluid restriction.

474. The answer is A (1, 2, 3). *(Federman, p 143. Gardner, ed 2. pp 476, 500, 571.)* The most common cause of ambiguous genitalia in female infants is congenital adrenal hyperplasia (21-hydroxylase deficiency). Maternal ingestion of androgens or progestins, the latter usually prescribed because of a threatened abortion, also may virilize a female fetus. True hermaphroditism, which is due to the presence of both ovarian and testicular tissue in the same individual, is a rare cause. Infants who have neonatal Cushing's syndrome present with massive obesity, plethora, and thinning of the skin but no evidence of virilization.

475. The answer is C (2, 4). *(Gardner, ed 2. p 565.)* Patients with testicular feminization, a genetic disorder transmitted as an X-linked recessive trait, are genetic males (karyotype 46,XY) with normal female external genitalia. The syndrome is caused by peripheral androgen resistance due to an abnormality of receptors within the cytosol; as a result, androgen translocation into the nucleus, a crucial step in mediating androgen action, fails to occur. Diagnosis is made either during infancy or childhood when testicular tissue is found in a hernial sac at herniorrhaphy or after puberty when affected individuals present with primary amenorrhea. Well-developed vasa deferentia and epididymes are usually present; and although there is no uterus, rudimentary müllerian elements may be discovered. At puberty, individuals with testicular feminization undergo normal female breast development and may grow small amounts of sexual hair.

476. The answer is B (1, 3). *(Gardner, ed 2. p 138. Rudolph, ed 16. p 698. Williams, ed 5. p 86.)* Children with diabetes mellitus in early stages classically present with polyuria, polydipsia, and polyphagia. Later on, anorexia rather than polyphagia is a frequent complaint. Central diabetes insipidus is caused by a deficiency of vasopressin (antidiuretic hormone). Because the renal collecting tubules are impermeable to water, hypotonic urine is formed. Polyuria, thirst, polydipsia, and anorexia are characteristic. Children with nephrogenic diabetes insipidus become symptomatic shortly after birth. Phosphate diabetes (hypophosphatemic rickets) presents with the characteristic signs and symptoms of rickets and not with polyuria and polydipsia.

477. The answer is A (1, 2, 3). *(Gardner, ed 2. p 226.)* Infants with congenital hypothyroidism may not manifest any symptoms or signs in the early weeks of life. Patients with secondary or tertiary hypothyroidism will have a normal (lower limit of the assay) concentration of thyroid-stimulating hormone and low levels of thyroxine. Most of the thyroid hormone in the circulation is protein bound, predominantly to thyroxine-binding globulin and thyroxine-binding prealbumin. Only the unbound (free) fraction is metabolically active; it regulates the pituitary secretion of thyroid-stimulating hormone by a negative feedback mechanism. In thyroxine-binding globulin deficiency, a hereditary disorder transmitted as an X-linked dominant trait, total thyroxine concentration is low although free thyroxine concentration is normal. Individuals who have this disorder have a normal metabolic rate and normal serum concentration of thyroid-stimulating hormone. This infant does not have primary hypothyroidism, in which one would expect a low level of thyroxine and a **high** concentration of thyroid-stimulating hormone.

478. The answer is E (all). *(Gardner, ed 2. p 103.)* Tall stature in children usually is familial and cannot be traced to an underlying physiologic or metabolic abnormality. Causes of nonfamilial tall stature include pituitary gigantism (growth hormone excess), cerebral gigantism, Marfan's syndrome, homocystinuria, and chromosomal disorders, including karyotypes 47,XXY (Klinefelter's syndrome) and 47,XYY. Although boys rarely complain of tall stature, excessive height may pose psychosocial problems for girls. The use of estrogens to accelerate epiphyseal closure and reduce final adult height in girls has been advocated in the past. However, in view of the possible carcinogenicity of estrogens, this therapy must be used with caution.

479. The answer is B (1, 3). *(Stanbury, ed 4. p 206.)* In the presence of a normal pituitary gland, a deficiency of thyroid hormones causes an elevation in thyroid-stimulating hormone levels and enlargement of the thyroid gland. Five familial disorders of thyroid hormone synthesis, including peroxidase deficiency, iodide transport defect, failure of iodotyrosine coupling, failure of iodotyrosine deiodinase activity, and altered thyroglobulin synthesis, cause goiter and hypothyroidism in neonates. In addition, maternal ingestion of goitrogens (e.g., iodide or antithyroid drugs), which cross the placenta, may cause neonatal hypothyroidism. Deficiency of thyroid-stimulating hormone may produce neonatal hypothyroidism but not gland enlargement. Thyroid hormone does not cross the placenta, and therefore, maternal ingestion would be neither beneficial nor harmful to a fetus.

480. The answer is B (1, 3). *(DeLuca, Annu Rev Biochem 45:631, 1976.)* Ergocalciferol (vitamin D_2) and cholecalciferol (vitamin D_3) are hydroxylated in hepatic mitochondria to form 25-hydroxy vitamin D. The rate of conversion is controlled by the concentration of 25-hydroxy vitamin D. A second hydroxylation takes place in the kidney, forming either the metabolically active compound 1,25-dihydroxy vitamin D or inactive 24,25-dihydroxy vitamin D. Formation of 1,25-dihydroxy vitamin D, the rate-limiting step in the metabolism of the vitamin, is enhanced by parathormone and low plasma phosphorus levels and is inhibited by high concentrations of calcium and phosphorus. The active form of vitamin D promotes calcium absorption in the small intestine and promotes calcium resorption from bone.

481. The answer is A (1, 2, 3). *(Senior, J Pediatr 82:555, 1973.)* In the immediate postabsorptive state, glycogen stores are metabolized to meet energy requirements. In fasting, however, as the supply of glycogen diminishes, the body must gradually switch to lipid metabolism. Accordingly, insulin concentration is diminished and lipolysis and ketogenesis are enhanced. Serum free fatty acids and ketones are at high levels and are used as fuel. Glucose utilization diminishes and glucose concentration is maintained at a level commensurate with the ability of the body to use alternate fuels.

482. The answer is A (1, 2, 3). *(DeGroot, pp 1184-1185.)* Cushing's disease is caused by increased secretion of adrenocorticotropic hormone by the pituitary. Trans-sphenoidal removal of the adenoma, if present, is the treatment of choice. However, this is not always possible, and other methods of therapy must be considered. Irradiation of the pituitary, either by conventional means or by proton beam, has been reported to cure some patients. A number of patients may require total hypophysectomy, and those who do not respond must have total adrenalectomy. Partial adrenalectomy is no longer recommended.

483-487. The answers are: 483-A, 484-E, 485-D, 486-B, 487-D. *(Harrison, pp 84, 117, 219, 258. Williams, ed 5. p 764.)* Vitamin D-resistant rickets is caused by a genetic abnormality in the renal tubular absorption of phosphate with resultant hyperphosphaturia and hypophosphatemia. No other renal tubular abnormality is present. The intestinal absorption of phosphate is also abnormal and calcium absorption from the gut may be secondarily affected. Calcium concentration is usually normal. The disorder is transmitted as an X-linked dominant trait.

Patients with pseudohypoparathyroidism have the same chemical abnormality (low Ca, high PO_4) as those with hypoparathyroidism. They are distinguished from the latter group by their phenotypic features and high serum concentration of parathormone. The basic abnormality in these patients is the unresponsiveness of the renal tubules to parathyroid hormone. They are classified into two groups depending on the site of the defect. Type I patients have failure to generate cyclic AMP and do not have an increase in urinary concentration of cyclic AMP or phosphate in response to parathyroid hormone. Type II patients have a defect in the renal tubules which causes failure to respond to high concentrations of cyclic AMP. These patients, if given parathyroid hormone, have increased urinary excretion of cyclic AMP but not of phosphate.

Osteogenesis imperfecta is a genetic disorder transmitted as an autosomal recessive (severe form) or, more commonly, autosomal dominant (mild form) trait. The basic defect is an abnormality in the production and composition of the matrix of bone cells. Serum calcium and phosphate concentrations are normal.

Hyperparathyroidism is rare in children. In response to high concentrations of parathyroid hormone there is increased bone resorption. In the kidney there is increased excretion of phosphate and enhanced formation of 1,25-dihydroxy vitamin D. Increased formation of 1,25-dihydroxy vitamin D in turn enhances the absorption of calcium and, secondarily, of phosphorus from the gut. The net effect is hypercalcemia and hypophosphatemia.

Medullary carcinoma of thyroid arises from the C cells of the thyroid. These tumors secrete excessive amounts of calcitonin and accordingly the concentration of this hormone in the blood is increased. Despite elevated levels of calcitonin, the serum concentration of calcium and of phosphorus is usually normal.

488-493. The answers are: 488-E, 489-A, 490-B, 491-E, 492-E, 493-B. *(Gardner, ed 2. pp 500, 1324, 1333. Wilkins, ed 3. p 262. Williams, ed 5. pp 255, 730.)* The Prader-Willi syndrome is a disorder consisting of hypotonia, hypogonadism, hyperphagia, and varying degrees of mental retardation. Children affected by this sydrome exhibit little movement in utero and are hypotonic during the neonatal period. Feeding difficulties and failure to thrive may be the presenting complaints in the first year; later, obesity becomes the most common presenting complaint. The enormous food intake of affected children is thought to be due to a defect in the satiety center in the hypothalamus. Stringent caloric restriction is the only known treatment.

Laurence-Moon-Biedl syndrome is transmitted as an autosomal recessive trait. Obesity, mental retardation, hypogonadism, polydactyly, and retinitis pigmentosa with night blindness are the principal findings in affected children. There is no known effective treatment.

The initial complaint in Cushing's syndrome may be obesity. Accumulation of fat in the face, neck, and trunk causes the characteristic "buffalo hump" and "moon" facies. Characteristic features include growth failure, muscle wasting, thinning of the skin, plethora, and hypertension. The bone age of affected patients is retarded, and osteoporosis may be present. The disorder results from an excess of glucocorticoids that may be caused by a primary adrenal abnormality (adenoma or carcinoma) or secondary hypercortisolism, which may be due to excess adrenocorticotropin. Exogenous glucocorticoids administered in supraphysiologic doses for a prolonged period of time will produce a similar picture in normal subjects.

Pseudohypoparathyroidism is a familial disorder probably transmitted as an X-linked dominant trait. Affected patients have biochemical findings (low serum calcium and high serum phosphorus levels) similar to those associated with hypoparathyroidism, but they also have high levels of endogenous parathormone; in addition, exogenous parathormone fails to increase their phosphate excretion or raise their serum calcium level. The defect in these patients appears to be either at the hormone receptor site or in the adenylate cyclase-

Endocrine, Metabolic, and Genetic Disorders 241

cyclic AMP system. The symptoms of pseudohypoparathyroidism are due to hypocalcemia. Affected children are short, round-faced, and mildly retarded. Metacarpals and metatarsals are shortened, and metastatic calcifications, basal ganglia calcifications, and cataracts may be present. The current treatment consists of large doses of vitamin D and reduction of the phosphate load.

Frohlich's syndrome was described originally in an obese boy with sexual infantilism and shortness of stature but is no longer used as a diagnostic term.

494-500. The answers are: **494-A, 495-E, 496-E, 497-D, 498-B, 499-A, 500-B.** *(Gardner, ed 2. pp 138, 145, 478, 511. Williams, ed 5. pp 91, 605, 942.)* In the salt-losing variety of 21-hydroxylase deficiency, the synthesis of both mineralocorticoids (e.g., aldosterone) and cortisol is impaired. Aldosterone deficiency impairs the exchange of potassium for sodium in the distal renal tubule. Affected patients have hyponatremia and hyperkalemia. Dehydration, hypotension, and shock may be present.

In the absence of vasopressin, renal collecting tubules are impermeable to water, resulting in the excretion of hypotonic urine. Patients with diabetes insipidus present with polyuria and polydipsia. Net loss of water leads to dehydration and hemoconcentration and, therefore, to relatively high serum concentrations of sodium and potassium. Patients with nephrogenic diabetes insipidus have similar laboratory findings. This genetic disorder is unresponsive to antidiuretic hormone (ADH). These patients are unable to concentrate their urine and present in the neonatal period with hypernatremic dehydration.

In hyperaldosteronism, renal tubular sodium-potassium exchange is enhanced. Hypokalemia, hypernatremia, hyperchloremia, and alkalosis are the usual findings. Primary hyperaldosteronism (Conn's syndrome) is very rare in children.

The hallmark of the syndrome of inappropriate secretion of antidiuretic hormone is the coexistence of hyponatremia, overhydration, and inappropriately high concentrations of sodium in the urine. Levels of serum potassium that are slightly lower than normal are the consequence of dilution and secondary hyperaldosteronism.

Addison's disease is associated with a combined deficiency of glucocorticoids and mineralocorticoids. Resorption of sodium and excretion of potassium and hydrogen ions are impaired at the level of the distal renal tubules. Sodium loss results in loss of water and depletion of blood volume. Individuals with compensated Addison's disease may have relatively normal physical and laboratory findings; Addisonian crisis, however, characteristically produces hyponatremia, hyperkalemia, and shock. The pathophysiology of the serum electrolyte abnormalities in this disorder is the same as in the salt-losing variety of adrenogenital syndrome.

Patients with a deficiency of glucose-6-phosphatase (von Gierke's disease) are, as a rule, hyperlipemic. Increased triglyceride concentration in the serum decreases the volume and solute content of the aqueous compartment. Because electrolytes are present only in the aqueous compartment of the serum but are expressed in milliequivalents per liter of serum as a whole, the concentrations of sodium and potassium are factitiously low in these patients.

Bibliography

Alpert E: Pathogenesis of arthritis associated with viral hepatitis. *N Engl J Med* 285:185-189, 1971.

American Academy of Pediatrics, Committee on Nutrition: Iron supplementation for infants. *Pediatrics* 58:765, 1976.

Avery GB (ed): *Neonatology: Pathophysiology and Management of the Newborn.* Philadelphia, JB Lippincott, 1975.

Baraff LJ, Wilkins J, Wehrle PF: The role of antibiotics, immunization, and adenoviruses in pertussis. *Pediatrics* 61:224-230, 1978.

Behrman RE: *Neonatal-Perinatal Medicine: Diseases of the Fetus and Infant,* 2nd ed. St. Louis, CV Mosby, 1977.

Bell WE, McCormick WF: *Increased Intracranial Pressure in Children,* 2nd ed., vol 8. Philadelphia, WB Saunders, 1978.

Bell WE, McCormick WF: *Neurologic Infections in Children,* vol 12. Philadelphia, WB Saunders, 1975.

Bowman JM: *Current Problems in Pediatric Hematology.* New York: Grune & Stratton, 1975.

Braunwald E: *Heart Disease: A Textbook of Cardiovascular Medicine.* Philadelphia, WB Saunders, 1980.

Brooke MH: *A Clinician's View of Neuromuscular Diseases.* Baltimore, Williams & Wilkins, 1977.

Browne TB: Valproic acid. *N Engl J Med* 302:661-665, 1980.

Burks J: Iron deficiency in an eskimo village. *J Pediatr* 88:224-226, 1976.

Caffey J, et al: *Pediatric X-Ray Diagnosis,* 7th ed. Chicago, Year Book Medical, 1978.

Calderon R: Myotonic dystrophy: a neglected cause of mental retardation. *J Pediatr* 68:423-431, 1966.

Cornblath M, Schwartz R: *Disorders of Carbohydrate Metabolism in Infancy,* 2nd ed. Philadelphia, WB Saunders, 1976.

Dallman PR: Iron deficiency in infancy and childhood. *Report of the International Nutritional Anemia Consultative Group (INACG),* 1979.

D'Angio GJ: Wilms' tumor: an update. *Cancer* 45:1791-1798, 1980.

DeGroot LJ (ed): *Endocrinology.* New York, Grune & Stratton, 1979.

DeGroot LJ, Stanbury JB: *The Thyroid Diseases,* 4th ed. New York, John Wiley, 1975.

DeLuca HF, Schnoes HK: Metabolism and mechanism of action of vitamin D. *Annu Rev Biochem* 45:631, 1976.

Denny FW, Clyde WA Jr, Glezen WP: *Mycoplasma pneumoniae* disease: clinical spectrum, pathophysiology, epidemiology, and control. *J Infect Dis* 123:74, 1971.

DeVivo DC, Keating JP, Haymond MW: Acute encephalopathy with fatty infiltration of the viscera. *Pediatr Clin North Am* 23:527-540, 1976.

Dillon HC: Impetigo contagiosa: suppurative and non-suppurative complications. *Am J Dis Child* 115:530-541, 1968.

Dodge PR: Myotonic dystrophy in infancy and childhood. *Pediatrics* 35:3-19, 1965.

Dodge PR, Swartz MN: Bacterial meningitis—a review of selected aspects. *N Engl J Med* 272:954-960, 1003-1010, 1965.

Dubowitz V: *Muscle Disorders in Childhood,* vol 16. Philadelphia, WB Saunders, 1978.

Evans AE: A review of 17 IV-S neuroblastoma patients at the Children's Hospital of Philadelphia. *Cancer* 45:833-839, 1980.

Evans AE, Angio GJ, Koop CE: Diagnosis and treatment of neuroblastoma. *Pediatr Clin North Am* 23:161-170, 1976.

Faerø O, Kastrup KW, Nielson EL, et al: Successful prophylaxis of febrile convulsions with phenobarbital. *Epilepsia* 13:279-285, 1972.

Feder HM Jr: Occult pneumococcal bacteremia and the febrile infant and young child—a clinical review. *Clin Pediatr* 19:457-462, 1980.

Federman DD: *Abnormal Sexual Development.* Philadelphia, WB Saunders, 1967.

Feldman WE: Effect of ampicillin and chloramphenicol against *Hemophilus influenzae. Pediatrics* 61:406-409, 1978.

Fishman RA: *Cerebrospinal Fluid in Diseases of the Nervous System.* Philadelphia, WB Saunders, 1980.

Forfar J, Nelson M: Epidemiology of drugs taken by pregnant women—drugs that may affect the fetus adversely. *Clin Pharmacol Ther* 14:639-641, 1973.

Friedman WF, Lesch M, Sonnenblick EH (eds): *Neonatal Heart Disease.* New York, Grune & Stratton, 1973.

Bibliography 245

Gangarosa E, Merson M: Epidemiologic assessment of the relevance of the so-called enteropathogenic serogroups of *Escherichia coli* in diarrhea. *N Engl J Med* 296:1210-1213, 1977.

Gardner LI: *Endocrine and Genetic Diseases of Childhood and Adolescence*, 2nd ed. Philadelphia, WB Saunders, 1975.

Gellis SS (ed): *Year Book of Pediatrics.* Chicago, Year Book Medical, 1978.

Goldman P, Peppercorn MA: Drug therapy: sulfasalazine. *N Engl J Med* 293:20-23, 1975.

Greenberger N: Medium chain triglycerides, physiological considerations and clinical implications. *N Engl J Med* 280:1045-1058, 1969.

Greseon NT, Kirkpatrick JA, Girdang BR, et al: Gastric antral narrowing in chronic granulomatous disease of childhood. *Pediatrics* 54:456, 1974.

Haller JS, Wolpert SM, Rabe BF, et al: Cystic lesions of the posterior fossa in infants: a comparison of the clinical, radiological and pathological findings in Dandy-Walker syndrome and extra-axial cysts. *Neurology* 21:494-506, 1971.

Harrison HE, Harrison HC: *Disorders of Calcium and Phosphate Metabolism in Childhood and Adolescence.* Philadelphia, WB Saunders, 1979.

Higby DJ: Granulocyte transfusions: current status. *Blood* 55:2-8, 1980.

Hoekelman RA, et al (eds): *Principles of Pediatrics: Health Care of the Young.* New York, McGraw-Hill, 1978.

Hopkins CC, Dismukes WE, Glick TH, et al: Surveillance of paralytic poliomyelitis in the United States. *JAMA* 210:694-700, 1969.

Hurst JW, et al (eds): *The Heart,* 4th ed. New York, McGraw-Hill, 1978.

Hymes K, Schur PH, Karpatkin S: Heavy-chain subclass of round antiplatelet IgG in autoimmune thrombocytopenic purpura. *Blood* 56:84-87, 1980.

Illingsworth RS: *The Development of the Infant and Young Child: Abnormal and Normal,* 7th ed. New York, Longman, 1980.

Isler W: *Clinics in Developmental Medicine.* New York, JB Lippincott, 1971.

Isselbacher KJ, et al (eds): *Harrison's Principles of Internal Medicine,* 9th ed. New York, McGraw-Hill, 1980.

Jaffe N (ed): *Bone Tumors in Children,* vol 2. Littleton, Mass., PSG Publishing, 1979.

Jennett B: *Epilepsy After Non-Missile Head Injuries,* 2nd ed. Chicago, Year Book Medical, 1975.

Kaplan HS: Hodgkin's disease: unfolding concepts concerning its nature, management, and prognosis. *Cancer* 45:2439-2474, 1980.

Kato HK, Koike S, Yokoyama T: Kawasaki disease: effect of treatment on coronary artery involvement. *Pediatrics* 63:175-179, 1979.

Katz SL: Ampicillin-resistant *Hemophilus influenzae* type b: a status report. *Pediatrics* 55:6-8, 1975.

Keith JD, Rowe RD, Vlad P: *Heart Disease in Infancy and Childhood,* 3rd ed. New York, Macmillan, 1978.

Kelly DH, Shannon DC: Periodic breathing in infants with near-miss sudden infant death syndrome. *Pediatrics* 63:355-360, 1979.

Kerr DN, Harrison CV, Sherlock S, et al: Congenital hepatic fibrosis. *Q J Med* 30:91-117, 1961.

Klaus MH, Fanaroff AA: *Care of the High Risk Neonate,* 2nd ed. Philadelphia, WB Saunders, 1980.

Klein JO: Current usage of antimicrobial combinations in pediatrics. *Pediatr Clin North Am* 21:443-456, 1974.

Kohl S: *Yersinia enterocolitica* infections in children. *Pediatr Clin North Am* 26:433-443, 1979.

Krugman S, Ward R, Katz SC: *Infectious Diseases of Children,* 7th ed. St. Louis, CV Mosby, 1980.

Lacey JR, Penty JK: *Infantile Spasms.* New York, Raven Press, 1976.

Lampkin BC, McWilliams MB, Mauer AM: Cell kinetics and chemotherapy in acute leukemia. *Semin Hematol* 9:211-223, 1972.

Levine PH: Efficacy of self-therapy in hemophilia. *N Engl J Med* 291:1381-1384, 1974.

Lightsey AL Jr, Koenig HM, McMillan R, et al: Platelet-associated immunoglobulin G in childhood idiopathic thrombocytopenic purpura. *J Pediatr* 94:201-204, 1979.

Lindenbaum J: Megaloblastic anemia and neutrophil hypersegmentation. *Br J Haematol* 44:511-513, 1980.

Lipton JM, Nathan DG: Aplastic and hypoplastic anemia. *Pediatr Clin North Am* 27:217-235, 1980.

Lumicao GG, Heggie AD: Chlamydial infections. *Pediatr Clin North Am* 26:269-282, 1979.

Lux SE, Wolfe LC: Inherited disorders of the red cell membrane skeleton. *Pediatr Clin North Am* 27:463-486, 1980.

Mathis RK, Andres JM, Walker WA: Liver disease in infants. Part II: Hepatic disease states. *J Pediatr* 90:864-880, 1977.

Bibliography

Mauer AM: Therapy of acute lymphoblastic leukemia in childhood. *Blood* 56:1-10, 1980.

McRae DL: Observations on craniolacunia. *Acta Radiol (Diagn)* 5:55-64, 1966.

Meissner HC, Smith AL: The current status of chloramphenicol. *Pediatrics* 64:348-356, 1979.

Menkes JH: *Textbook of Child Neurology,* 2nd ed. Philadelphia, Lea & Febiger, 1980.

Montpetit VJ, Anderman F, Carpenter S, et al: Subacute necrotizing encephalomyelopathy. *Brain* 94:1-30, 1971.

Nadas AS, Fyler DC: *Pediatric Cardiology,* 3rd ed. Philadelphia, WB Saunders, 1972.

Nathan DG, Oski FA: *Hematology of Infancy and Childhood,* 2nd ed. Philadelphia, WB Saunders, 1981.

Necheles TF, Rai US, Valaes T: The role of hemolysis in neonatal hyperbilirubinemia as reflected in carboxyhemoglobin levels. *Acta Paediatr* 65: 361-367, 1976.

Nelson KB, Ellenberg JH: Predictors of epilepsy in children who have experienced febrile seizures. *N Engl J Med* 295:1029-1033, 1976.

Neville BG: Central nervous system involvement in leukemia. *Dev Med Child Neurol* 14:75-78, 1972.

Oski FA, Jaffe ER, Miecher PA: *Monograph: Current Problems in Pediatric Hematology.* New York, Grune & Stratton, 1975.

Oski FA, Stockman JA: Anemia due to inadequate iron sources or poor iron utilization. *Pediatr Clin North Am* 27:237-253, 1980.

Oski FA, Stockman JA: *The Year Book of Pediatrics.* Chicago, Year Book Medical, 1979.

Partin JD: Mitochondrial ultra-structure in Reye's syndrome. *N Engl J Med* 285:1139-1143, 1971.

Patterson MJ, Hafeez A: Group B streptococci in human disease. *Bacteriol Rev* 40:774-792, 1976.

Perloff JK: *The Clinical Recognition of Congenital Heart Disease,* 2nd ed. Philadelphia, WB Saunders, 1978.

Peter G, Smith AL: Group A streptococcal infections of the skin and pharynx. *N Engl J Med* 297:311-317, 365-370, 1977.

Philip AGS, Hewitt JR: Early diagnosis of neonatal sepsis. *Pediatrics* 65:1036-1041, 1980.

Pincus JH: Subacute necrotizing encephalopathy (Leigh's disease): a consideration of clinical features and etiology. *Dev Med Child Neurol* 14:87-101, 1972.

Piomelli S, Brickman A, Carlos E: Rapid diagnosis of iron deficiency by measurement of FEP/hemoglobin ratio. *Pediatrics* 57:136-141, 1976.

Piomelli S, Yachnin S: *Current Topics in Hematology,* vol 1. New York, Alan R. Liss, 1978.

Pollack JD: *Reye's Syndrome.* New York, Grune & Stratton, 1975.

Price RA, Jamieson PA: The central nervous system in childhood leukemia. II. Subacute leucoencephalopathy. *Cancer* 35:306-318, 1975.

Prince AS, Neu HC: Antibiotic-associated pseudomembranous colitis in children. *Pediatr Clin North Am* 26:261-268, 1979.

Rabe EF: Skull transillumination in infants. *GP* 36:78, 1967.

Reye RD: Encephalopathy and fatty degeneration of the viscera: a disease entity in childhood. *Lancet* 2:749-757, 1963.

Robinson SJ: Diagnosis of congenital heart disease. *Cardiovasc Clin* 2:75-95, 1970.

Root AW, Harrison HE: Recent advances in calcium metabolism. *J Pediatr* 88: 1-18, 177-179, 1976.

Rose AL, Lumbroso CT: Neonatal seizure states. *Pediatrics* 45:404-425, 1970.

Rubenstein L, Herman MM, Long TF, et al: Disseminated necrotizing leucoencephalopathy: a complication of treated central nervous system leukemia and lymphoma. *Cancer* 35:291-305, 1975.

Rudolph AM, et al (eds): *Pediatrics*, 16th ed. New York, Appleton-Century-Crofts, 1977.

Rutherford CJ: The decision to perform staging laparotomy in symptomatic Hodgkin's disease. *Br J Haematol* 45:2439-2474, 1980.

Saarinen UM: Serum ferritin in assessment of iron nutrition in healthy infants. *Acta Paediatr Scand* 67:745, 1978.

Sabesin SM, Koff RS: Pathogenesis of experimental viral hepatitis. *N Engl J Med* 290:944-950, 996-1002, 1974.

Sanford JP: Legionnaires' disease—the first thousand days. *N Engl J Med* 300: 654-656, 1979.

Schaffer AJ, Avery ME: *Diseases of the Newborn,* 4th ed. Philadelphia, WB Saunders, 1977.

Schapiro RL: *Clinical Radiology of the Pediatric Abdomen Gastrointestinal Tract.* Baltimore, University Park Press, 1976.

Scharli A, Sieber WK, Kiesewetter WB: Hypertrophic pyloric stenosis at Children's Hospital of Pittsburgh from 1912 to 1967: a critical review. *J Pediatr Surg* 4:108-114, 1969.

Schiff L: *Diseases of the Liver*, 4th ed. Philadelphia, JB Lippincott, 1975.

Schmidt RP, Wilder BJ: *Epilepsy: A Clinical Textbook.* Philadelphia, FA Davis, 1968.

Schwartz E: *Monograph: Hemoglobinopathies in Children*, vol III. Littleton, Mass., PSG Publishing, 1980.

Scriver CR, Rosenberg LE: *Amino Acid Metabolism and Its Disorders.* Philadelphia, WB Saunders, 1973.

Senior B: Ketotic hypoglycemia. A tale (tail) of Gauss? *J Pediatr* 82:555-556, 1973.

Senior B, Sadeghi-Nejad A: The glycogenoses and other inherited disorders of carbohydrate metabolism. *Clin Perinatol* 3:79, 1976.

Seto DSY: Viral hepatitis. *Pediatr Clin North Am* 26:305-314, 1979.

Shumway CN: Iron deficiency in children. *Pediatr Clin North Am* 19:855, 1972.

Silverman A, Roy CC, Cozzetto FJ: *Pediatric Clinical Gastroenterology*, 2nd ed. St. Louis, CV Mosby, 1975.

Simone JV: The treatment of acute lymphoblastic leukemia. *Br J Haematol* 45:1-4, 1980.

Singer WD, Rabe EF, Haller JS: The effect of ACTH therapy upon infantile spasms. *J Pediatr* 96:485-489, 1980.

Sleisenger MH, Fordtran JS: *Gastrointestinal Disease: Pathophysiology, Diagnosis, Management*, 2nd ed. Philadelphia, WB Saunders, 1978.

Smith DW: *Recognizable Patterns of Human Malformation: Genetic, Embryologic and Clinical Aspects,* 2nd ed. Philadelphia, WB Saunders, 1976.

Stanbury JB, Wyngaarden JB, Fredrickson DS: *The Metabolic Basis of Inherited Disease,* 4th ed. New York, McGraw-Hill, 1978.

Steinhoff MC: Rotavirus: the first five years. *J Pediatr* 96:611-622, 1980.

Stirling ML: Minimum effective dose of intermediate factor VIII concentrate in hemophiliacs on home therapy. *Lancet* 1:813-814, 1979.

Sullivan DW: Hereditary spherocytosis. *Pediatr Ann* 9:38-42, 1980.

Suzuki H, White JJ, el-Shafie M, et al: Nonoperative diagnosis of Hirschsprung's disease in neonates. *Pediatrics* 51:188-191, 1973.

Swaiman KF, Wright FS: *The Practice of Pediatric Neurology.* St. Louis, CV Mosby, 1975.

Swensen O, Sherman JO, Fisher JH: Diagnosis of congenital megacolon: an analysis of 501 patients. *J Pediatr Surg* 8:587-594, 1973.

Taylor-Robinson D, McCormack WM: The genital mycoplasmas. *N Engl J Med* 302:1003-1010, 1063-1067, 1980.

Tipple, MA, Been MO, Saxon EM: Clinical characteristics of the afebrile pneumonia associated with *Chlamydia trachomatis* infection in infants less than 6 months of age. *Pediatrics* 63:192-197, 1979.

Torphy DD, Bond WW: *Campylobacter fetus* infections in children. *Pediatrics* 64:896-903, 1979.

Trier JS: Diagnostic value per oral biopsy of the proximal small intestine. *N Engl J Med* 285:1470, 1973.

Ulshen MH, Rollo JL: Pathogenesis of *Escherichia coli* gastroenteritis in man — another mechanism. *N Engl J Med* 302:99-101, 1980.

Vaughan VC III, McKay RJ, Behrman RE: *Nelson Textbook of Pediatrics,* 11th ed. Philadelphia, WB Saunders, 1979.

Vietti TJ, Valerioti FA: Conceptual basis for use of chemotherapeutic agents and their pharmacology. *Pediatr Clin North Am* 23:67-92, 1976.

Walton JN: *Disorders of Voluntary Muscle,* 3rd ed. New York, Longman, 1974.

Watson H (ed): *Paediatric Cardiology.* St. Louis, CV Mosby, 1968.

Wilkins L: *The Diagnosis and Treatment of Endocrine Disorders in Childhood and Adolescence,* 3rd ed. Springfield, CC Thomas, 1966.

Williams RH (ed): *Textbook of Endocrinology,* 5th ed. Philadelphia, WB Saunders, 1974.

Williams WJ, et al: *Hematology,* 2nd ed. New York, McGraw-Hill, 1977.

Wilson, HD, Eichenwald HF: Sepsis neonatorum. *Pediatr Clin North Am* 21: 571-581, 1974.

Woodruff CW, Wright SW, Wright RP: The role of fresh cow's milk in iron deficiency. II. Comparison of fresh cow's milk with a prepared formula. *Am J Dis Child* 124:26-30, 1972.

Yow MD, Katz SL: *Red Book,* 18th ed. Evanston, Illinois, American Academy of Pediatrics, Report of the Committee on Infectious Diseases, 1977.

Zieve L: Pathogenesis of hepatic coma. *Arch Intern Med* 118:211-223, 1966.

ASHEVILLE-BUNCOMBE TECHNICAL INSTITUTE
DEPT. OF COMMUNITY COLLEGES
LIBRARIES

DISCARDED

JUN 26 2025

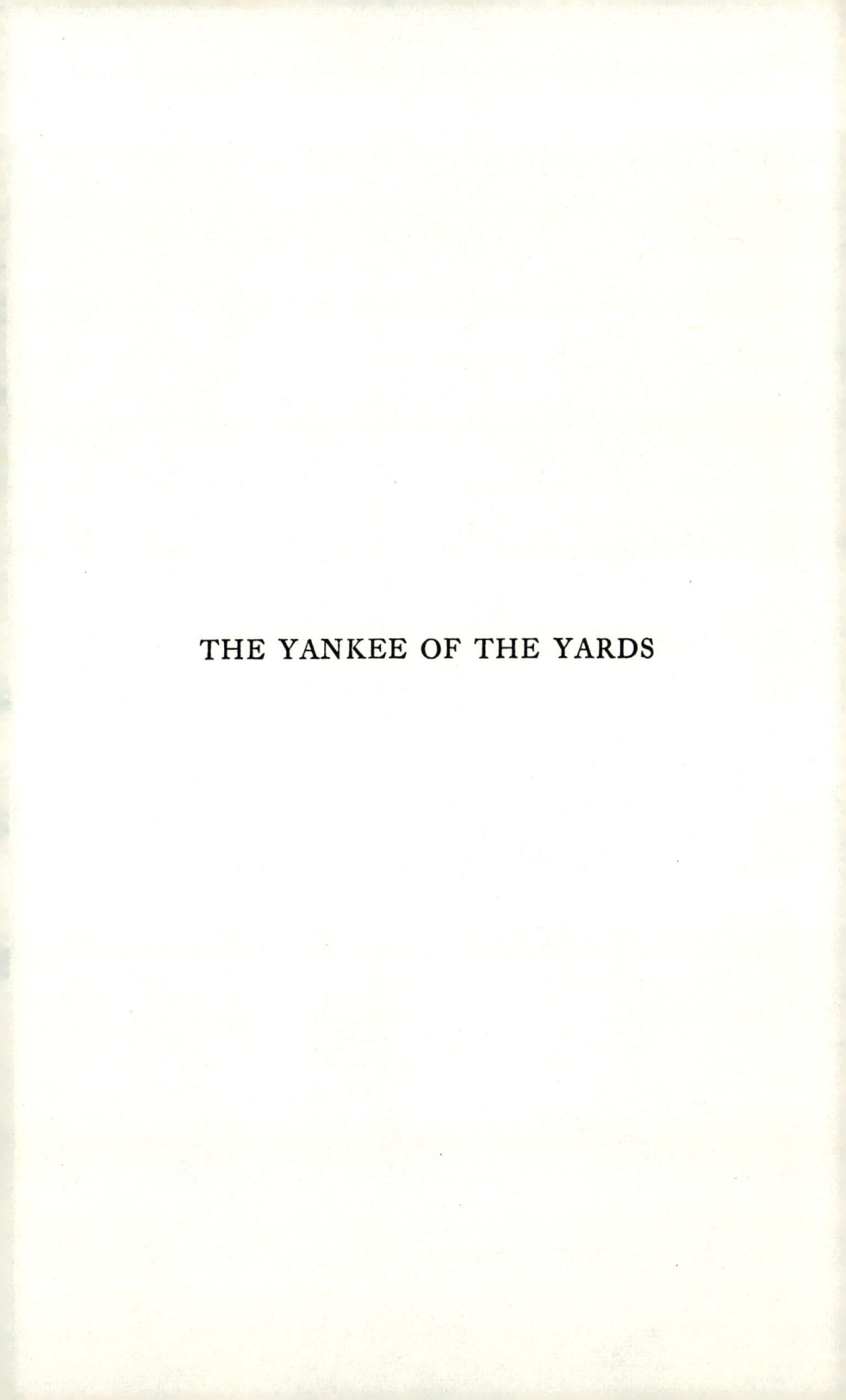

THE YANKEE OF THE YARDS

SWIFT & COMPANY

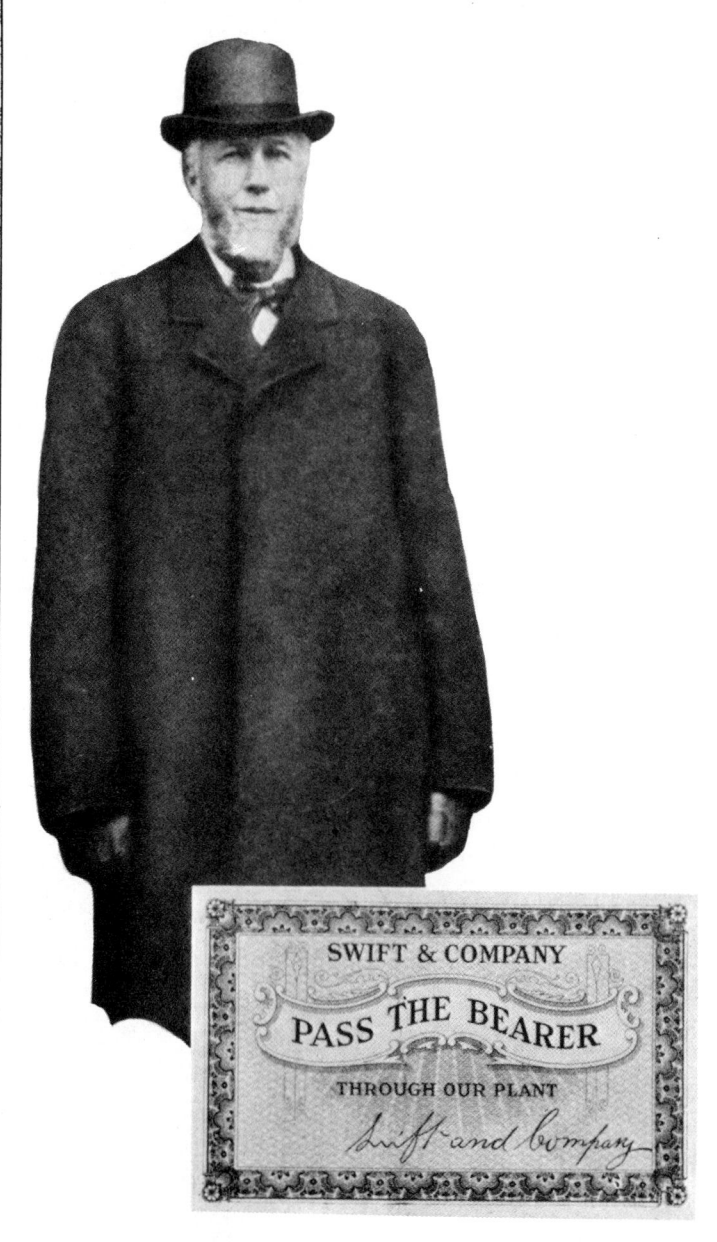

PASS THE BEARER

THROUGH OUR PLANT

Swift and Company

GUSTAVUS FRANKLIN SWIFT ABOUT 1902. A PASS
CARD FOR VISITORS ABOUT THAT TIME.

THE YANKEE OF THE YARDS

THE BIOGRAPHY OF GUSTAVUS FRANKLIN SWIFT

By
LOUIS F. SWIFT
IN COLLABORATION WITH
ARTHUR VAN VLISSINGEN, JR.

◆

AMS PRESS
NEW YORK

Reprinted from the edition of 1927, Chicago
First AMS EDITION published 1970
Manufactured in the United States of America

Library of Congress Catalog Card Number: 78-112003
SBN: 404-06309-8

AMS PRESS, INC.
New York, N. Y. 10003

FOREWORD

SHEER accident has swept many men to that slight height above their fellows which the world calls fame or attainment or success. At their sides stand others who reached the same place by ceaseless work and native shrewdness.

For this reason the life stories of most outstanding men lack interest except to the unimaginative who worship success for its own sake. Accidents which turn out well make dull tales, toiling plodders make still duller.

Rare indeed is the man who attains preeminence with the steady, irresistible thrust—who leaves in those who started with him a sense that his progress was inevitable, that one could no more have stopped him than an Alpine glacier or a Sierra cascade. Such a man, to be sure, combines ability and gluttony for work. But to these sober, uninteresting virtues their owner has the good fortune to add being born at a time and place which make his every stroke count for two or ten or ten thousand times the strokes of men who came before or will come after. Every circumstance from his birth to his grave seems calculated to give him a lead over his fellows. Every apparent misfortune turns out to be his lucky chance.

So it was with the first Vanderbilt. Rockefeller and Ford are subsequent examples in the field of

American industry. And had young Bonaparte been born fifteen years after he was, he would have been a child instead of a lieutenant when France burst into fire. For all his military genius and burning ambition he would probably have served his country as a pompous little colonel of the Guards, while the world went ways far different from those history records.

What created of a corporal an emperor, of these other men the chief commercial figures of their times? For want of a better name we call it destiny, that motive power which makes life interesting—and which makes interesting lives. For it smacks of destiny when force and industry and shrewdness are found in conjunction, with all the auspices favorable to their most effective use.

Destiny it was which presided at the birth of a boy in a Cape Cod village ninety-odd years ago. He was not to change the world's maps, nor make military history. Instead, he was the human instrument by which destiny transformed the world's sources and supplies of an essential class of foodstuffs. From a start which at first glance seems inauspicious, he built a knowledge and an ability that were to serve him well when circumstances called them into full play.

A younger son of a large family on a sandy, unfertile farm in the dreadful '40s, he did not have much of a chance; yet—his elder brothers were butchers and from them he learned the ins and outs of the trade on which he built. New England was a long way from the plains which sent it cattle; still—here a trade current was first felt which lent its strength to the young butcher's brawny blows on Fortune's door. Chicago in the '70s was a sprawling city with little to recommend it to his energies except a plentiful supply of cattle from the western plains. The Yankee left its "Yards" the undisputed meat-packing center of the hungry world.

That he accomplished so much may be surprising, but it is not necessarily of great interest. That he gained great wealth in the process is neither surprising nor worth more than passing comment. That he worked hard, was honest, practiced the homely copybook virtues is neither here nor there.

The salty, spicy fact is that destiny swept him on to accomplishment extraordinary in any one man's career, that his abilities and the world's changing needs came together to produce a career as exceptional as it is interesting. His battles and his victories were in the field of business. It is this, and not the material success he attained, which makes the chronicle of his life a chronicle of commerce.

For destiny, that spinner of men's threads of life, decreed that business should be his skein. . . . .

CONTENTS

Foreword iii

I
"A Dollar Wasted" 3

II
"We Cannot Fail!" 24

III
Just Right or All Wrong 46

IV
Taking the East 65

V
Many a Minute 82

VI
"I Vote No!" 102

VII
He Had to Spread Out 117

VIII
"I Raise Better Men" 138

IX
The Forbidden Yardstick 158

X
Fight When You Must 178

XI

NEVER STAY BEATEN 193

INDEX 213

ILLUSTRATIONS

Gustavus Franklin Swift, about 1902. A pass card for visitors about that time.................... *Frontispiece*	
Union Stockyards of Chicago in 1865..................	10
The slaughterhouse at Barnstable. In the circle, the wagon that G. F. Swift drove when he sold his meats from door to door..............................	50
Longhorns came from the plains of Texas................	72
Edwin C. Swift. D. M. Anthony.....................	78
Louis F. Swift......................................	90
The old Live Stock Exchange Building, Chicago..........	114
Sally Sears Crowell Swift, mother of G. F. Swift. William Swift, father of G. F. Swift......................	120
Wellington Leavitt, dean of the cattle buyers, who became associated with G. F. Swift about 1875, the Prince of Wales, and Louis F. Swift riding through "the Yards" October 13, 1924..............................	128
G. F. Swift, about 1885............................	132
Union Stockyards, Chicago, 1927.....................	154
The farm house at Barnstable. G. F. Swift's accounts, 1859-60, recording sales of meat from his butcher cart.	174
The original windlass used by G. F. Swift for hoisting steer after killing — Barnstable, 1861-1869. The original bull-ring used by G. F. Swift for pulling animal down for slaughter..................................	196

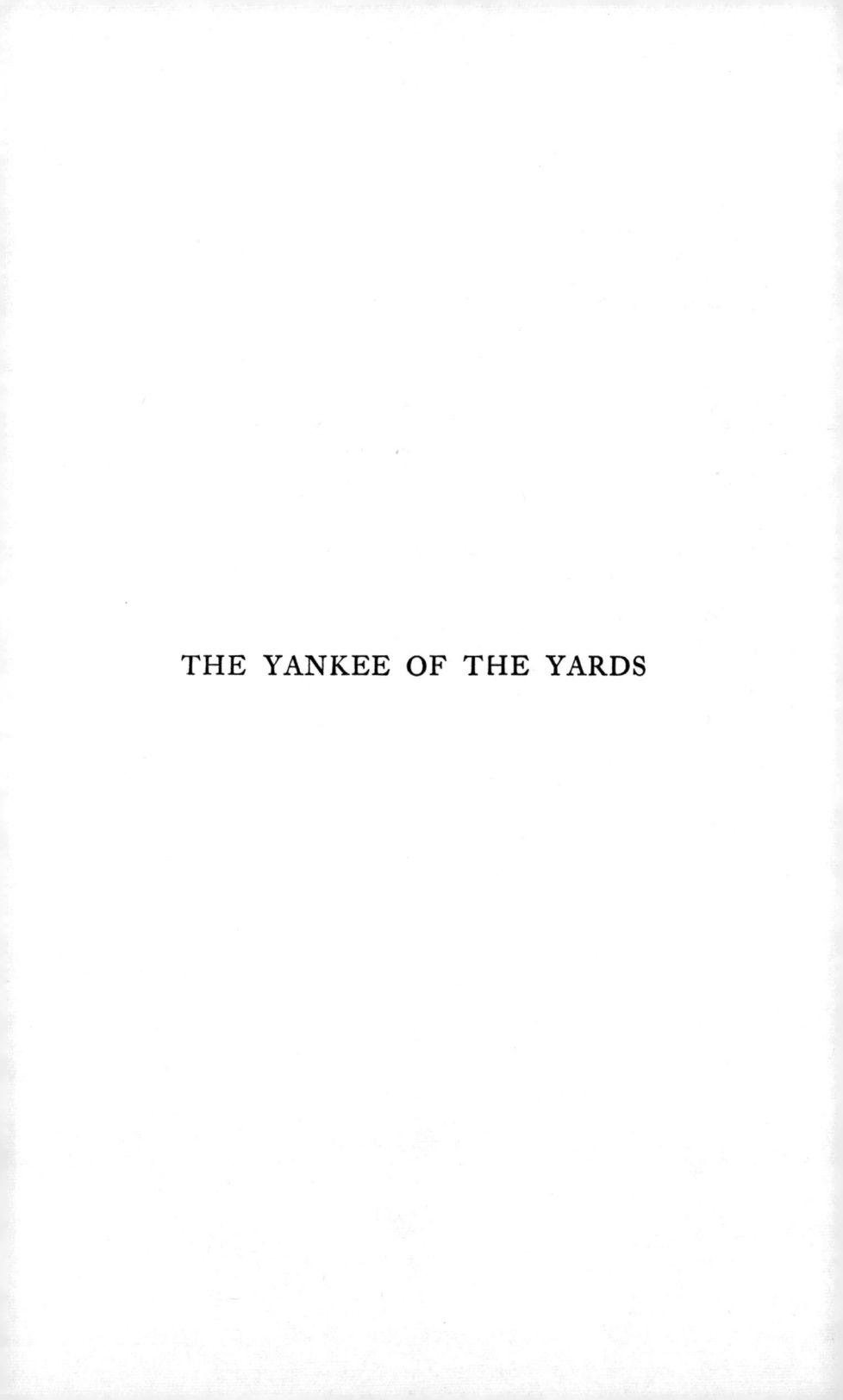

THE YANKEE OF THE YARDS

CHAPTER I

"A DOLLAR WASTED...."

ANYONE whose work kept him on the bank of Chicago's old "Bubbly Creek back of the Yards" was not to be envied his job in the 1880s and '90s. The marvel was that he would hold the job. For where today a boulevard is building astride a huge tiled channel, thirty years ago there ran a malodorous open sewer.

In his turn the workman had something to marvel at: the regularity with which another man visited this unattractive locality. The frequent visitor was a tall bearded man above middle age. He invariably wore a dark suit with a tail coat, and usually a stiff hat. His stoop suggested desk work. His bearing suggested authority. To the knees he had the appearance of a business proprietor fresh from his private office.

At the knees his appearance shifted abruptly. The tailored trousers disappeared into a plebeian pair of top-boots. The cowhide bore unmistakable traces of wear outside the counting room. Plainly the visitor was not one who devoted his time exclusively to papers and meetings and that nebulous science called management.

This man was my father, Gustavus Franklin Swift.

Even after Swift & Company was well established on a large scale, he would frequently visit the bank of Bubbly Creek. He had, in fact, gone to the trouble of finding out where the company's sewer emptied into Old Bubbly; this point was his invariable objective.

It was not a pleasant place to visit. In those days sewage disposal was more direct than scientific. One might have pardoned the head of a large business for avoiding it altogether.

But down to Bubbly Creek father would go, and scrutinize the sewer outlet for a few minutes every once in a while. He was on the lookout for waste. If he saw any fat coming out, that evidenced waste in the packing house. Briskly he would head for the superintendent's office. And before the episode was closed, someone would smart.

His long suit was keeping expenses down. Next in his interest, perhaps, came developing by-products—which is another form of the same thing. Low expenses and maximum return from every pound of the live animal are what made G. F. Swift a leader in the new industry of which he was a founder. For even at the start of his career as a Chicago packer, when margins were not narrowed down as they have been since, he recognized that waste and accomplishment are incompatible. A dollar wasted is gone forever—with no one the better off for its going.

It was his constant seeking after ways to save—a frugality engendered and inbred by ancestors who for two hundred and fifty years had fought a none too equal battle with the miserly sands of Cape Cod—which led the Yankee from Massachusetts and out to the stockyards of Chicago. It was his never-failing creed of economy which built under his leadership a concern that today does a manufacturing business second in volume only to United States Steel.

Truly it may be said, and with little room for dispute, that his sharp eye for the pennies and nickels and dimes founded a compact, economically efficient industry to supplant a scattered assortment of inefficient, uneconomic small units. The proof of the economic service he performed is in the large financial success, on the narrowest of profit margins, of the business unit he built.

Through his years of working with live stock and meat products and packing he had accumulated a fund of experience—sometimes it seemed to a harassed department head that father's experience must be principally a knowledge of where to look for leaks of money or material. His watchfulness—of which his frequent visits to Bubbly Creek were typical—taught every good man in the organization the need for not wasting a penny. Few pennies, consequently, were wasted.

First thing every morning at the office would come the question, "Any hogs die during the night?" If any had died, there was trouble—enough trouble so that the loss did not occur again soon. He knew that hogs, if they have plenty of room, do not smother. Eventually everyone who had anything to do with the company's hogs knew the same thing. So the hogs were kept in roomy, uncrowded pens—and few were lost from this source.

It was the eye for waste which brought Gustavus Swift from the East to Chicago in 1875. Glamour enveloped the cattle business of fifty and sixty years ago. These were the picturesque days of longhorn herds plodding in fogs of dust across the Great Plains.

Wide-hatted cowmen flanked the herds, yipping and swinging their ropes to drive the strays back into line.

Hundreds of miles the steers were herded, to the end of steel where venturesome railroads pushed their pioneering lines into the West. At the railroad the cattle were driven aboard slatted cars and hauled to the East of concentrated populations which demanded beef above the local ability to supply.

The animals were shipped to central live-stock markets. One of these was at Brighton, just outside Boston; another at Albany; another at Buffalo. At these stockyards the animals were sold and shipped to the slaughterers.

An amount of the glamour of the cattle ranges surrounded even the stockyards—diluted glamour, but glamour nevertheless. For here cattlemen rode from pen to pen, bartered on horseback, and in tall cowhide boots swaggered the streets of the cities.

But beyond the stockyards was little of the glamourous. Unsanitary conditions, thriftless practices, unsound customs prevailed on every hand.

Each community had its little slaughterhouse. Animals beyond the local supply were shipped from the nearest stockyards. They were slaughtered by the local butchers, who sold the meat before it had time to spoil. Refrigerators for keeping meat were almost unknown.

The abattoir was literally a shambles. Meat and hides were the products. Livers, hearts, tongues all went unweighed to the meat market man who bought a whole carcass of beef. Everything else was waste, or at best was used as an unwholesome ration for a sty of "slaughterhouse hogs."[1]

Into this hodge-podge of small, dirty, wasteful local businesses came the Cape Cod Yankee who was to upset practically every idea which had been accepted in the trade since its inception. His acquaintance with meats and live stock had begun in 1855, at the age of fourteen, when he went to work for his brother, a local butcher. It had continued, and grown, through the different phases of slaughterer, local dealer, export cattle shipper, and wholesale meat dealer until at thirty-five he was partner in two large, well-established firms and sole owner of a third,

---

[1] The improvements in sanitation and the development of inspection methods constituted one of G. F. Swift's notable contributions to the preparation of meats for human consumption. His methods, scientifically worked out in the light of scientific discoveries, formed a basis for the inspection and control exercised by the Bureau of Animal Industry of the United States Government. This supervision is extended to over nine hundred packers today, principally those engaged in interstate commerce.

local and smaller enterprise. His interests had spread from Cape Cod to Albany and Buffalo. His firms did business in eastern Massachusetts as well as abroad. He was, as they say down Cape Cod way, getting on in the world.

But Gustavus Franklin Swift was never content simply to get on. Always he saw opportunities ahead for eliminating waste, thereby getting more business and making more money for himself.

At first he saw the waste of buying cattle which had passed through the hands of too many middlemen and against which too many charges had accumulated. He went west to buy the cattle nearer their source, to eliminate these extra charges.

Then he began to think about the waste of shipping the whole animal east instead of shipping only the parts which were needed there. It was not alone the freight on the sixty per cent inedible portion— though that was a tempting saving if it could be attained. But also in shipping the cattle east they were bruised too much. They shrank in weight too much. The expense of feeding in transit was too much. It was all waste—and to my father any waste was too much!

Father was the man who began to slaughter cattle at Chicago, and to ship the beef east. At first this was confined to the winter months. Then, through the refrigerator car's development, it became an all-year business. And thereby the greatest saving possible in producing meat from animals had become a reality. This saving from that time on meant cheaper meat for the consumer, higher prices for the cattleman—and the birth of a great industry.

It was not, of course, as simple as all that. There were years of venturing, years of back-breaking, heart-breaking, spirit-breaking work. There were in those early years times when if G. F. Swift's debts had been measured against his assets he would have been unquestionably insolvent.

But his frugality in the management of his business overcame these handicaps—and left him eventually in command of one of the greatest businesses of the world.

How the refrigerator car and the beef cooler were perfected is a story in itself. Through many a summer's night at his plant he alternately eyed the thermometer in his single beef cooler and ordered his men to shovel more salt and ice, faster.

Through many years, before the Interstate Commerce Act was passed, he fought single-handed a railroad association which would not haul his dressed beef at a rate he could pay.

How he wore down the eastern public's prejudice against western dressed beef is of itself an epic of selling.

With all of these major problems to handle, however, he never overlooked the economies of operation and the need to develop every possible revenue from the materials passing through his hands. If he had lost sight of this, then Swift & Company could hardly have survived the early years to remain in business successfully today.

In the free-and-easy days of slaughtering in New England, for example, the slaughterer saved, besides the meat and the hide, only the head, feet, tripe, heart, liver, and tongue. The head, feet, and tripe constituted a "set," and a set was sold separately. If the customer bought a whole carcass, he received free a heart, tongue, and liver.

On the outskirts of the larger slaughterhouses, such as that of Anthony, Swift & Company at Fall River, there grew up the establishments of people, who, while the slaughterers blindly followed the age-old customs, made money out of what the meat men threw away. The butchers were glad to have this "rubbish" carted off, for disposing of it was difficult.

The by-products people made a good thing of it. The big firm in the trade which included such products as neat's foot oil, tripe, and so on was also operating extensively in some of the materials which it did not have to pay for because they were not included in the sets which had a market value.

Shortly after my father came to Chicago and began operating on the larger scale which characterized most of the Chicago dressed-meat establishments, he was instrumental in developing paying outlets for other by-products. By-products revenue is what developed his business.

A man was brought on from Fall River who contracted for sausage casings at a stipulated figure per

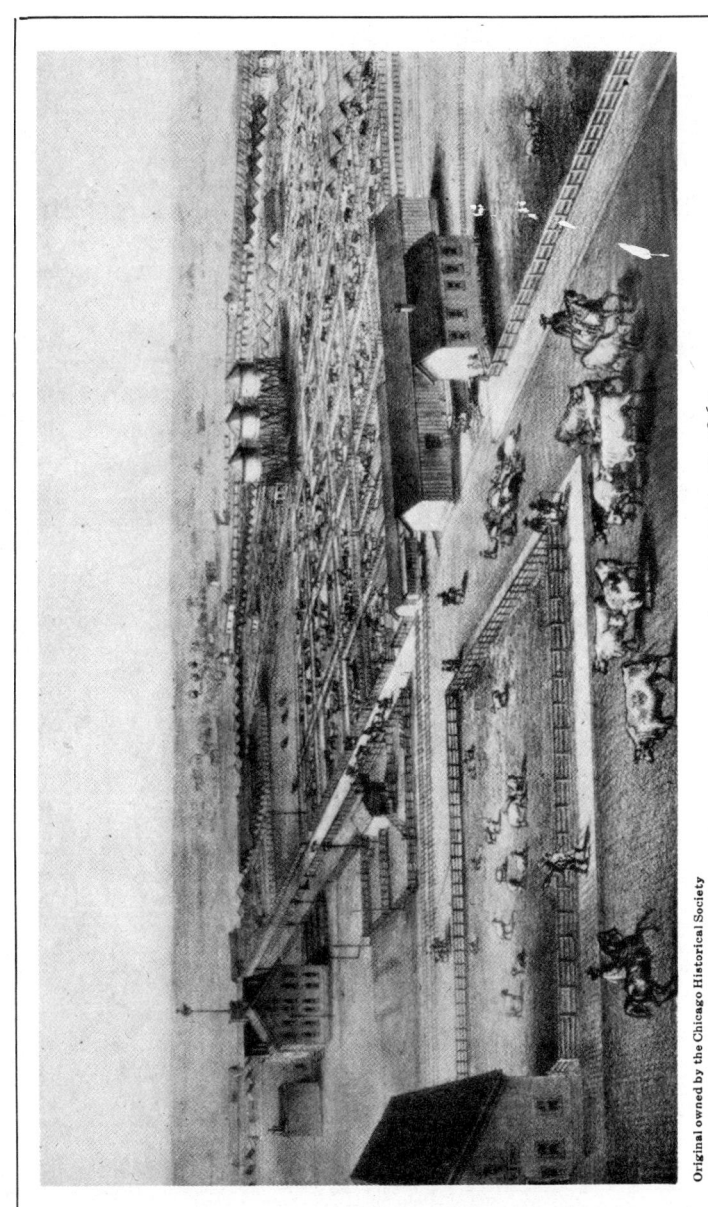

UNION STOCKYARDS OF CHICAGO IN 1865.

Original owned by the Chicago Historical Society

carcass. Blood and tankage became a source of fertilizer. We made a hobby, almost, of fertilizer and a few years later of oleomargarine. In our early days at Chicago, by-products people bought the sets, the blood and tankage, and the shin-bones for knife handles. Peddlers were encouraged who came to buy livers and sell them from their wagons in the poorer parts of town. What livers could not be disposed of in more profitable ways were tanked. Nothing was given away—this would have been waste.

G. F. Swift knew, by Cape Cod instinct, that no enterprise can grow soundly and survive the lean days which always come, unless it blocks off every possible source of waste. Even though a customer might be induced to buy a whole carcass instead of only three quarters, by "throwing in" heart, liver, and tongue, it would not increase that customer's sale of meat. His retail customers could be counted on to eat just the same amount of meat; and if he bought the smaller quantity he would simply have to come back that much sooner to replenish his stock. Hence, if the heart, liver, and tongue could be sold separately, and made to yield some of the money the new packer needed so urgently, then certainly they must yield it.

Before he had finished with the process, he was using everything from the animal to produce a profit. In fact, the hackneyed remark that Chicago packers use every part of the hog but the squeal probably had its inception in a remark my father once made, when the by-products utilization was complete, that "Now we use all of the hog except his grunt."

Not that Swift & Company was the only one to do anything along the lines of by-products. All of the sizable packers were at work on the problem. The keen competition among them all, and especially among the larger concerns, forced down prices and forced down margins. Unless one kept abreast of the others in by-products utilization, then that laggard inevitably went under.

G. F. Swift was without question the aggressor in this war for extra sources of revenue. He was never satisfied with his business. He knew he could get more if he could crowd his prices below the rest of the field without sacrificing his profit. Out of this continual pushing for sales by cutting his costs, he built his own business to a place of preeminence.

After the stage of selling raw materials to others to make products from, came the stage where our own people did the jobs themselves and thus crowded costs down a little more.

New lines were entered; by-products were split into further by-products; and out of it all, the public benefited as well as we did.

Along with the development of by-products revenue—ahead of it, in fact, for it required no development of processes—he practiced this creed of keeping every expense at rock-bottom. Swift & Company had a reputation wherever it was known, as a thrifty, compact, well-managed business. There were no little cracks in the walls which permitted anything to get away undetected.

One of father's especial ways to hold down expense was to avoid alterations which, while desirable, were not necessary. He hated to see mechanics at work around any of his properties. The sight of a man with a hammer or a saw or a trowel was a red flag to him.

"Whenever you see a lot of mechanics at work anywhere you are in charge, fire 'em," were the instructions he once gave a man whom he had placed over a considerable section of the company's properties.

"But sometimes they are needed, Mr. Swift," protested the department head.

"They'll find their way back, then," he disposed of this argument. "They're a luxury. We can't afford luxuries. It isn't only the high wages you pay 'em—it's the lumber and nails and brick and hardware they use, too. No, sir, when you see a gang of 'em around and you don't know that you have to have 'em, be on the safe side and fire 'em. That's the way I always work it."

After all, there is little question that his ideas were fundamentally right in regard to holding down expenses. Given an enterprise which has an economic reason for its existence, then if you stop every leak, that enterprise is bound to be in good shape. It is the leaks which ruin more basically sound businesses than any other cause. For one business man who watches expenses carefully, there are five who are careless. And of fifty who are careful, not more than one really keeps his organization keyed up to the importance of waste as did G. F. Swift.

He was visiting the St. Joseph plant back in the '90s, shortly after it had been built. As he was going over the plant with the manager, he noticed a place where car loaders had spiked a loading runway to the dock. When the runway had been removed, the nails had been left sticking up from the planking.

"Nice dock you have there," he observed casually.

"Yes, fine, isn't it?" agreed the manager.

"But look at those nails"—pointing to them. "You won't have a dock if you let 'em do that."

They walked along and father began looking at some other parts of the plant with the superintendent, who had been a few feet behind all the while. The manager meanwhile encountered one of the office boys in the yard and sent word by him to the loading foreman that those nails must be removed within five minutes.

On the way back, the chief led the party quite casually along the loading dock. This time he was with the superintendent. And while he appeared to be unaware, the manager saw him looking for the nails and scraping about a bit with his foot in the vain effort to find them. Finally the rest of the party was allowed to go on its way, while the manager was taken to the cooler to look at the beef.

Together they looked over the carcasses for

perhaps ten minutes without a word. Then: "Did you have those nails pulled out?"

"Yes, Mr. Swift."

"Well," plaintively, "I wish you wouldn't have things fixed up until after I'm off the plant. How do you think I'm going to make everybody look alive about these things if you get 'em fixed up before I have a chance to tell the other men about them?"

When the St. Joseph plant was being built, he would go there about once a month. Ostensibly his visits were to check up on the general progress of construction. There was a vigorous idea among some of the men in charge of construction, however, that he came out quite as much to see that everyone was working as hard as he should.

He appeared one mid-morning at construction headquarters. No one had known that he was in St. Joseph. But from his comments it was apparent that he had arrived early and had been on a self-conducted tour of the plant.

"There's a gang of carpenters over on the hog-house," was his opening shot. "Of about twenty men, not more than half a dozen are really working. I think you need a new foreman for them, to get the work out of 'em. And something is the matter with the bricklaying gang; they haven't got enough hodcarriers to keep the masons busy. Somebody better take care of that in a hurry. If more of the bosses were out on the job instead of in the office, this plant would go up for a whole lot less money."

After that, there was less chair warming!

Whenever he visited a branch house or plant, he went without warning. Generally he came in the back way and got his eyes full of what was going on, before ever he looked up the men in charge.

Watchmen were almost a hobby with him. He wanted them alert, on the job, and not to be talked out of doing their duty. One story which has almost become a classic among the men who knew him has to do with a visit he made to the East St. Louis plant.

He appeared at the back gate one morning and tried to walk past. "Here," challenged the watchman, "where are you going?"

"Isn't this Swift & Company's plant?" he inquired.

"Yes, but you can't come in this way. Have to go around the front," directed the watchman.

"I'm going in this way," he declared, to see what the watchman would do.

"No, you're not," the man contradicted him.

"I certainly am. It's shorter to go through than to go around."

"You won't go through this gate," the watchman announced flatly. "Now, get along out of here."

"Say, do you know who I am? I'm G. F. Swift."

"I don't care who you are. My orders are that nobody comes through here unless it's part of his job. You can't go through here, even if you are Mr. Swift—and I don't think you are."

"What's your name?"

"Bateman."

"All right, Bateman, you'll hear more of this." And he started for the front gate.

A few minutes later he appeared at the manager's desk. He apparently had something on his mind, and he was not long getting it off. "You've got a watchman named Bateman on the back gate?"

"Yes, sir."

"Mighty good man. He wouldn't let me in. Better raise his wages. A man like that will save us a whole lot more than he costs."

There was another time when, in the sweet pickle cellar at Chicago, a new watchman found him poking into the barrels and examining the meats. The watchman ordered him out.

"All right," said the chief, without identifying himself. But as soon as the watchman's back was turned he resumed his looking.

In a minute the watchman returned. "Here, I told you you can't do that. You'll have to go out, right away." So, with all apparent grace, the founder of the business started out.

But on the way he saw something else which attracted his attention. It was not thirty seconds before the employee had him by the arm—a valiant thing to do, since father towered well above six feet while the watchman was a scant five feet six. "Look here," was the man's ultimatum. "I've told you to get out of here, twice. And you're still hanging around. Now get out before I put you out."

Again the boss did as he was told—but this time

he went all the way. Within the week that employee was getting two dollars more in every pay envelope. And father never tired of telling the story. To his mind, it illustrated the very qualities of carefulness and persistence which he most desired in his men.

One characteristic which seemed almost a peculiarity, though actually it was a necessity in conserving his attention for the jobs that needed him most, was his disinclination to talk about departments which were making a profit. "I have no time to talk about that," he would point out to anyone who might undertake it. "I want to talk about the ones that are losing. I have no time for the others."

No detail was too small to be worth watching, if it bore on the subject of waste. He used to keep an eye out for Swift wagons on the streets and when he saw a meat wagon, one quick glance told him whether the meat was properly covered.

If it was not, he was out in the street in a jump. The driver was called down off his seat, then and there to be shown exactly how meat should be covered. It is said that he never had to stop the same man twice—and in later years he rarely had to stop any wagons. Swift meat went out completely covered by the tarpaulin. Everyone who had anything to do with the teaming had heard it too often to forget it.

When the business was getting started, he used to check over every detail himself. One plant man tells of being called up to the chief's desk about the

"A DOLLAR WASTED...." 19

amount of beef which had been put into a car. "See here," he was taken to task, "your sheets show so much beef put into car number thus-and-so for this branch house. The branch house sales sheets show three hundred and fifty pounds more beef sold out of that car than you say you put in it. That means one beef went in without being tallied. We can't have that sort of thing happening. It might not have been shipped to one of our own branches." He watched everything as closely as that.

A good many years later, when he could no longer check all things himself, he still insisted on seeing the facts of every claim. Always he had on his desk several claim sheets with the name in each instance of the employee who had made the error. And until the business had grown far beyond the point where anyone else might have relinquished this, he used to talk personally with every man who made one of these errors. The interviews were usually none too pleasant—yet they were talks where the man was taught rather than threatened. And anyone who was called in because he made a claim error took away from G. F. Swift's desk a comprehension of why errors and wastes cannot be allowed, if a business is to go ahead to success and profit.

Once, on a visit to a western plant, he headed straight for the oil house when the superintendent started out with him to go over the place. As soon as he was in the oil house, he asked that the sewer board be taken up. And the sewer, sure enough, revealed a loss of oil stock. He followed up the line until he came to the cooler from which this sewer drained. His inspection showed the tierces were leaky.

The foreman was sent for. But he was not given simply a general reprimand on the subject of waste. He was told, besides the fact that the oil was worth money, that a shipment from this plant to Rotterdam had arrived with many of the tierces empty. He heard about the freight, both rail and ocean. He heard about the effect which a shipment of this sort has on a customer who is expecting the shipment for immediate use. Altogether it was a lesson in business which any foreman might be glad of the opportunity to receive.

An amusing sequel was that several months afterwards on father's next visit to this plant word got ahead of him to the foreman. So the foreman shut off the sewer, had it cleaned out and then forgot to open it again.

Once more the visitor came in and had the floor board lifted. And to his astonishment he found the sewer not only free from oil, but also free from the water it should have been carrying. This time the lecture was not so restrained in tone.

In his zeal for eliminating the needless expenses, he would spare himself no more than anyone else. In going through a hog killing department one day, he had to climb up a dirty ladder. He soiled his hands, and an overzealous boy who accompanied the party to carry the frocks handed the chief a piece of cheesecloth to wipe his hands.

The boss examined the cloth with interest. "What did it cost? How much is in it?" he demanded.

"A cent and three-quarters a yard," the superintendent told him. "There are about four yards of it in that piece."

"Thank you, I will use my own handkerchief," was the instant decision. "I think you should see that the company's supplies are not wasted."

He was always teaching. His aim was not to make a man feel bad for something which had gone to waste, but rather to avoid the possibility of repeating any similar loss. Whether it was a lump of coal which he saw projecting from the cinders in the yard, or whether it was seven cents worth of cheesecloth, he always commented because he wanted his men to realize the importance of the trifles.

One result was expressed in his own words, "I don't have to go out and hire very many managers. I can raise better than I can hire." It is noteworthy that today, twenty-odd years after his death, most of the men in positions of high responsibility are men who were trained directly under the founder of the business.

His plan assured him soundly trained managers. Another important result, from his point of view, was that it avoided the tendency to five-figured salaries, which his business could not afford in the early days.

A man who has been brought up from the ranks through all of the different stages in one company is almost certain to be a better man for that company than a man who is hired from the outside. Moreover, such a man realizes that he has invested a great deal of his time in the employing company, just as it has in him. He recognizes that loyalty is mutual and that there is on him an obligation to the company just as the company has an obligation to him.

Such a man is a living refutation of the theory that the only currency which can enter into the employee-employer relation is that of cash down at the moment. He recognizes that the man who has come up through the ranks has a greater opportunity to be worth a big salary and a big responsibility in future than has the outsider. And in the long run, he is right.

My father inspired this loyalty in his men. They knew him as the man who had taught them what they knew about the business, the man who had built the business and had given them correspondingly more opportunity for advancement than if the company had gone ahead with less phenomenal strides.

They had seen him recognize, in a material way, the employer's obligation to his men. They acknowledged their obligation to him, as well as their personal loyalty to him as a man.

It was well for him and for the business that they did. For despite the years of unparalleled prosperity which had come to the company after it had gained a bit of headway, there was coming a lean time. The business had grown fast. If it had failed to come through the times of trouble, the verdict must be that it had grown too fast. As it is, one must say that it had grown to the absolute limit of safety.

CHAPTER II

"WE CANNOT FAIL!"

FROM his first transaction as a boy until some time after the wearing days of 1893, my father never had enough cash to handle his volume of business comfortably.

It was not that he did not have during most of this time a good deal of capital to work with. Rather, his vision of the opportunities in his business ran far ahead of the money which the business earned him. And his daring led him to expand abreast of his vision rather than abreast of his cash.

He was a born expansionist. But if he had lacked this tendency, his first few years of shipping beef east in refrigerator cars would have implanted it in him. For, just as soon as he had succeeded in delivering his Chicago-dressed beef all sweet and edible in the hungry centers of the East, he was able to undersell everyone else.

No one could haul live cattle east, slaughter them there, and sell the meat for anything like what it was costing us to lay down Chicago beef at the same point. We were not paying freight on the inedible portions of the animals, nor feeding them for another thousand miles of railroad journey and standing a heavy shrinkage in shipment to boot.

The first working capital which G. F. Swift had was the twenty-five dollars his father gave him when he was sixteen to serve the double purpose of keeping him from going to Boston for a job and of setting him up in the meat business. He got this twenty-five dollars in 1855. He expanded it to a good deal more by shrewd trading and hard work.

In 1873 he was "well fixed," as the New England idiom has it. And despite that panic year's losses to the three firms in which he had interests, he was getting on in the world.

Yet within three years, so thoroughly was he convinced of the opportunities ahead, he shifted his scene of operations to Chicago from eastern Massachusetts. Shifted his ideas from eastern slaughtering to Chicago-dressed beef. And held so firmly to these ideas that his Boston partner, James A. Hathaway, forced a dissolution of their partnership.

Hathaway was the financial man, Gustavus Swift the live-stock man, of the firm of Hathaway & Swift. Its operations had been financially comfortable because Hathaway had both money and belief in his younger partner's ability.

But when it came to so radical a change as my father proposed, the older man would have none of it. Partnership dissolved, my father received his share shortly after he came to Chicago.

The proceeds to him were a little more than thirty thousand dollars. It was all the money he had, and it did not look to him to be very much. He had been operating three sizable businesses—and even in those days live cattle cost about one thousand dollars a car.

He had no illusions that he could work comfortably on this amount of money. But he did not let this fact deter him.

No one saw fit to give him much competition in the early days at Chicago. The general attitude around the Yards was that if the Yankee newcomer was allowed enough rope he would hang himself. His logical competitors, the big Chicago concerns engaged in pork packing and in the local fresh meat business—the concerns which were his real competitors when their owners finally saw how wholly right were his ideas—let him have so much rope that instead of hanging himself he obtained a substantial lead.

The savings through dressing beef in Chicago instead of shipping live cattle east constituted so large a sum per head that Swift beef, which was better than locally slaughtered beef, could be sold below the market and still leave a handsome margin. Once the plan was working, we made money at a great rate.

Obviously he could not count on the rest of the world to leave him this rich field. Some day the other members of the industry would realize what was going on. And forthwith they would enter into competition to obtain a share of the eastern business.

Under these circumstances my father did the only

thing thinkable. He went to any length to expand his business while he had the field to himself.

He borrowed every cent he could to build more refrigerator cars, to extend his plant, to establish his distributing machinery in the East. Every cent his business yielded went back into it again.

Friends in the East, former associates and competitors, were induced to buy shares in his enterprise. And so it was that by the time the big Chicago pork packers awakened to the profit for them in fresh beef he was intrenched as firmly as they. Financially, that is. In the beef business he had a head start which was never to be lost.

But his head start was stalwartly contested. The other concerns, once they entered the race, worked for business. There was plenty to be had—what the local slaughterers of the East had had but could no longer hold against the economically invulnerable competition from Chicago.

Our problem was finding the money to build the equipment necessary for getting the business which was to be had. Obviously, if we were first on the ground in a given territory we should always be the big factor there while the other concerns would be merely our competitors. And father was a great one for being the big factor in anything he touched.

On April 1, 1885, Swift & Company was incorporated for $300,000. On December 1, 1886, the capital stock was increased to $3,000,000—the inventory showed that the plant was worth it. December

1, 1891, saw an increase to $5,000,000. Shortly afterwards still more stock was sold, for a total capitalization of $7,500,000.

The first issue of stock had gone pretty much to eastern friends and associates—wholesale meat dealers, retail butchers, and live-stock shippers for export. After a short while, Swift shares were universally recognized as desirable securities. They were always sold directly by the company to investors, merely by announcing the new issue and giving "rights" to the shareholders of record. Every share of stock ever sold by the company has been sold for its par value.

When the panic of 1893 swept down upon the man in charge of the business, as it swept down upon all the commerce of the nation, he was not ready for it. He was at the height of his last big period of expanding the business. Swift plants were springing up along the Missouri River—for if it was good to dress beef at Chicago and save hauling live cattle a thousand miles, was it not better to dress it at Kansas City and save fifteen hundred? The new plants increased the earnings, but also they increased the capital requirements. Hence when the panic came, money was tight with us.

My father had always regarded his credit, and rightly so, as unquestionably his greatest asset. When a loan came due, he always had the money on the spot—and he usually asked for a renewal immediately after he had paid.

His credit was wonderfully good. No wonder.

In the first place he had been building, from his earliest days, this unbroken record of prompt payment. Then there was his history of commercial success. And not least of all was his personality.

Anyone meeting Gustavus F. Swift was at once impressed with the fundamental honesty of him. It was in his face, in his manner, in his whole personality. One knew, instinctively, that here was a man to be trusted to any extreme. And besides his whole air of honesty, there was no question that he was substantial. Physically, he was over six feet and weighed about a hundred and ninety. There was no suggestion of fatness about him; he was bone and muscle. His whole appearance was enough to lend money on!

When he first came to the Chicago Yards, the East was his source of all funds. Chiefly they were derived from cattle and meat sources, from men who knew him in the stockyards and meat centers of New England. And through these people he was able to get substantial lines of credit from eastern banks, both through personal calls and by correspondence. Swift paper was, in 1893, scattered throughout the East; almost every bank in New England and New York State had some.

The large banks, too, in Chicago and other centers had Swift notes in more substantial amounts. Yet even at this time he felt himself held back by the lack of money. He *was* so held back; his vision raced ahead so fast that the money could not keep pace. His maxim was to borrow all the money anyone would lend him. He never turned down the offer of a loan. The business was growing too fast for that.

The business was, it may parenthetically be admitted, growing at a rate faster than was altogether conservative. As I have said, he was a natural-born expansionist. And for years all of his training had been for more expansion, and then still more beyond that.

We went into the panic, in May of 1893, owing about $10,000,000 to the banks—a tidy sum in those days. Forthwith the banks evinced the greatest desire to collect their loans and not to renew them.

Here was the test of G. F. Swift's policy. Could he pay off these loans, accumulate enough new borrowed money in hard times to carry on his business, and emerge unscathed? Or would he find himself in financial difficulties which must result in money loss, perhaps even in loss of the management of the business? These questions were very real—for in 1893 ten million dollars was not a sum to be bandied lightly about, nor for that matter is it today.

Those who knew my father best say that in his life were dozens of occasions when almost anyone else in the world would have quit, but when he fought his way through the difficulties by sheer grit. Of all of these occasions, 1893 takes first place.

For several months then, he literally did not know two days in advance just where he was going to get the money with which to meet his obligations. Times were hard, hard as ever they had been in the memory of man. Collections came only through everlasting persistence and even then they could not be relied on. Several times the day was saved by expedients which could have been devised by no one less determined than was Gustavus F. Swift that his business would not fail to meet its obligations, and promptly.

Off and on, rumors became current that Swift and Company had failed or was about to fail. Always this was the signal for another lot of creditors to descend for assurances. And always they received the assurances that all was well, just as they always received their money on the dot.

The president of one Chicago bank heard these rumors and became badly worried. So he called at the office, bearing a statement showing all of Swift & Company's notes in his bank with amounts and due dates. The head of the business looked over the list. Then he said:

"I am sorry, sir, that you put your bookkeeper to the trouble of making out this long statement. Are any of these notes due?"

"No, Mr. Swift. But I am worried about the rumors I have heard about Swift & Company's financial condition."

"I have always thought it was a pretty good man who could pay his debts when they came due," declared my father. "And I have a record of always having paid every debt when it came due. These notes will all be paid when they come due, but I can't pay you before then. You will get your money on time." And he did.

Gustavus Franklin Swift believed in the destiny of his business. He sincerely believed that it could not fail, for he would not let it. A dozen or more times that summer the company could not have met its obligations except for the superhuman efforts of its founder.

Practically every department head of the company had lent the company his lifetime savings on a note endorsed by G. F. Swift. Many of the subordinate employees had lent their money, too. Some of these loans were well up into five figures; others were of only a few hundreds of dollars. But every one of them was made voluntarily. The men knew their chief needed cash, so they brought him what they could.

The aggregate of these loans by employees was large. The margin of safety by which the company escaped disaster was, several times, extremely narrow—much narrower than the margin given by the loans of employees. If Swift people had not lent their own money, the business might not have come through.

Small loans were made not only by employees but also by outside friends and associates. Many a livestock commission man in the yards had lent ten thousand or even twenty-five thousand dollars on an endorsed note. Every cent of the family's was in the business then.

But my father gathered in money not only from these logical sources; he also brought in some goodly sums from places of which no one else might have thought. One morning, bright and early, he sent for the department head in charge of ice houses and icing stations. "Do you know A. S. Piper?" he demanded.

"Yes, I know him rather well."

"I see by the paper that he had a big fire in one of his ice houses. The paper says it was fully insured, and that it was worth a hundred thousand dollars."

"Yes, I think the ice house was worth fully one hundred thousand dollars, Mr. Swift And Mr. Piper would not slip up on a question like insurance."

"Hm-m," his boss concluded. "That hundred thousand is too much money for him to have."

"He can handle one hundred thousand dollars very intelligently, Mr. Swift."

"He can't handle it as well as I can," was the retort. "Can you get him to come to my office?"

Within an hour or two the department head had Mr. Piper in the big front office. And then, as the eyewitness has since recounted the story, was displayed an urbane, an almost ingratiating manner which seldom came to the surface.

"I have heard a great deal about you, Mr. Piper," he told his visitor. "Lots of people will no doubt come to you about this hundred thousand dollars which the fire insurance companies will pay you.

The place for it is with Swift & Company, at six per cent interest. I will give you a demand note, and will endorse it personally. Then you can get your money when you want it."

He got the money! The department head ushered Mr. Piper to his carriage, and returned to his own desk. An hour or two later his chief sent for him. "I suppose you thought I wouldn't get that money," he chuckled.

"Yes, sir, that's exactly what I thought."

"Well, I had to have it. I suppose that if you needed that hundred thousand, you'd just sit around and say you couldn't get it."

"I don't know, Mr. Swift. I probably would have tried."

"I'll tell you, young man, you've never needed money the way I needed that money. If you had, you'd know just how I felt about it. You'd have got it too."

Every morning during these times of stress there was laid on his desk a sheet showing estimated money requirements and estimated receipts. Those documents were the storm center of the business.

The estimated requirements were inelastic. If a note came due, it came due and that was all there was to it. Live stock had to be purchased, for customers must be supplied with fresh meat.

Estimated receipts were, however, highly elastic. Their natural elasticity consisted principally of their tendency to shrink. Customers were not paying their bills as promptly as in other times; many of them were in straits which resulted in their eventual failure.

To offset this natural shortage was my father's big task. For only too often the estimated receipts fell perilously short of the requirements, and the actual receipts fell short of the estimates. Then it was that he accomplished strokes such as the hundred-thousand-dollar loan from A. S. Piper.

His task was complicated by the thick-flying rumors of bankruptcy. One prominent company in the industry had failed. Bankers sat on the edges of their chairs, awaiting the next failure.

And because Swift & Company had expanded so fast and was spread out so thin, it seemed the logical candidate.

G. F. Swift's handling of the whole situation revealed to the pessimistic bankers a consummate financial skill of which they had never suspected him. For the whole summer, while the panic raged, he drove coolly along the edge of a cliff above it. Sometimes he had one wheel part-way over. If ever he had lost his head, if ever he had become careless, he must have crashed squarely into it. How he ran along tranquilly, getting the money somehow on the day he had to have it and meeting every obligation on the dot, is one of the wonder points in business history. Certainly it was the height of his accomplishment.

Tranquilly? Almost always. But there were one

or two occasions when even his outward tranquility was disturbed.

One of these was at the time when the ticker tape from the Chicago Board of Trade carried the message that Swift & Company had failed. Inside half an hour he was on the floor of the board, a place he had probably not been half a dozen times in his life. He strode in the door, walked to a table and rapped on it with that hard, heavy fist of his. Everyone looked up except a few traders off in a far corner, so he called, "Attention! Attention!"

By this time he had the floor. He raised his voice so that everyone could hear clearly what he had to say: "It is reported that Swift & Company has failed. Swift & Company has not failed. Swift & Company cannot fail!" He walked out in a dead silence which held for thirty seconds after he was gone.

Another time he got word that a meeting of bankers had been called to consider just what steps should be taken to put an end to all this uncertainty and to plan concerted demands at once so heavy he could not possibly meet them.

Twenty minutes later any passer-by on Michigan Avenue might have seen him whipping his carriage horse through the crowded traffic as though he had the street to himself. The least surprised man present, he walked into the midst of the bankers' meeting which had gathered to bury the business.

He opened up without wasting any time: "You gentlemen think you might be better off by bringing financial pressure to bear on us. I'm sorry, gentlemen, but we have to have more money, not less. It is up to you to lend it to us. If we don't get it, we go down—and a good many of you go down with us."

Before he left the meeting, he had increased his line of credit—and on terms which permitted of no future harassment. The bankers who had met to call his loans increased them!

Yet nothing can make me believe that if he had failed with these men, my father would not have succeeded in raising enough money somewhere or other to meet any demands which could be made on him. When he told the Board of Trade, "Swift & Company cannot fail," he was telling what he felt to be the truth. When he told the bankers, "If we don't get more money, we go down," he was telling what he knew they believed and what would therefore give him the greatest leverage on them for increased loans.

Periodically, even today, one hears or reads how this or that packer poured millions of dollars into Swift & Company in 1893 in order to save a gigantic failure. To the man who does not know the competitive situation which existed at that time, this may sound reasonable. To anyone who was in the heart of the industry at that time it is ridiculous. If we had gone out of existence, or had even suspended operations, it would have meant millions of dollars in increased annual sales to each of the large packers. That statement should make the situation clear.

Actually, during the whole period, Swift & Company had exactly one bit of assistance from another packer. When he saw ahead a shortage of money rather more stringent than even the regular daily crisis, father arranged that Morris & Company should pay for Swift & Company's purchases of live stock in the Chicago stockyards for a period of not exceeding one week.

As it worked out, Morris & Company paid for two days' purchases by Swift & Company on the Chicago market—a sum not over one hundred thousand dollars at the most. On the third day the "estimated receipts" were bettered by the actual receipts, and Morris & Company was repaid in full on that day.

This was not a situation where Swift & Company would have fallen by the wayside if the hundred thousand dollars had not been forthcoming. A simple way, but less desirable, would have been to suspend purchasing live stock for a day or two and shut down the packing house.

Not only did we weather the storm, but also we operated continuously throughout—though at a reduced rate of production because of the need for liquidating inventories. My father insisted that he had to keep the packing houses open, even though money was so hard to get. He declared he would not willingly be caught short of product—and he wasn't.

But there was a time in '93 when the shelves were almost bare of all stock—by-products, glue, hides, wool, pickled and smoked meats—everything that could be sold for cash. The head of the business kept firmly to the idea that if you needed money, there was no point in holding goods in an effort to avoid a loss. He needed money right then more than he needed anything else; he sold off everything which would yield money. This is how he provided the funds to pay off those banks which were clamoring for cash.

At the beginning of the panic, in May, we owed about ten million dollars to banks. By September, when the worst of the storm was past, the bank loans had been reduced to one million—and this was in the banks which had proved themselves ready and willing to believe in G. F. Swift. Given another month of the panic, he unquestionably could have liquidated every cent of bank indebtedness. As it was, the actual accomplishment was a feat little short of unbelievable.

Yet, except for the one or two occasions when anyone would have lapsed from tranquility, he handled the whole job quietly, comfortably, and efficiently. It was World's Fair year and the house was full of visitors all summer. On a Saturday morning in June he called in his chief clerk in charge of banking matters and announced, "I am going away. I don't want to see you again until Monday." And he went out to his buggy.

Within half an hour the head of one of the large downtown banks telephoned. He wanted to talk with the chief; but after failing to get him, or one of several other people, he talked with the financial clerk. "There is a rumor downtown that Swift & Company has failed and I must get hold of Mr. Swift very quickly," he told the employee. "Even if he is away, you find him and get this word to him."

The clerk had a feeling that his boss was at the World's Fair. So he set out for the Midway, and walked around looking for the familiar tall figure. Finally, at about 1:30, he found him.

His boss listened to his excited story. Then he smiled. "I said I didn't want to see you until Monday. I meant it. The bank is closed, isn't it, until Monday? All right, we'll answer them on Monday." With no more ado he continued on his way.

For while he was tremendously concerned about his firm's credit, he would never allow anyone else's excitement to stampede him. He personally instructed the handful of employees in the banking department that the duty of the department and of everyone in it was to keep the company's credit good. He kept his finger on all of it.

Long after he was running a large and widely ramified business, after he had relinquished to subordinates duties which are supremely important, he still held to the details of the credit structure. He signed all notes, warehouse receipts, and other documents of like nature. He was able to present a full statement of the company's financial condition from the records which he maintained.

One evening early in the panic year the president

of a large bank wrote asking for a statement of his assets and liabilities—something which was a good deal less freely given out by all concerns then than now. The request arrived by messenger after office hours.

Next morning he appeared at the bank with a statement made out in his own writing. The statement showed that while the firm owed a large sum, it was a long way from insolvency. He went over the statement with the bank president and left it with him.

Then he went to another bank and to another, until he had been to all five of the banks where he had considerable amounts borrowed. To each bank president, after the first, he said just about this: "You did not ask for this, but another bank did. I gave it a statement and I want to deal fairly. I have brought you one also. I hope it will be satisfactory."

He afterwards explained to someone who questioned the wisdom of this move: "There's no use in trying to deal with a banker and not letting him know how you stand. If I had not always worked that way, I would not have received as good support as I did receive from the banks during the panic. And if I had not submitted that statement when the first bank asked for it, there probably would have been a good deal harder situation a little later on than actually ever developed."

Years before, when he was doing much of his own cattle-buying, the market broke in the East—this was in the very early days when he was still shipping cattle, before he was slaughtering in Chicago. He saw an opportunity, with the consequent cheap prices in the Chicago Yards, to get hold of a great many cattle and start them rolling eastward while everyone else at Chicago was holding off in trepidation. That would mean a nice profit the next week, when the cattle could be sold in a strong eastern market.

So he bought and bought and bought some more. His weight tickets, which are a form of document constituting a sight draft payable at the buyer's bank, came rolling into the National Livestock Bank in great quantities.

Levi B. Doud was president of the bank. When the flood of tickets reached a disturbing height, he sent a boy out to bring in G. F. Swift. But that gentleman did not come to the bank. Instead, he kept right on buying cattle. A second boy failed to bring him in and a third. So Doud got on his horse and hunted up the recalcitrant customer. He found him on horseback, at the cattle pens.

"You're buying a lot of cattle, Mr. Swift," was his greeting.

"I know it," agreed my father. "Weigh 'em," he said to a live-stock commission man he was with, to indicate that he was buying this lot too.

"To tell you the truth, your tickets have overdrawn your credit. I'm worrying about you, Mr. Swift."

"Glad to hear it," declared his customer heartily. "I was worrying a little myself until now, but there's no use of two of us worrying. I'm not worrying any more. Good-by, Mr. Doud. I've got to go over and look at some cattle." And he rode away.

That was perhaps a method not to be advocated in dealing with bankers generally. But he knew his man. In '93, he was on the ragged edge of his credit with Levi B. Doud almost every day.

A good many times during a few months his weight tickets represented a large share of the money in the National Livestock Bank. He would be far overdrawn at night. But Doud knew him as well as he knew Doud. There was a world of mutual confidence, after all the years of dealing.

So, after 3:00 p.m., when the day's tickets were in, G. F. Swift and his chief clerk would go over to see Doud. The three would sit down and figure out just where they stood. Then, somehow or other, they would devise a way to leave Swift's account in satisfactory shape overnight. Next day, bright and early, part of the morning mail receipts of money would be deposited—and all was well again until three o'clock.

There were key banks of this kind to which he looked for considerable sums and unusual helpfulness. But a large bulk of his financial safety lay in the fact that Swift paper was scattered in small pieces all through the East, which at that time was the only money-lending section of the country. Hardly a bank east of Ohio and north of Virginia which did not have a Swift note or two—whether it was a large bank with five hundred thousand dollars or a small bank with fifteen hundred. But in the widely scattered indebtedness lay an unlikelihood of its all being called at the same time.

The financial and credit-building methods all had to be developed by my father from his own experience and common sense. He had no skilled financial man until L. A. Carton, an established dealer in commercial paper, came in as treasurer along in the latter part of 1893. By that time, G. F. Swift had had about all he wanted of financing for the rest of his life. So he brought in L. A. Carton as a man he could depend on to take over this important job.

L. A. Carton's unusual ability in financing was of very real value from the start. He aided his chief both by taking off his overburdened shoulders the whole responsibility of the corporation's finance and by bringing to this work his specialized financial skill.

There is little question that we had been expanding rather faster than was altogether wise when safety is considered—though this is contrary to the views of Carton that my father's knowledge of every factor in the industry was so great that what to others seemed too fast an expansion really was not. But L. A. Carton, with his skill in corporation finance, saw that thenceforth it might be preferable to go more slowly. He began to exert a conservative influence.

The bigness of his financial operations had come upon father so fast that he hardly realized their magnitude until the panic of 1893 struck. One of the old-timers among the executives often tells how his chief remarked to him, on the first day that the business reached the new high-water mark of one hundred head of cattle, "If I could only kill a hundred cattle a day regularly, that would be about as big a business as I could ask." Yet in less than six months the killing gang was not allowed to start work in the morning unless a hundred cattle were on hand.

To this same man, G. F. Swift remarked when Swift & Company was incorporated for three hundred thousand dollars in 1885, "It seems like an awful lot of money, but we may need it yet." Just twenty months later the capitalization was increased to three millions—because it was needed.

It was the great speed of growth which caught him unawares in 1893. He knew more money was needed for capital. A new issue of stock was offered to the stockholders.

But it did not go. They were already feeling the pinch of the approaching panic. So was begun the long, hard fight which could not really be counted as over until the banks opened their credit resources once more and the new stock issue cleared out in a hurry.

If G. F. Swift had not done everything exactly right, all the way through those stormy months, he must have gone under. But he did everything exactly right. This was a characteristic of his—and a characteristic of the men who made good with him.

CHAPTER III

JUST RIGHT OR ALL WRONG

MANY a man of equal ability has left behind to witness his prowess no such structure as my father left. I have no doubt that many such men have consciously chosen not to. As between a career of undivided attention to business and a life rounded out by a catholicity of interests, they have selected the broader. For them it means greater contentment.

No such choice was thinkable to G. F. Swift. With never a backward look of regret for those pleasures of life which by his choice he perforce left untasted, he unhesitatingly elected to be master of his own business. The cost was more than other men might willingly pay. His whole mind and heart and strength went into building up his packing enterprise. Church and family alone excepted, he had little time or inclination left for outside interests.

Had he been less than unusually able, he could not have succeeded so well in accomplishing his purpose. Yet ability could not by itself have done what he did. His thoroughness was the source of his magic-working dissatisfaction with half measures. Father could not be happy if anything with which he was connected functioned short of one hundred per cent.

Whether it was the way the beef was dressed, or

the salt slush left on icy walks by a careless plant engineer—he would go to the root of the trouble and do his best to correct it for all time to come. On both of these subjects I have heard him deliver repeated lectures to employees. And I cite them not because they were hobbies, but as random selections to typify the range over which his attention wandered.

He was a crank on doing things right, or at least some of his men thought him so. Actually, of course, he had so complete a comprehension of every detail from buying the cattle to running a wholesale market that he saw not only the error but also the ultimate consequence of it.

He recognized that no business can ever attain perfection in all of its operations. But he was determined that his own should come as close to that goal as could any. It is my sincere conviction that he carried his determination over into the realm of accomplishment.

When he found grease in the East St. Louis plant's oil-house sewer, he visualized the irate oleomargarine maker in Rotterdam sputtering guttural expletives because many casks of the shipment he had counted on to keep his plant running had leaked themselves empty in transit. When he observed an Austrian bruise-trimmer doing slovenly work at Kansas City, he appreciated how this must lower the customer's opinion of Swift beef—and to him it made no difference whether that quarter of beef was destined for the epicure of Beacon Hill or the Italian family of South Boston. The inividual error, which to the man on the job was of tiny consequence, in his chief's mind translated itself into losing a good customer—and losing thousands of good customers if the error should continue.

To the oil-house foreman or the bruise-trimmer's boss, my father doubtless seemed an unreasonable old gentleman who made a tremendous fuss about very little. On every subsequent visit to East St. Louis he lifted the sewer board of the oil-house cooler. Quite as unvaryingly on each inspection in Kansas City he stopped to watch the way the knife sliced out the bruises. Since he continued checking up on these operations several times a year for the rest of his life, to many of his people they doubtless seemed like hobbies of his.

Basically, of course, he comprehended a fundamental commercial truth: If everything is done right, if errors are held below the errors of competitors, and if a business serves an economic end, then it must prosper. He schooled himself to do everything absolutely right, and to expect the same of everyone else.

Perhaps the one point where he laid the most emphasis on having everything done absolutely right was in cleanliness. He insisted on cleanliness both because he liked it—it fitted in with his ideas of doing things right—and because it cut down spoilage materially.

The most noticeable improvement of the Chicago packing houses over the old local slaughterhouses was in cleanliness and sanitation. And father was the leader in this respect.

He had learned the lesson when he was a local retail dealer in meats back East. In those days when refrigeration was little employed, if at all, in the preservation of fresh meats, he had found out that meat which is handled fastidiously and kept in well-scrubbed containers does not spoil so quickly as when it is handled in slovenly fashion.

The principle, of course, is universal. There is less loss in handling steel or coal, just as with meat, if it is kept in a clean, orderly, well-planned way. In handling perishable foodstuffs this is outstandingly important.

But cleanliness cannot be obtained without eternal watchfulness. Dirt will accumulate if vigilance is relaxed. And the average human being seldom considers it worth while to keep up the fight.

Proof that it pays had come to him—rather he had worked it out—at Clinton, Massachusetts. After his original start with twenty-five dollars, nineteen of which bought a heifer and yielded a profit of ten dollars, he had scraped together a little capital for working funds—it was far from a fortune. It took him fourteen years from that start to save up enough money to carry out any plan at all extensive.

His first ambitious enterprise was opening a large retail meat market at Clinton. This was a move from sandy, sparse Cape Cod to the richer, more populous hinterland.

There were already here two or three small meat markets serving the local mill hands. They served, that is, by carrying a meagre stock of meats which they kept in their ice boxes—for by 1869 refrigeration was coming a little more generally into use. When a customer stated a desire for a given cut, the market man disappeared into the murky recesses and emerged either with a piece of meat from which he cut what was desired, or else with the information that he did not have the requested variety in stock.

There was no attractive display and no effort at cleanliness beyond what common sense dictated would save on meat spoilage. There was a deal of greasiness and little of daintiness.

My father, in his trips around New England buying and selling cattle, had done his best to sate his unquenchable inquisitiveness about anything bearing on the meat trade. He had consequently noticed that in the larger cities like Worcester and Providence and Boston the prosperous meat dealers were those who made their stores pleasant and their service nice.

So in his new Clinton market he put into effect all of his ideas which seemed practical from among those he had observed and he added a number of others he had never seen tried. Perhaps the larger cities had meat markets as attractive as his at Clinton. Certainly no other towns of that size had its equal, in quality or size.

To Swift's Market came wives of the hungry mill hands who made Bigelow Carpets and Lancaster

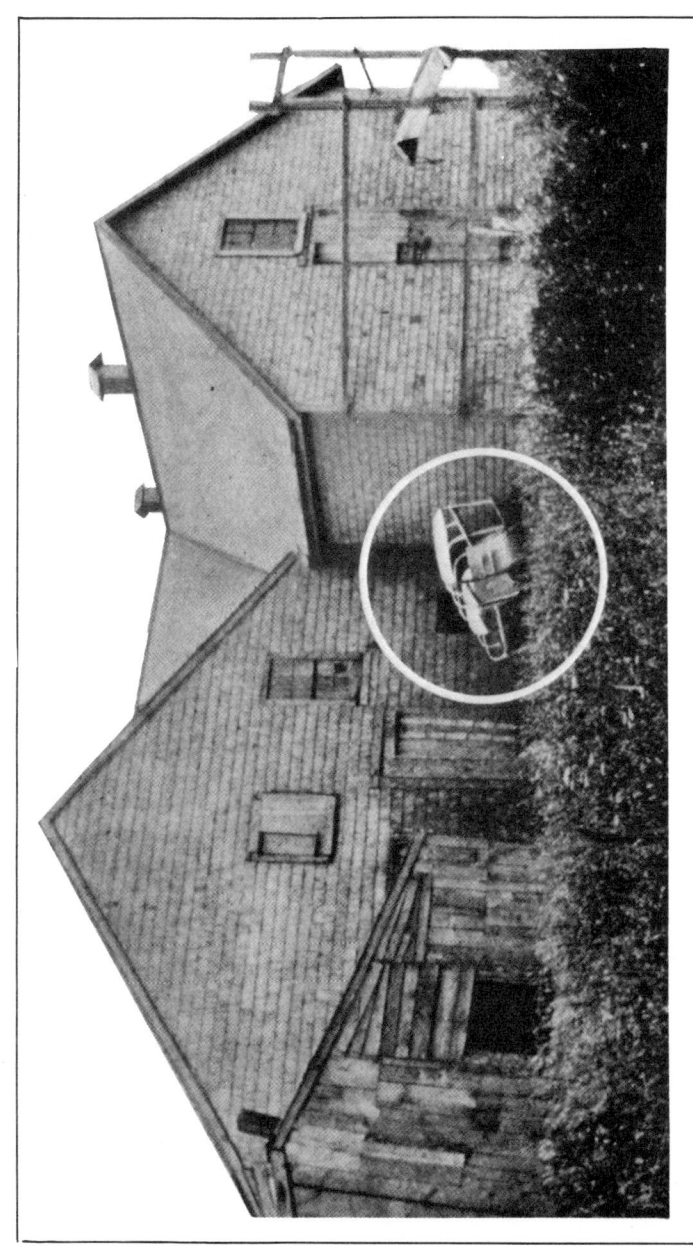

THE SLAUGHTERHOUSE AT BARNSTABLE. IN CIRCLE, THE WAGON THAT G. F. SWIFT DROVE WHEN HE SOLD HIS MEATS FROM DOOR TO DOOR.

JUST RIGHT OR ALL WRONG 51

Ginghams. They liked the cleanliness of the place—the clean windows, the clean floors covered with clean, fresh sawdust, the neatly scrubbed butcher blocks and counters. They were a bit awed by the white marble trays on which cuts of meat were displayed—but not too awed to buy the meat.

For the proprietor of this store deserved his reputation of being a finicky meat seller. He insisted then, just as he insisted all of his life thereafter, that "good enough" was never good enough. He wanted everything right, every iota of it. If it was not, then someone was in trouble.

The natives were not used to this nicety of handling meat, nor were they used to seeing cuts of meat on display. Father displayed those cuts which he most needed to dispose of. People who came in bought them as a matter of course. And right here is where he learned some of the fundamentals which were to prove of utmost value in later years when Swift's Market at Clinton was but a memory and Swift & Company at Chicago was taking all of his attention. The fundamentals of selling which he had been developing in his earlier career and which had been shaping themselves in his mind came into their clear-cut shapes at Clinton. How he used them to develop one of the world's largest businesses must be reserved for a subsequent chapter.

From the store he had men operating three meat wagons which daily sold over regular routes. His own experience back on Cape Cod had included driving a meat cart or two with himself as sole proprietor. Now, however, he was hiring others to do this for him.

The carts were doing a business of perhaps twenty-five dollars a day apiece. The market was doing about fifty a day over the counter. And if you question whether thirty-five to forty thousand dollars a year was a substantial volume for a small-town meat dealer in those days, ask some old New England housewife what her mother paid for meat about 1870. For fifteen cents a good-sized family could have a meat meal; for twenty-five cents the table could carry generous helpings of the choicest beef ribs or loins.

Principally it was cleanliness and the will to do things right which had made the Clinton market such a success. These fundamentals are quite as important today—more important, even—in any business which deals with the general public. Standards have gone up. The show market at Clinton would be an altogether ordinary market in any city of the same size today. Any man who wants to stand out above competition must set new standards, just as my father set new standards when he opened the Clinton market.

That is why he made a good profit regularly out of the Clinton business. He always maintained that if an operation was performed correctly, we made money by it. Often after we had undertaken some activity which lost money for us and kept on losing money, he would say: "We lose because we haven't learned yet how to do it. When we know how to do it right, we'll begin to make it pay. But you can't expect to make money when you do a thing wrong."

So he was always checking up, always looking for things that were not being done exactly right. When he inspected a plant—and this was frequent in his routine—he would not let anyone go ahead of him. He did not want it known that he was on the way.

He never looked at the big, showy things for cleanliness. He looked in corners, down sewers, under benches, and in the least well lighted parts of coolers.

When he found something wrong, sarcasm was his working tool for getting it corrected. "I think you ought to hang an electric light on that so you could see it," he told the foreman in charge of a beef cooler when he found a long, heavy cobweb swinging down from the ceiling.

"Do you think tallow's going down?" he inquired of his brother Nat, in charge of the mutton cooler at the Chicago wholesale market. Nat's frock was very greasy.

"I don't know," responded Nathaniel.

"Well, I think it's going up. If I was you, I'd fry out that frock right away. It's a chance to make a good bit of money."

There was another time, when a new foreman could not lay his hands on a clean white frock promptly after word reached him by grapevine telegraph that "G. F." was on the way. So he slipped out of his dirty frock, and donned a new tan overcoat of fashionable cut.

"Do you work here?" was the first question.

"Yes, sir; I'm the foreman."

"I guess you didn't come down to stay all day," he commented.

The foreman needed no further hint. Off came his new coat. He went through the department without a frock. And today, risen to plant superintendent, he testifies that not since then has he ever mislaid his frock—nor ever worn a dirty one. That sort of thing, multiplied by thousands, is a contribution which father left us and which will never be outgrown. For the men he trained are training others in the same ways; and his lessons are thus passed on direct from one business generation to the next.

It was back before the days of concrete floors that he stopped, suspiciously eyed the planking, and asked the foreman of the killing floor at Kansas City: "How do you keep these floors clean?"

"We scrub them with soap every night, and once a week with sal soda," answered the foreman.

"We advertise cleanliness," observed his chief. "Use sal soda every night," he directed the plant superintendent who was going through with him. And the foreman, still active on a like job, remarks, "G. F. was the greatest man for sal soda ever I see!"

On this same killing floor, on the same visit, he called the foreman's attention to a negro cattle skinner who always put his foot on the inside of the hide. No one saw anything wrong with that. "Wait until they hoist the carcass," urged the president.

Sure enough, in the process the footprint from the inside of the hide—harmless enough in that place—"offset" onto the carcass when it was hoisted. It looked for all the world as if someone had been standing on the carcass. And it was not a sanitary practice.

No one had ever noticed this before, though the negro said he had been doing it ever since he came to work a year and a half before. Only a man with complete grasp of every detail of a complex business could have seen why this was bad practice. Father saw in passing what had escaped the men who spent full time right there. And with his passion for cleanliness and for having everything done shipshape, he corrected the situation at once.

One time back in the '90s while I was out of town, he took occasion every afternoon for weeks on end to call in a youngster who worked under me. Daily he lectured him about the crumbs of suet on the outside of carcasses dressed in this youngster's department. Finally the young man succeeded in getting everyone to brush off the crumbs of suet. It was years after the employee became manager of one of our largest plants that he discovered for himself why the old gentleman was so vehement about this. The broken tissues of the crumbs of suet allow mold spores to get a start, and thus to depreciate the carcass. G. F. Swift probably did not know this specifically. But he knew that anything perfectly clean and orderly kept longer than the same thing when mussy. The suet crumbs did not belong on the carcasses, hence he fussed about it until he got the beef coming through right.

In the early days he fired a floorsman at Chicago for having dirty arms—always a pet irritation to him. But this floorsman was a skilled workman. So the superintendent hired him back two years after, thinking that it had all been forgotten.

Three days afterwards father was going through the plant. "Isn't that the man I fired for dirty arms a year or so ago?"

"Yes, Mr. Swift."

"All right, fire him again. When I fire anybody, I want him to stay fired until I vote on him." Dirtiness around the plant was an unforgivable sin.

On every loading platform of our plants stood a tripe keg. The boy who swept off the platform had as part of his duty to pick up any fat which might fall off the carcasses and put it in the tripe keg before someone crushed it under foot. Never did father cross a shipping platform without looking up and down for these bits of crotch fat. If one was found flattened against the planking, the foreman and the boy both heard of it. For when this was overlooked, it crossed two of his prime ideas—it was dirty and it was wasteful. Either was a misdemeanor—the combination constituted a major crime.

Everything connected with the handling of his

goods was just right or else it was all wrong. He allowed no middle ground.

For example, he never failed to look over the beef coolers. It was part of his routine every time he visited a plant. He would don a frock and spend half an hour or so squinting down the long rows of beef carcasses. He paid particular attention to the neck fat and how it was trimmed. It must be trimmed to exactly the right conformation to look pleasing, but there must not be a hair's breadth extra trimmed off. Fat on the carcass was worth the carcass or quarter price. Trimmed off, it was tankage, or, at best, oleo oil.

If he saw a carcass which looked wrong somehow as he squinted down the long row, he would examine it closely. If he saw a dark spot on the sawdust covering of the floor, there was bound to be trouble. Things must be clean; things must be done right. Anything else called for a reprimand.

When it came to the cuts, his inspection was likewise of the closest. Beef ribs are very desirable and bring a high price. Chuck is not so highly thought of by the American housewife and therefore is less in demand. When a carcass is cut absolutely right, it yields nine per cent rib and twenty-six per cent chuck. If the cut is made at the wrong place, the carcass will yield perhaps eight per cent rib and twenty-seven per cent chuck. He never lost an opportunity to point out to a foreman what it cost to do this wrong.

For father was a teacher, along with his insistence on doing everything right. I remember when I was nine or ten years old, back in Massachusetts, how he used to get me up sometimes before daylight to help him butcher a steer. My part was to hold the lantern.

Boylike, I would become so interested in some side line of activity that I would forget my part of the job. He never used to lose his temper, even though the lantern would go into eclipse just at the moment when he most needed its light. Instead he would say: "You'll want to know some day how to do what I'm doing now. Hold the lantern so that you can see. Then I can see, too."

He knew how to buy cattle and how to pick cattle buyers. He knew that the only way to buy cattle was by the most painstaking care and that the only way to check up on the results was to look over the cattle as they came to the skinning floor.

When father first came to Chicago, everyone used to laugh at his habit of riding a low Texas pony which left his legs dangling almost to the ground. He would ride around on his low-slung steed buying his cattle and caring little what anyone else might think. He knew why he was doing it and he knew he was right.

In the first place, he could let himself into a cattle pen without bothering to get off his horse—or without taking a boy around with him to do this job. But more important still, he was down at about the

JUST RIGHT OR ALL WRONG

level of the cattle's backs. He could reach over and feel the butts of the cattle to see whether there was any fat there. A great many wise jokes were made about this habit of his.

Finally, however, someone inquired just why he felt the rump of every beef animal he bought. "Back where I ship these cattle to, they're bought that way. That's how I sell 'em, and how I buy 'em." He was simply applying at Chicago the test which he knew each animal would have to meet when it reached Brighton or Albany. And when his cattle brought a better price in those markets than did other shippers' cattle, this was the reason. He always tried to find out the right way to do a thing, and then he followed out this right procedure unfailingly.

There were dozens, yes hundreds, of points which he had settled as the best way of doing a thing, and on which he checked up by personal observation at every opportunity. Sometimes he could not demonstrate the right way. Nevertheless he knew what the wrong way was and what the right.

He stopped one day in the Chicago packing house to show one of his old-time New England butchers how to split a bullock. It was years since he had personally wielded a cleaver and his hand had lost its cunning. He did it clumsily and made a poor job of it. "Now, then, that's not how to do it," he explained to the old-timer, "but you know how it should be done. Do it the right way. If a thing's worth doing at all, it's worth doing right."

If a thing's worth doing at all, it's worth doing right. This was father's creed and pretty nearly the whole set of rules he ran by. He repeated that copybook maxim thousands of times, to thousands of different people who worked for him. And he said it each time with the simple faith and conviction which made the other man appreciate the basic truth in the hackneyed words.

Every detail of the business was at his finger tips. He knew cattle-dressing, for example, as well as any one I have ever encountered. He insisted on prompt sticking to prevent dark meat. He always looked into the carcass to see that no skirt meat had been cut away with the viscera—for it is easy to lose a quarter-pound of meat per animal in this way, which really means something in the course of a day.

At St. Joseph a new method had been devised for performing an operation in splitting a hog—it consisted of using shears instead of a knife to split the aitch-bone, and is nowadays standard procedure. But at that time it had just been devised and was to be tested out at Chicago in my father's presence.

So at the appointed time he walked to the spot in the plant where the test was to be conducted. The hogs were in improper shape. Someone had scalded them and had left the hair on. Without a word he picked up a knife and began taking off the hair. Everybody else turned to and inside a few minutes the hogs were scraped.

Then he walked back to the place where he could

see best and the others prepared for the test. The plant functionaries were all there. They showed him the new operation, explained to him its advantages, and awaited his verdict.

Not a word had he said from the time he saw the hogs hanging there. He had simply worked and listened.

Now when the others had finished talking and hung on his decision as to whether the new method should be considered standard henceforth, he said, to their surprise:

"You know, when you're dressing hogs you ought to take the hair off; you ought, ought to take the hair off. Never ought to leave a hog like that." And he walked back to his office without a word about the new method of cutting the aitch-bone.

He was much more concerned about maintaining a right method than about adopting a new method. Therein he showed that common sense which distinguished his ways of working from those of so many men of greater apparent brilliance. Once he had a good method established he never allowed anyone, himself included, to overlook it. He was ready to supplant it at any time if a better method came his way. But he avoided that common failing of being so busy with new-hatched plans that he overlooked the old, tested, profitable methods.

His everlasting desire that things be done right was in no sense confined to his business. He felt exactly the same way in everything he came in contact with and used to go out of his way to see that things were done as they should be.

Father was not at all averse to doing them, if need be. He went to church regularly. I do not believe that he ever arose less than half a dozen times during a service to raise or lower a window or two. He wanted the ventilation of the church just right, just as he wanted every one of his refrigerator cars scrubbed out and cleaned with live steam between trips. It was not that he wanted to be officious— though I dare say a good many people thought him so in this respect. Rather it was his desire that the ventilation be right. Since the church could employ no corps of workmen to do the job, he was willing to do it himself.

He was always inveighing against a style which was current for several years of wearing black hats in the summer time. "You ought not to wear a black hat in the summer," he would tell his employees— or a caller from outside, perhaps someone he had never seen before that day. "Black draws the sun. You ought to wear a light hat." Again, it was not his desire to be meddlesome but rather his feeling that everything ought to be absolutely right all of the time. If it was not, if he saw anything which was not as it should be, it made him so uncomfortable that he tried to set it right.

At Omaha those men who drove their own horses to work (this was in the late '90s) maintained a horse shed with a boy in charge of their horses. My

JUST RIGHT OR ALL WRONG 63

father's natural inquisitiveness led him thither one day and he did not think that everything was as it should be. "Your horses aren't looking very good. Better give 'em a bran mash once in a while," he directed.

It was almost a year later that he made his next visit to the Omaha plant. As soon as he was through in the office and on the plant he headed for the horse shed. The same boy was on the job. "Your horses look better than last time I saw them," was his comment. "Guess those bran mashes helped 'em along." He had trained himself never to forget anything until he had seen it to a successful conclusion. Even when he was running one of the world's largest businesses he could not overlook the condition of the horses he had noticed a year before.

It was the same way whether he was checking up on the loss of horse blankets at one of the Chicago wholesale markets or making sure that the standard shade of paint was being used on all Swift properties. In both instances he was interested in having things exactly right and also in saving money. But he was even more concerned with the rightness than he was with the saving.

In overseas selling, especially in England, he ran into trade abuses which could not be tolerated by his standards. He made, altogether, more than twenty trips across to get them cleared up.

When he started at it, American-dressed meats had no show to be sold either attractively or economically.

Before he had finished with the job, American meats were going to Great Britain by the shipload and he was realizing the real value of his products. Moreover, a great deal more of his beef was being sold there than of locally raised beef.

He used to get up at three o'clock every morning in London to go over into Smithfield Market and check up on what was being done with his product. He would row with any marketman who tried to perpetuate a trade abuse. And eventually he cleaned the situation up. He was quite as interested in accomplishing this because it was right as because it gave him another profitable market—though he did not discount the market, at that.

Father's knowledge of every part of the business and his attention to the most minute details was one of the secrets of his operating success. While the microscopic eye was his for scrutinizing little things, he had the telescopic eye for surveying big things. And he never put on the wrong lens!

CHAPTER IV

TAKING THE EAST

"YOU never made any money on business you didn't do."

This was the idea which governed my father's whole activity. If you did a good job of selling, you had a chance to make money—you *made* money, assuming your business was competently managed. But if you did not sell, then you stood no chance to make it.

"You don't make a profit on shortages," was another of his maxims. Every morning he carefully looked over the previous day's orders which could not be filled completely because we hadn't the goods in stock to ship.

I still follow this custom. Shortages may readily cut two per cent or even more off the total sales. And when we are working every day to build up our volume at a profit, I see little sense in throwing away trade.

As long as a manager sold plenty, G. F. Swift stood by him—even if he made no money. Failure to make money on a big enough trade simply showed that a condition existed which could with thought be corrected.

But failure to sell put the man in a hole. If he did

not sell when his job was selling, then someone soon replaced him.

Whenever he faced the job of breaking in where he had had no trade, father was a plunger. He would quickly take a chance to lose a lot of money if that was the key to getting a big trade quickly.

When he decided to sell Chicago-dressed beef in New York City, he hired a man there—and forthwith shipped him a car of beef, followed by another a week later. Then in a few days he went to New York.

"How are you making out?" was the first question he shot at the salesman.

"Awfully bad, Mr. Swift. I lost you a thousand dollars on each of those two cars."

In these early days two thousand dollars was a whole lot of money to father. But he never blinked an eye. "All right. You'll do better next week, won't you?"

"I hope so, Mr. Swift. I hate to promise." The salesman was a conscientious, hard-working fellow.

"Well, I'm going to ship you three cars next week. Sell it somehow."

With the knowledge that he could count on a boss determined to sell beef in New York regardless, the man succeeded in disposing of those three cars at a smaller loss than his previous record. The week after, he just about broke even.

Very soon he was making a little money on each car he handled; he was handling a goodly number of cars each week. His trade grew so that it wiped out the red-ink figures within a few weeks more. In less than six months we were an important factor in the New York market—at a profit.

"If you're going to lose money, lose it. But don't let 'em nose you out." This was my father's standard policy and his standard advice: to the pioneer New York man; to the man in charge of our British beef business; to his brother Edwin, who handled the eastern sales after a few years; to me when I was starting the pork and provision ends of the business a few years later.

"Don't let 'em nose you out." It is about as good advice as can be given to any man anywhere.

After the first two or three cars of Chicago-dressed beef had been quickly and profitably sold in Lowell, Massachusetts, the local market men agreed to buy no more Swift beef—and bound their bargain by posting cash forfeits. So the next car we shipped ran against a figurative stone wall.

The evening of the first day a telegram came from the Lowell agent: "Local butchers combined agreeing buy no Chicago beef. No sale for beef in Lowell. Shall I ship the car to Lawrence or where?"

"Sell it in Lowell," his chief wired laconically.

Next evening came another telegram: "No sales today. Where shall I sell it?"

Again the answer: "Sell it in Lowell."

The Lowell experience was by no means unique. Our agents in the East were having none too easy a time of it in many instances. They met with opposition, frequently well-organized opposition.

Nearly every agent was applying from time to time for permission to ship his beef elsewhere. Chicago-dressed beef was never going to be established anywhere if the agents were allowed to give up. My father put a stop to it, nor permitted any exceptions.

Next day anyone in Lowell could buy Swift beef at the price he offered. That day the car was sold out.

Within less than a week the chief arrived in Lowell. In rapid succession he bought a lot, obtained a switch track, and had lumber delivered to the site. Next day a branch-house market was being erected.

Before the market was opened, one of the outstanding local dealers called on him. "I was in the combination against you," the native began. "But I'd like to handle Swift beef as your local agent."

"We lost five hundred dollars on a car of beef because of your boycott," he was told. "If you assume that loss, I'll be glad to have you as my partner in this market." The deal was closed right then. G. F. Swift would not be nosed out, but he thought no less of the man who tried it.

That was typical—except for the boycott—of how he broke into many an eastern town. Usually he began by having his beef sold out of the car, or from the platform on a switch track. Then, if he could, he would get local wholesale dealers to handle the beef. Sometimes he had to put in salaried men because he could not find the sort of local dealer to whom he would entrust the job.

When Chicago-dressed beef began coming on the market, the East had a real prejudice against it. To be sure, it had better edible qualities, by reason of hanging in refrigeration for several days after slaughter, than had the fresh-killed beef the easterners had been eating.

But the idea of eating meat a week or more after it had been killed met with a nasty-nice horror. There was about as much sense in avoiding Chicago-dressed beef as there would have been if the reformers a few years before had succeeded in doing away with sanitary plumbing in residences. Each was a marked improvement over the old order. Yet each was guilty of the original sin of newness.

While he had hard situations to meet in some places, in many others he was able to get the most desirable agents merely for the asking. His reputation as a business man and as a meat man was enviable throughout New England. Even though he had been away several years, his reputation held its old gleam. G. F. Swift's word that his product was good and marketable was enough for most of his friends.

He always went to the best possible local man. If this man could not be obtained as agent, then an employee got the job.

"There's no use handling poor stuff or dealing with the wrong sort of people," father used to explain. "There are enough people who want good stuff and who will deal honestly, to give us all the business we can handle." This was his guiding principle in picking men or live stock.

He simply wore off the prejudice against western beef—where he could, by diplomacy. Where diplomacy proved inadequate, he resorted to open warfare.

In Fitchburg, for example, Lowe & Sons was the leading firm of meat dealers. As soon as he was able to furnish Chicago-dressed beef in winter—this was eighteen months before the first successful warm-weather shipment was delivered at Fall River—father called on the elder Lowe.

Lowe not only refused the agency, he was downright unpleasant about it. "I wouldn't sell a pound of your beef if Fitchburg was starving," he vehemently declared.

"All right, I'll feed Fitchburg myself," was the retort.

So my eldest uncle, William Swift, went to Fitchburg as our agent. "G. F." was a natural trader; but William had trading, old-fashioned Yankee trading, down to a fine art. His original keenness in this direction had been sharpened up by infinite practice and observation. He would swap horses or jack-knives—and never to my knowledge did he get the worse of a trade.

If a market man would let William Swift supply a quarter or a side or a carcass of western beef, he would trade for a calf or a sheep or a barrel of pork—then sell the swapped stuff for cash. If a customer who had bought on credit showed signs of weakening, he would back up a wagon and load up enough pork or any other portable assets there might be to square accounts.

William Swift supplied competition which was real competition. He cleaned up the local business at a profit, nor left much for the Lowes. It was not long before the old established firm of Lowe & Sons had retired from business, leaving the field pretty much to Swift beef.

But here, once more, father joined forces with the enemy after the defeat. Three of the Lowe boys came to Chicago and went to work for him. After a few years they went back home to Fitchburg and started in again, handling Swift products exclusively. Until about fifty years after the historic encounter between G. F. Swift and the elder Lowe, a Lowe was managing Swift & Company's Fitchburg branch house.

G. F. Swift when he was going after trade would always give a competitor a chance to join with him. "If you'll handle my beef, we'll be partners. If you won't handle my beef, I'll put it in against you." This was the squarest kind of competition. And if it came to competition, my father always won. He had the mighty advantage of economics on his side.

Beyond even his ability as a packer was his ability as a trader. He was, to be sure, a superlative manufacturer in his chosen field. But it was as a trader that he excelled.

"The best cattle always sell first," was one of his

maxims. Another was, "Sell off the odds and ends first. You can always sell the top pieces."

He believed a good man sold what was hard to sell. He emphasized on every occasion that anyone can sell beef tenderloins and rib roasts if his customer has the money—but it takes real ability to sell a chuck pot-roast to a customer who wants to buy porterhouse steak. "See that row of houses over there?" he inquired of one of his managers with whom he was in 1900 revisiting Sandwich, the Cape Cod home town of his youth. "That's where I used to peddle meat. Many a time the women came out of those houses to buy—and usually I sold 'em what I had the most of," he ended with a chuckle.

When Texas longhorns were coming into the stockyards in quantity, they were not in high esteem. Texas beef was not the most easily salable. Yet we of course slaughtered our share.

My father visited the Cleveland branch house once and saw perhaps two hundred Texas cattle in the cooler. "You needn't say a word about those cattle," he told the manager. "I can tell all about 'em. They're on your mind, aren't they?"

"You bet they are."

"If I had those cattle on my mind, I wouldn't have 'em there by tonight. I'd have 'em on somebody else's mind by tonight."

"I'd have to sell them at a ridiculous price, Mr. Swift."

"I'd have 'em off *my* mind."

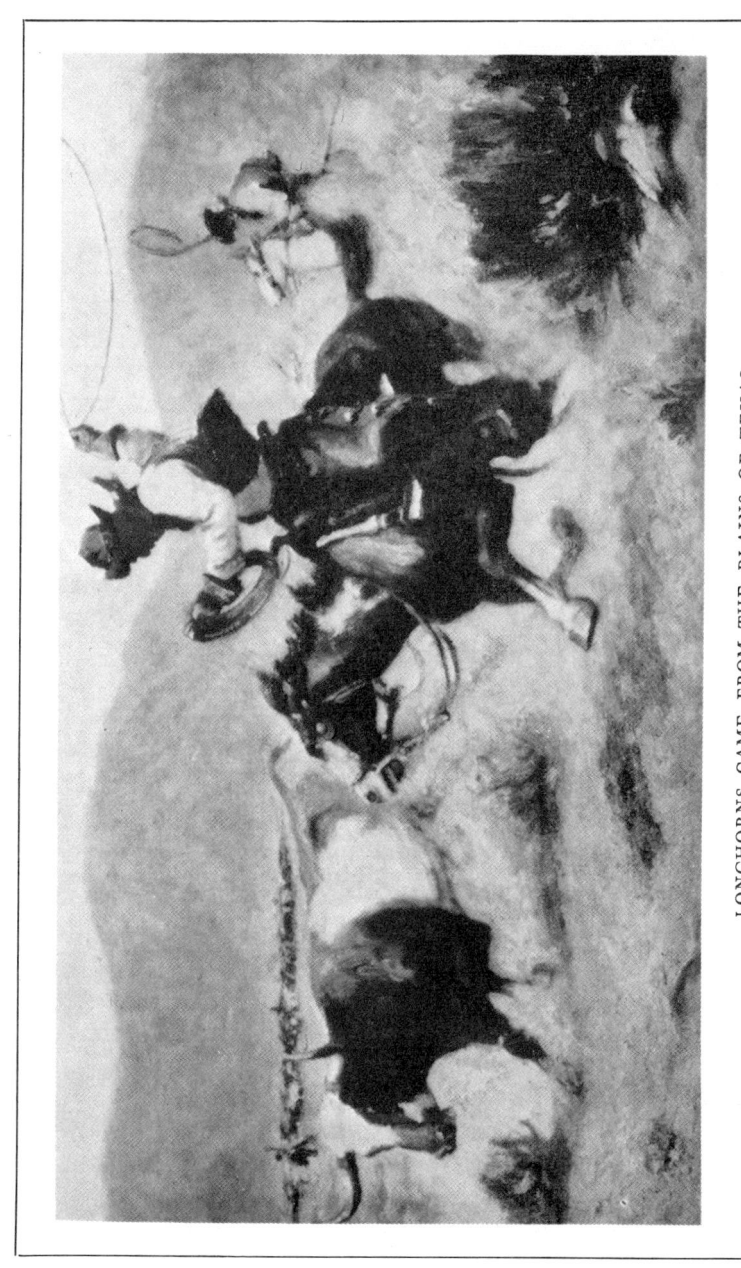

LONGHORNS CAME FROM THE PLAINS OF TEXAS.

Next day he wired from Buffalo: "How many of those cattle are left?"

"No cattle left," the Cleveland manager telegraphed back. His men were seldom slow to take his hints.

G. F. Swift never believed in holding to a thing because selling it might bring a loss. For one thing, fresh meat is perishable. And again, he believed that the best way to make money is to keep turning over goods and capital. He developed a technique which kept his goods moving at a rate far faster than was needed to avoid spoilage. I doubt whether he could have built up his tremendous business in so short a time otherwise. As it was, he was kept scratching for funds to run his business. Because he made every dollar do the work of ten, he expanded much faster than he otherwise could have.

Yet with all of his desire to sell and then sell some more, he kept warning his people not to overload a customer: "Never try to sell a customer more of anything than he can get rid of quickly. Try to sell him what he needs, and then he'll come back. He'll be a better customer in the end."

Similarly he held that smaller customers should not be discriminated against in price. "It isn't wise to make extra low prices to big customers on large quantities," was the way he told it. "Encourage the small customer. Maybe some day he'll be a big customer."

And when he made a price, it stuck. Whether he was selling or buying, he stood by his price.

It was based on worth as he saw it. Father would not change his price unless conditions changed. And often it angered him to have someone come back to him with another offer.

One of his fundamentals of selling he proved out in his retail market at Clinton, back before he came to Chicago. He had driven a retail cart on Cape Cod, selling to housewives meat which he had slaughtered. Then he had come to Brighton market, near Boston, to buy his cattle and drive them to Barnstable for slaughtering. Next he devised the plan of doing his slaughtering at Brighton, selling the meat along the way as he drove home to Barnstable.

He saw the chance to branch out as a cattle buyer. He would buy cattle from the farmers who raised a cow or two for market, drive them to Brighton, and sell them there.

By the time he had developed through fourteen or fifteen years of these varying but related experiences, he opened his market at Clinton. The success of this market has already been described, but one phase of it deserves more than casual attention. For one of the methods he devised there to sell meat to housewives who entered the shop was carried over into selling meat at wholesale when we had wholesale markets stretched from coast to coast.

The meat-market men who had the Clinton trade before father opened his store there used to keep their meat in the ice box. Nothing was on display.

Father had learned, years before, that he had to sell

off the plate and chuck and round if he was to make his profits from the animal. And he had developed the knack of convincing his retail customers that these were the parts they should buy—if at the time it was the sort of meat he had the most of. He knew that the ribs and loins take care of selling themselves.

So when he opened his Clinton market he displayed tempting cuts of meat where customers could not fail to see them. His store was clean in every detail, no one could take exception to having the meats outside the cooler.

He made a point of displaying most prominently those cuts which he needed to sell. The sirloin-steak customer could be depended upon to insist on getting sirloin steak. But a woman who came in undecided, and whose pocketbook was thin, would profit both herself and the store by buying one of the less popular cuts.

The plan worked—worked beautifully. Not only did customers buy the meat he wanted to sell, but also six times out of ten they bought more than they had intended buying. It was exactly the principle of store display which has subsequently been employed by progressive retail merchants. The five- and ten-cent store chains are the prominent examples of using this plan. Store display is the mainspring of their success.

In pursuing his idea of store display, father discovered that if you cut them up, you sell more cattle in a day. (The same thing applies, of course, to every other kind of animal. But in the early days at Chicago he dealt only in beef. Mutton and pork came later.)

When a retail meat dealer enters our wholesale market to buy something, he is probably aware that he has a good-sized stock of meats in his ice box. If he sees in the wholesale cooler row upon row of whole carcasses, or even of quarters, he simply remembers the general condition of his stock and buys nothing beyond what he came in to get.

But if he sees instead a large assortment of cuts in the foreground, with the larger pieces in the background, he begins to particularize in his mind. "I've got too many rounds left," he may think. "But I'm getting pretty low on ribs. Better buy some, so I won't be running out." We make the additional sale, which likewise helps him to keep his stock better balanced and his customers satisfied because they find at his store exactly what they want.

"Cut it up and scatter the pieces," the chief would direct the manager of a branch house where a cooler of beef was not moving well. "The more you cut, the more you sell." The advantage of the small sale now instead of the large sale later is obvious. And there is the benefit to the dealer who is better able to turn his stock when he buys cuts instead of quarters. "If they won't buy a whole carcass," father would tell a man whose sales were slow, "maybe they'll buy a cut."

Inertia militates against doing things this way. It is hard work to cut up beef carcasses into cuts for display. The unambitious manager hated to go to all this trouble. But after his chief had jumped him for it a few times and he had seen for himself how rapidly meat sold in cuts when the carcasses from which the cuts came had not been selling, even the laziest manager learned the wisdom of the plan.

Once father dropped in to see a man who had recently left us to take charge of another packer's St. Louis wholesale market. There was a big selection of cuts on hand in the cooler, well displayed and thoroughly attractive.

"Nice lot of cuts you've got here, Halloway," commented his former boss. "Don't know when I've ever seen a better line of cuts in a cooler."

"I don't think you ever did, Mr. Swift," replied Halloway. "But it's your idea, and it's doing just what you always said it would. You told me once, years ago, that you literally cut your way into the beef business any place you opened a market. I'm trying to cut my way into it for these people here in St. Louis. You taught me that, Mr. Swift. And I'll tell you, we're cutting our way in."

"Cut it up and scatter it out." This was one of the principles which made sales for my father and which worked quite as well for him in other lines of activity. I have already told how he placed Swift financial paper in the hands of every small bank which wanted it. This was an application of the same theory, one of the best ideas which was ever devised in our financing. The country banks got accustomed to having Swift paper, in small pieces. They learned it was safe stuff to have, and when a pinch came they held to it as if it were government bonds.

His financial policies and his sales policies touched in at least one other important point. He intermeshed so completely the financial interests of many important distributors with the interests of Swift & Company that there was no question that we had adequate, enthusiastic sales representation.

His chief assistance in this whole field of developing and insuring thorough distribution was his brother Edwin C. Swift. "E. C." was ten years younger and had been father's first lieutenant before father came to Chicago. He had managed the Clinton retail market after his elder brother's interests had ramified, when the larger affairs of Hathaway & Swift, and Anthony, Swift & Company, were claiming G. F. Swift's attention. After the Clinton retail market was sold, E. C. continued to run the wholesale business at Clinton.

But when G. F. Swift's whole interest was transferred to the Chicago business and its development through the early stages of slaughtering in the West and shipping to the East, E. C. and he had parted. E. C. wanted to see the country. He had gone to the Pacific Coast, and what had become of him there no one in the family knew. Letters sent to his last address at San Francisco came back unclaimed.

Once the technical problems of the young enterprise had been met at Chicago, there came the need

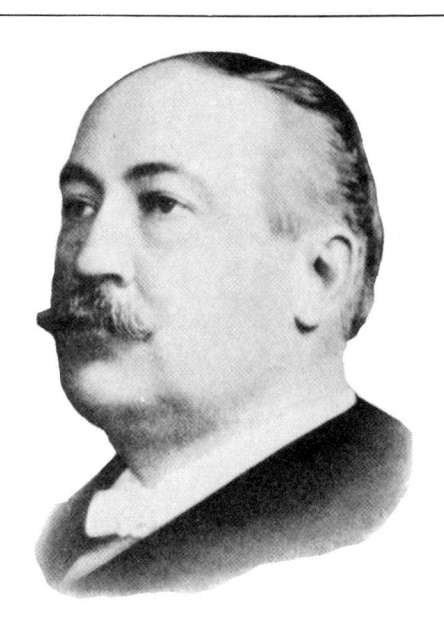

EDWIN C. SWIFT

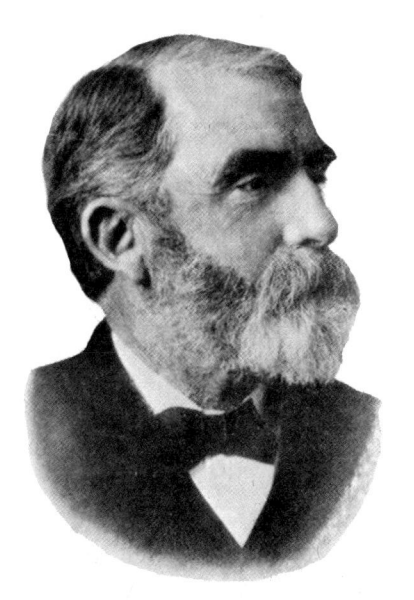

D. M. ANTHONY

for developing eastern trade just as fast as was humanly possible. Father could not carry the whole load; he could not be both in Chicago running his company and in New England building up its trade. He spent as much time in the East as he could, but it was not enough, and he knew it.

So he naturally thought of his brother Edwin. Edwin knew father's ways of working, was trustworthy and energetic, was a good mixer. In short, Edwin was exactly the man to take charge of eastern affairs.

But where was E. C.? No one knew. G. F. determined to find him, for he never let any ordinary difficulties stop him.

So he sent for a relative who was working at Chicago and who knew Edwin well. He gave him a comparatively large sum of money and directed: "I want you to find Edwin. Here is the last address we had for him, in San Francisco. You'll have to trace him from there. But you must find him. And when you find him, bring him to me at once. I must have him come here to see me."

After a good deal of amateur detective work in San Francisco, the relative found Edwin C. Swift's name on the pay roll of a railroad contractor. The gang was engineering a railroad eastward across the mountains, several hundred miles from San Francisco. The messenger set out to find the gang, and succeeded after several weeks of hard travel.

"What does Stave want of me?" was the first

question Edwin asked after the messenger had told him he was wanted.

"I don't know, Bub. But I know he told me to bring you without fail, that he had to see you in Chicago. You know he wouldn't have gone to all this length to hunt you up if he hadn't meant it."

"But I'm bound here by a contract," protested E. C. "I can't leave this job. And I like it here, anyhow."

The messenger stuck to it. He kept after E. C. for two weeks or so, and finally persuaded him to make the change. It took a while longer to find a man to replace him, but eventually they started eastward. Sharing one horse to Ogden, two hundred miles away from their start, they there boarded a train and came to Chicago in comparative comfort.

When the brothers had talked, E. C. saw that the opportunity in the East was just his sort of job. So he took it on and became a partner. He was then twenty-nine, my father thirty-nine. Between them they developed trade at a rate which actually surprised them both.

When E. C. Swift joined us at this time the parent concern was known as G. F. Swift & Company. In the East it was selling as Swift Brothers. And it was not so long afterwards that the whole business was incorporated as Swift & Company, with three hundred thousand dollars capital stock—in less than two years to be increased to three millions.

Father had personally gone into partnership with

many of the eastern dealers who became his local agents. He and Edwin C. Swift sold a good deal of the stock to many of the eastern dealers who became his local agents, key men in the East. Thus with part of the agency owned by G. F. Swift and with the more important agents heavy stockholders in the company, there were built up outlets which gave unquestioned loyalty and enthusiasm.

This solidarity of interest meant that our sales went up at an almost unbelievable rate. The important men at the yards had not believed it possible for father to succeed in dressing his meat at Chicago and selling it in the great consuming centers. They had been content to go ahead with their own affairs of smoking and salting pork, or of selling dressed beef locally around Chicago.

While they were waiting for their Yankee competition to fail, G. F. and E. C. built up a fresh meat business such as no one had ever dreamed of. The brothers put their whole minds, hearts, and strength into its development. By the time the other packers realized what was taking place, our slaughtering and shipping fresh beef and mutton had reached a point which gave us a tremendous lead. In this chosen field, the others could never catch up.

CHAPTER V

MANY A MINUTE ....

BY HIS last-minute, hair-breadth methods of doing, he saved more time than most men have altogether." This statement was made by a man who worked closely with my father for a long term of years.

It brings out, as well as can be brought out, one of his personal working methods which accounts for a great share of what G. F. Swift accomplished. It was largely through applying his energies without a waste motion or minute that he built up a large and profitable business in a comparatively short time.

I have known rather closely a good many business men who have made large successes. Most of them have been personally efficient.

They have applied their energies in ways that brought large results.

But I have yet to see anyone whose methods of working could compare with my father's. He made every minute, every idea count. He centered his thought and his time on his work. Swift & Company was the almost inevitable result.

Not a business man of his day or this day but could profit by adopting bodily many of G. F. Swift's working methods. They were sound and fundamentally simple. Literally, he saved more time than any other man I have ever known.

Out of this characteristic has grown a whole fund of stories—most of them true—about how he saved a minute here and five minutes there. Any old-timer in the Chicago stockyards can reel them off and can usually testify that he personally witnessed part of them.

Every Swift employee during G. F. Swift's lifetime knew, for instance, that if he ever saw the chief's horse and buggy pulled up at a railroad crossing, deserted, it was his duty to get in and drive to the barn with it. And almost every employee whose duties took him outside performed this task on one occasion or another.

The reason was that thus the boss saved time. Then, as now, long freight trains poked through the yards—and showed that perverse tendency of freight trains to stop on crossings. When a freight train halted G. F. Swift at a crossing, he looked to see whether the caboose was about to pass. If it was not, and he was near where he was going, out he jumped, climbed through the freight train, and left his horse beside the track to be put away by the first of his employees who happened along.

If, on the other hand, he was a long way from his destination and a long train was passing, he sometimes managed to signal the engineer to stop the train. He would step between the cars on the crossing, uncouple them and signal the engineer to pull up a few feet. Then he would drive through, couple up the train again, and be on his way. He would spend a minute or two at hard work any time in order to save a five-minute wait.

He never started for a destination until the eleventh hour. But he always got there on time. His chases after the "dummy," the train which used to be the only fast transportation between the Yards and the Loop, have yielded a crop of stories which might make a minor epic.

One man tells of an occasion when G. F. summoned him to Chicago from a Missouri city. Their talk was to start on the train which father had to take to a downtown meeting. And the visitor occupied a chair in the private office until they should be ready to start.

At ten minutes before train time the man from the information desk walked into the office and said, "Dummy leaves in ten minutes, Mr. Swift." There was no sign from the busy man at the desk. In one minute the clerk entered and said, "Only nine minutes now for the dummy." Thereafter he entered every minute with his reminder. Finally he said, "Only four minutes now, Mr. Swift. You'll miss the dummy."

"I'll miss no dummy," retorted his chief, leaping into action. With two or three motions he had gathered up his hat, his coat, the papers he needed. "Come on," he shouted to the astonished visitor—and down the stairs they fled three steps at a time. The buggy was waiting at the door, with a boy holding the horse's bridle. As G. F. Swift came out the door the horse, experienced at these affairs, started off at a run with the two men swinging into their seats as best they could.

"I never want such a wild ride again," declares the man who was the unwilling participant. "We went through all that traffic without even slowing up. Mr. Swift never picked up the reins, just left them on the dash. As we swung up to the station, the conductor was starting the train. 'Come on,' Mr. Swift cried, and jumped to the ground before the horse had even slowed up. I scrambled after, and somehow we managed to catch the train which by this time was a few yards down the track. 'Well, I didn't miss the dummy, did I?' the chief remarked triumphantly, and we settled down to our business. With him it was apparently all in the day's work."

On one such occasion the horse swung the buggy into a telegraph pole and wrecked it. Father had a dozen close shaves in his wild rides to catch the dummy. Yet he never missed it. And since he did not allow himself to become in the least ruffled by his hurry, he lost nothing to offset the time that he saved in this way.

When he went to catch a street car, his driver was never allowed to stop for the first car. Instead, the horse was speeded up and the next street car ahead overtaken. Then the car was stopped and the passenger got aboard—one car ahead of where he would have been if he had followed the conventional practice.

His time saving was not always spectacular, but it was always at work. He never used two minutes for any job if one would suffice. He never idled away the minute he had saved. In handling mail, for instance, he plowed through prodigious quantities by methods which would serve as well for almost any man in a position where he could plan his own office arrangements.

He was the best correspondent in our offices. His letters said everything that needed to be said on the subject at hand. Yet they contained never a useless phrase. And particularly if they were concerned with other than business affairs, as some of them must inevitably be, he cut off all the fringe and trimmings. He went terribly to the point.

I recall a letter written him by a friend who took perhaps a page and a half to weigh the pros and cons of the candidates in the pending presidential election. He ended by asking father's opinion as to who would be elected. The answer has stuck in my mind as a masterpiece of brevity in letter writing. It went:

"I am guessing that Mr. McKinley will be elected. You have the same privilege."

Time was the great element in his life. There was nowhere near enough of it to let him do all the things he wanted to do. He had no patience with anyone or anything which wasted time, his time in particular. His files, for example, had to be in charge of a mature man. It was no job for an office boy in those days when boys commonly handled files. His files had to give up to him anything he wanted, and at once. Let thirty seconds elapse between the time he called for a letter or document and the time it was placed on his desk—someone heard from it, heard from it strongly enough so that the crime was not repeated.

This was not captiousness. It was common sense. He had no overdeveloped sense of personal dignity. He required no kow-towing. But when he wanted something he wanted it without wasting any of the fleeting minutes of his busy day.

He wrote his letters on a half sheet of paper. He wanted others to be as considerate in writing to him. He abhorred receiving long letters. Going through his morning mail he would come to a long letter. Some few of his managers used to write voluminous letters, despite his best efforts to break them of the habit. "What does it say, what does it say?" he would demand impatiently, tossing the letter to his secretary. The secretary as a regular part of his duties boiled down long letters and returned them to his chief with a one- or two-paragraph summary. Father never read the original unless the summary indicated some point on which he wanted the fullest information.

He did not care about having things fixed up to look nice at the expense of his time. Once, at the height of his money troubles of 1893, he called for a list of the notes outstanding. He wanted it right away and could do nothing until he had it. So he stood watching the employee who was making out the list. Halfway through, a credit slip was placed on the clerk's desk as notification that one of the notes had been paid. It happened to be a note which had already been listed. So the clerk got out an eraser and began to correct the report.

"Put down the net, put down the net," father almost shouted when he saw what the clerk was doing. "I want the net, I don't want it pretty." He heartily disliked any duplication of work for appearances' sake.

Certainly he was right about it. Time is one asset which cannot be increased. And most of us waste tremendous quantities of it without getting a commensurate return. Nearly every business man devotes an inordinate amount of time to "keeping up appearances" and to idle talk which has no reason for taking up his minutes. The man who puts to one side all of the useless frills of the business day and keeps himself to the essential affairs quickly finds he has performed in one day not only that day's work but also a lot of back work which he has been intending for weeks to get at, but "hasn't had time for." The time is there, but we waste it.

"When I realize the proportion of my time that I used to waste, it makes me feel as though I have misspent half my life," an acquaintance told me not long ago. He has in the course of twenty years or so built up one of the great manufacturing companies of the country. But he declares regretfully, "If I hadn't wasted time so lavishly all my life—excepting only the years when I was getting this business of mine started—I'd have had it ten years further along than it is right now." His situation differs from most men's only in that he recognizes his loss.

Using time to good advantage involves principally setting standards of what is worth taking time for and what is not—then holding up these self-imposed regulations. G. F. Swift believed that he did his best work only when he had had adequate sleep. So he left word, once the worst times of stress in the business were past, that he must not be awakened at night for any calls whatever.

A friend tells a story that one night continued telephone ringing awakened a servant. After she heard the message, she rapped on father's door until he responded. "They want to tell you that your packing house is burning down," the maid said.

"Tell them they can tell me about it at seven o'clock in the morning," was his reply, and back he went to sleep. He knew that nothing he could do would impede the fire. If it really was a serious fire, it might take serious planning next morning to meet the emergency. Very well. He would be in better condition to meet the emergency after a good night's sleep. So he got the sleep.

Another time, lightning struck the barn back of the house and it began to burn brightly. This was perhaps at ten o'clock, just before he was ready to go to bed. The barn was not far from his bedroom window.

With his superintendent, who lived down the street a way, he stood in the street and watched the firemen at work. They had the fire stopped, it was making no progress. He yawned, looked at his watch, and turned to the superintendent. "It's half past ten and I guess I'll go to bed," he remarked. "You and the firemen can get that fire put out, Foster. There's no reason why I should stay up." And with the flames still crackling, he went to bed and to sleep at once.

He was all for business all of the time. He kept long hours when there was occasion for them. In the early days when it was a struggle to make expenses and income balance he left the house at five o'clock every morning for the stockyards. At that time he bought all of the cattle we handled. He didn't need any help, nor could he afford the expense of hiring a cattle buyer. By the time he had to spend his full time in the office and the packing house, he had trained me into the cattle buying. For some time I did all of it. Then as I went on to other duties my five brothers followed me. It was some time before finally he brought on Wellington Leavitt from Brighton to be our head cattle buyer. By then the business had expanded to many times its original size.

Even after the business was well established and making good profits father did not altogether give

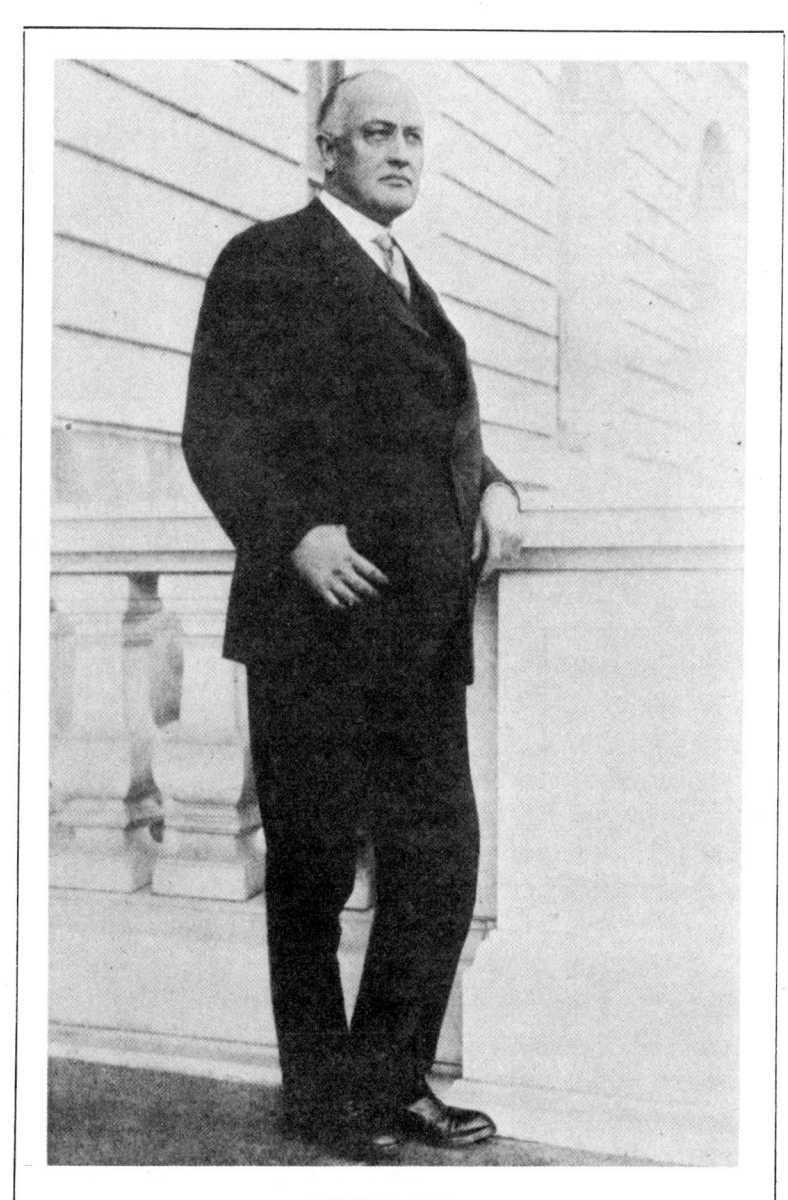

LOUIS F. SWIFT

up his early morning habits. We had a good deal of trouble with the treatment accorded our products by the English butchers during the first few years we were in the British markets. He made several trips to England to correct this difficulty.

During all of his time in London, three o'clock every morning saw him at Smithfield Market, the focus of the troubles. The rest of the day, after the Smithfield business was done, by nine or ten o'clock, he devoted to the more routine matters of our British agencies. His efforts cleared up a bad situation which might never have been cleared up without his early rising.

It was not only early in the morning but also late in the evening when we were getting a start in Chicago. He was not alone in this, the whole family worked with him. Mother was for many years the only bookkeeper he had. He and she used every night to make out the beef sheets, the shipping directions for next day's work. A little later the boys had the same job. The whole family, or that part of it which was sufficiently grown up to do so, worked every evening until ten or eleven o'clock.

"What time is it, Mr. Swift?" a workman inquired of him as he strode through a workroom in the days when a hundred men or so constituted the whole force.

"You'll know when the whistle blows!" snapped the boss, always in a hurry and in no temper to waste time to relieve a clock watcher's mind.

"When a clerk says he must leave the office because it is five o'clock, you'll never see his name over a front door," he has been quoted as saying. No wonder he had so little patience with the clock watcher.

His own life had shown him how necessary is hard work in getting a start. If it had not been for the terrific hours he put in, I doubt whether G. F. Swift could ever have got the start he did. He came to Chicago with thirty thousand dollars, which even then was altogether inadequate as capital for the smallest packing business. And broad as had been his experience in every side of the live-stock and meat business, he lacked first-hand knowledge of how to manage a large and complex organization.

The principal figures in Chicago packing on his arrival were Nelson Morris and Philip D. Armour. Armour, to be sure, arrived in Chicago the same year as did G. F. Swift. But he moved from Milwaukee, which had been his headquarters, because the Chicago branch of his business was rapidly becoming of more importance than the parent house at Milwaukee.

Both Armour and Morris had their organizations built and functioning. Behind them were records of successfully operating their large businesses. So their credit was ample.

This was a hard situation for the young Yankee to face in the yards. He never could have overcome the handicap if his entrenched competitors had realized from the start just how serious a problem he was bound to make for them. But even though he was allowed unmolested to continue on his way, he could never have accomplished what he did if it had not been for the long hours he worked and the intensive use to which he put those hours.

His taste was not at all for society. His church alone excepted, his entire interest was in his family and his business. For a good many years the two pretty much overlapped. His whole energy and most of his family's energy went into the business.

Long into the evenings, even after he no longer had routine work to do at home, he lived with it. He was a great man for continuing his day's occupation after dinner, unquestionably one of the things which wore him out.

No doubt there is a great difference between the types of man required to build a great business and to carry it on. He had to work as he did to build Swift & Company. After he had built it to a large and profitable institution, the habit of work was so strongly fastened on him that he could not shake it off.

The rest of us were fortunate. The period of worst struggle, once over, found us young enough to change our working methods to what accorded better with the requirements of the job. I have never since those early days yearned to live all my waking hours with the business. I have been willing to stay at the office as late as anything held me, of course.

But once a man gets away from his office, it strikes

me that he does better to get away from its worries. His free hours can set his mind off far enough so that when it comes back to work next morning it has gained some perspective on the job.

This applies to the established institution. The owner of an enterprise which is struggling up from a tiny start to attain its place in the economic scheme of things can seldom free himself of worries. A young business requires extra attention just as a child needs more care than an adult. But when it has come up to a sturdy youth, then it gets along better with less than excessive hours of attention. If the owner has broken off the overwork habit soon enough, he is of course a whole lot happier.

My father was self-reliant, as are practically all commercial pioneers. Moreover he wanted everyone around him to be self-reliant. He had little use for the employee who had to have instructions for every step in his day's work, or who did not know how to proceed in an emergency.

He believed in helping those who helped themselves. He used to urge along those of his children who showed any tendency to turn the other cheek. "Go after him; don't let him do that to you!" he would exhort one of the boys and stand by to see that his advice was taken.

The employee who required a lot of attention and waiting on did not interest him much. He carried the same feeling throughout. One morning as he was driving to the stockyards his horse slipped and fell on an icy corner. Half a dozen of horse dealers standing on the corner rushed to the rescue, intending to lift the horse to his feet.

"Let him alone, let him alone," my father protested. "If he can't get himself up, I don't want him." Presently the horse got up—a better horse for having taken care of himself.

Absolute honesty like G. F. Swift's is exceptional. Not only did he know that he was honest in all of his dealings, everyone who dealt with him experienced his honesty and felt perfect assurance in it as an unvarying characteristic. The extent to which some people with whom he did business relied on his honesty and fairness is almost unbelievable.

Consider one incident. In the days when great quantities of dressed beef were going from North American ports to Europe, we and a steamship company became involved in a dispute involving somewhere above one million dollars. Settled one way, the transaction would net the steamship line a million dollars less, Swift & Company a million dollars more. The individuals negotiating it were so far apart in their ideas that they simply could not agree on anything pointing toward a settlement.

It had all the ingredients of a fine lawsuit which would drag through the courts for years, yielding tremendous fees to the attorneys. And word of this went to the steamship line's principals in England.

These shipping men knew my father. They cabled back: "We will submit this to the personal arbitration of G. F. Swift." It was one of the most startling tributes to character that has ever come to my attention. His decision, granting some things to the steamship company and some to his own company and arriving at an award somewhere on middle ground, was the basis on which the ship owners settled without a question.

G. F. Swift's honesty was not of the sort which took advantage of excuses for not paying over something which belonged to somebody else. To a new employee who had brought him a question of refunding some money to a customer who did not even know it was owed him, father once said: "It isn't mine. I find when it's decided that money isn't mine, I don't have a very hard time finding whose it is." There's a whole practical sermon on honesty in that statement.

Let a Swift employee make a bad trade for the company—he heard from it strongly, from the chief in person. But once the trade was made, it had to be carried through. There was no trying to wriggle out of it. "Lord help you if you tried to get him out of a bad trade by short weight or lower quality!" remarked an old-timer in talking over this characteristic of his chief.

There was in charge of an important department a man who made an especially bad trade for the company on a tremendous contract. Then, some days after he had been told a few things about his chief's opinion of his business ability, he came around with the news that the contract had been canceled by the purchaser, a governmental institution.

We were never able to get to the bottom of just what had happened. It had all the earmarks of someone having cut a sharp corner to get us out of that contract, and there was just one person likely to want to do it. Not long after, this man was let go. But before he was fired, father had warned me about him. "You want to watch that fellow," he declared. "The kind of fellow that'll do that sort of thing for you will do it against you when it suits him to." Anything of a dishonest sort made him distrustful. That the man would cheat for us made him all the worse. Cheating has never been a Swift policy.

Father detested sham and "front." Anything savoring of lying was distinctly on his bad book. He used to spend evenings on end visiting with managers of branch houses and branch packing houses and with executives within the organization. The visit consisted usually of G. F. Swift's asking questions—innumerable questions—and of the visitor's trying to answer them. He would go back and forth over the same ground, coming to it from different directions and checking one set of answers against the others. If anyone attempted to temporize, or to bluff it out, the boss was after him. "Say you don't know, say you don't know," he would impatiently urge the victim of his inquisition. Once he had proved to his own satisfaction that the other man was not a liar, then he eased up on the questioning.

If he found the man was a liar, out of the company he went at the first good opportunity.

He would ask all manner of questions, many of them so technical that no man not an expert on the particular point could answer it. "What percentage of casings are you saving?" he asked one branch plant manager one night.

"I don't know."

"How many hogs does it take to make a bundle of casings?"

"I don't know." (No one not specializing on casings in a plant could possibly know, for it varies with the hogs.)

"Well, I think I'd know that if I were managing a packing house," he would admonish the honest man who said "I don't know." Probably G. F. Swift, with his passion for knowing everything about the business, would have known such statistics as those on casings. But no plant manager could be expected to know them.

"You never felt at ease with G. F. unless you knew him extremely well," is the way one plant manager expresses it. "He was always trying to pick you up. He would ask you questions he knew the answer to, to see if you knew. When he finally made up his mind that you knew a good deal, and wouldn't try to bluff him on the things you didn't know, he took you into his confidence. After that he let you alone with his questions."

His questions always had a definite point, however. He was always digging for something he felt he needed to know. "There's no use fooling ourselves," he would declare to a manager who might protest at the work involved in finding out some fact on which he had been keeping no record. "We might as well find out, then we'll know—and we can't fool ourselves."

"G. F. is the best auditor I ever saw," declared his brother Edwin C. Swift after a long trip with him through a number of branch houses neither of them had ever seen before. "He can get at the facts with questions quicker than anybody I ever knew. And after he gets through asking questions in a branch house, there's no need of going over the books. G. F. knows as much about it after an hour's questioning as an auditor could find out by checking the books for a week."

He was a great man for detail, despite his grasp of the big things in his line. He checked up on literally hundreds of things every time he visited a packing house or office of Swift & Company. One of his pet items was working temperature in the office.

On his way to the manager's office he always managed a look at the thermometer. Coming into the packing-house office in Kansas City one winter morning when the steam was hissing, he saw that the temperature was eighty. "It's a wonder your brains ain't cooked," was his greeting to the manager.

Another time he came into the South Omaha office

with the remark: "Good morning. Too hot in here."
"It's seventy in here, Mr. Swift."
"On what?"
"This"—holding up a thermometer on his desk.
"Is it reliable?"
"Yes, absolutely."
"These others out in the office say seventy-three, seventy-four, seventy-five."
"I know, but this one is right."
"Then what do you have 'em around for?" he protested.

"And you know," the man insists who had the inaccurate thermometers, "that's the first time it had occurred to me that I was not saving money by keeping those things in use!"

A summary of G. F. Swift's personal working methods would not be complete without reference to his thrifty Yankee ways—"his Cape Cod ways," as his managers jocularly called them. Two little incidents, showing opposite sides of his character as it could be seen in a straight business affair and in one tempered by sympathy for those in need, may help to sum up some of the reasons why he was able to build what he built.

His carriage boy usually went with him to hold his horse when he had to go to a meeting. Then at night father drove home, to have the horse available for coming to work next morning. When he dismissed the boy during the working day, he handed over a nickel for carfare to take the lad back to the plant. But when it was after hours he asked, "Going home or to the Yards?"

If the boy said, "Yards," then he got a nickel. If he said, "Home," he got none. Why? Because it would have cost him a nickel to get home from work anyhow. That was the frugal side of G. F. Swift.

Beef for export was shipped in muslin bags. These bags were always made by people who needed the money the work brought in. Chiefly they were made at home on ordinary sewing machines by widows of workmen from the stockyards. Father, because of his intimate knowledge of the circumstances of a great many back-of-the-Yards families, always insisted that he approve the list of those who were to get the work.

One day a man in the purchasing department came to the front office with a proposal that beef bags be made by concerns equipped for doing this sort of thing most economically. We could, it developed, save a good many thousands of dollars a year on beef bags and on the related jobs—which went to the same class of workers—of stringing tags for beef quarters.

"You keep out of this bag and tag business," father directed the employee. "That's something I'm running."

And until export of dressed meat shifted from North American to South American sources, the beef bags were made and the beef quarter tags strung by the widows back of the Yards.

CHAPTER VI

"I VOTE NO!"

MY FATHER doted on frequent reports from weak departments of his business. Not that he found actual pleasure in records which showed he was losing money. But the problems of turning a loser into a money maker involved activity and employing his best abilities. And above all else he preferred action.

He had been brought up on it. He would rather be on his horse buying cattle in the yards than sitting quietly at his desk. But when his business grew beyond the size which permitted him to buy the cattle and boss the skinners, he had to become a manager despite his preference.

His training had been where such things as reports were scarcely known. His beginnings had been small, his development had been through individual enterprises which were almost subvisible when compared to Swift & Company within five years of its start at Chicago. His inclinations naturally held to spreading his time over just as much as possible of the physical equipment of the business, in the idea that only thus could we hope to know what was going on.

But he quickly realized as the business sprang

up to unthought-of heights that he must work out other ways to keep a finger on and in its every activity.

So he became a devotee of reports—weekly reports. "You've got to know how you stand every week," he used to explain. "If you wait a month, maybe you're broke." So he doted on reports, detailed weekly and brought right up to the minute.

His reports came to him weekly as a matter of routine. They were never disposed of as routine, however. A report which can be treated by the executive as routine is a nonessential routine, and probably is better discontinued.

Above all else his favorite statistical diet was the reports of weak departments. His whole being enjoyed the sheer difficulty of going into a seat of trouble, digging out the facts, aligning them, and putting things right. So any losing department had to submit more frequent and more complete figures than did the rest of the business.

The man responsible for the loss had little rest while this persisted. G. F. Swift believed in frequent reminders and in prompt corrective measures. If a loss was not stopped quickly, then something drastic happened.

Once, for example, all the meat in pickle at the Kansas City plant went sour. This meant that we lost the money value of the meat and also the profits on orders we could not fill because of the curtailed supply.

The meat spoiled, of course, because a faulty cure was in use at this plant. Most packers under similar circumstances would have reprimanded the manager and the man in charge of curing so that the trouble would not recur.

Fundamentally, however, the trouble lay deeper than carelessness. The weakness was in the management for allowing to continue a condition which at the time was universal in the industry.

The cures for pork were all secret. The head man at each plant had his secret formula. By paying him a large salary, we obtained his services. These included supervising the curing and personally mixing the pickle. And of course the product of every plant was different. A Swift ham from Omaha was slightly different from a Swift ham from Chicago or St. Joseph or St. Paul or Kansas City.

The unfortunate happening at Kansas City brought sharply to father's mind the fundamental unsoundness of operating this way. So he called a meeting at Chicago of the principal men in the operating end of the business—managers, general superintendents, and so on.

When he had stated the problem, he asked for a vote. The problem was essentially that if we demanded that the formulas be given to the company the men who had the formulas would quit, leaving us in difficulties. Should we demand that they give up their formulas, or should we continue at the old way of doing?

Decidedly the men in that meeting were opposed to taking the bull by the horns. "No," voted each man. Then the chief spoke.

"You've all voted no, because you're afraid to face a little possible trouble. There's no use dodging trouble, if you've got to do things the wrong way to dodge it. You're wrong on this. I'm going to vote yes and it will be yes."

The meeting had, so it seemed to many of the men who gathered there, been called for no purpose. They thought the new rule might better have been promulgated by a general order from Chicago. But in this, too, they were wrong.

Father wanted to hear at first hand just what they thought about the proposed plan. He wanted them to convince him if they were right. Failing this he decreed that the cure used at each plant should be forwarded to Chicago, the best of the formulas selected and made standard for all plants. And by deciding this in the meeting he let those men who believed sincerely in his judgment see for themselves that he was basing his decision on a principle rather than on caprice.

It went through without a ripple. The men in charge of curing at each plant sent in their formulas, despite their many and lusty threats of quitting. The formulas were almost alike in ingredients and proportions. The standard formula was worked out from these. Only slightly modified through the experience of the years this formula is used today as the standard cure in preparing our pork products for market, including our Premium Brand of hams and bacon.

The meeting about secret formulas was not the only one which father ended by voting yes, when the rest of the meeting had voted unanimously no. Because he was dominant in the business, because his ideas generally prevailed—of this, more later—his people from time to time fell into the habit of voting on a business question as they believed he was going to vote.

I recall one meeting where everyone gathered, from his whole attitude, that the chief was in favor of the plan which was up for discussion. So, despite some transparent weaknesses in the idea, they voted yes. After everyone had voted—the votes were always polled singly—the chairman made his announcement:

"I vote no, and the noes have it. You men voted yes because you thought I would. I pay you for your real opinions, not to say what you think I think." It was a good object lesson. It ended the yessing for a good many months.

He was not arbitrary in making these decisions. He had confidence in himself bred of his conduct of the business. He knew the right turn of the road where most of his men must guess on a far less complete knowledge. No wonder he generally arrived at the destination while the rest were wondering what it was all about!

An old plant which had been purchased was to be

extended by adding a large unit. The manager came to Chicago with the plans.

One feature of the blueprints, an open floor for hanging freshly dressed hogs, attracted the unfavorable attention of practically everyone in the meeting. It seemed a needless expense, if not a positive impediment to economical operation. Father listened to the attacks for a while, then leaned back in his chair.

"What've you got to say to that, Johnny?" he inquired of the manager, the son of a Yankee who had come to the Chicago Yards with the original butcher gang from Assonet.

"We can use this open hanging floor for refrigeration three months a year," the manager pointed out—the plant was our farthest north to date. "And it has other technical advantages." He proceeded to enumerate them.

Before he had got well started on the advantages, his chief held up a hand to stop him. "Of course you're right," he decided. The meeting closed right then with the plans approved.

It was not that he wanted his own way regardless. His knowledge was so great that when a practical man was enumerating practical reasons, he absolutely knew. There was no use, therefore, in submitting the plan to further discussion by a number of others even though these others were, after himself, best fitted to judge.

A good deal may be said in favor of this type of meeting after all. It measures up to the ordinary conference as a means of bringing out opinions and information from everyone. And then it leaves the decision to the man best qualified to make it. It puts an automatic stop to buck passing and time wasting, which no business man of experience will deny are the principal products of many meetings. If the top man makes his decision the moment he has the facts at his disposal and then dismisses the meeting, it stops the time wasting before it has a chance to get started. The plan has not been wholly disregarded in our organization since father's time.

Knowledge of every detail of the business was the taproot of his way of managing. His technical knowledge was exhaustive, perhaps as great as that of any man the packing industry has known even to this day. His grasp of the facts of distribution, of transporting the products, of the current standing of company finances—in everything from buying cattle and icing cars all the way through where he would get another ten millions of capital and how he would use it—made him completely the master.

One reason for his mastery of the facts was the time he devoted to business, at the office, at the plants, and at home. Never have I known anyone gifted with such a quick mind who would put in such long hours at his job.

You can rarely talk with anyone who held a place of responsibility under G. F. Swift without there coming out: "I remember one evening G. F. had me over at his house and he asked me—" Hardly an evening that he did not have some of his people at the house talking business and cramming into his already exhaustive knowledge an added store on this point or that—and incidentally giving the employees the benefit of his knowledge and experience.

Talking business was his principal out-of-hours recreation, if it could be called out-of-hours—for he had no hours as working time is generally recognized. The waking day constituted his working hours and he worked at top speed all the while.

One old-timer, a plant man, tells how for weeks on end his chief had him at the house every evening until bedtime. This was in the early days, when the packing house developed new and difficult problems every few hours. Right after supper the plant man would arrive and for perhaps an hour they talked of the day's experience in workrooms and coolers.

Then, the subject temporarily exhausted, father would begin to talk about the export business which was at the time beginning to take shape in a small way but with infinite promise for the future. At least two or three hours he would talk exports to this man who knew slaughtering and dressing and shipping but who had not an ounce of first-hand knowledge on selling overseas.

"I suppose you think it's funny that I get you over here and tell you about all this export business and its troubles," was the explanation which came one night when the practical packer was almost drowsing in his chair from an overdose of exporting. "I'll tell you, I've got it on my mind. I've got to tell it to somebody, and it's got to be somebody I can trust. That's why you get it every night."

For many years we all lived on Emerald Avenue or a block or two away. And "we all" meant the Swifts and the whole management. If a man held a place of responsibility, he lived within easy reach.

The Emerald Avenue location was a neighborhood of better homes than now, of course. But it was never, at best, an especially attractive residence district. When finally G. F. Swift moved to Ellis Avenue, every man of the lot joyfully moved across town to that neighborhood.

A manager or superintendent was supposed to come to the house when he was sent for, no matter what the hour of day or night. And while father aimed to be a considerate man in all ways, he had no respect for idle time. If he wanted a superintendent at 9:30 of an evening for an hour's talk, he sent for him. It would not occur to him that the superintendent would have to be on the plant at 6:30 next morning and that the evening's talk would cut into the night's rest. To any one of his people a night's rest was of no consequence in comparison with supplying information to the chief.

On the evening after the big stockyards strike of 1884 had been broken, principally by father's stubborn stand against the strikers' demands, he called all his foremen to the house. "How many men stayed with you through the strike?" he asked each one. He kept them there until late in the evening discussing their records in holding their men. When he had finished, they had a new comprehension of the value of working with men in the way that wins loyalty.

He was always known as a pusher of men, but never as an inconsiderate driver by the men who remained with him long enough to get really acquainted with his ways. He worked hard himself, harder than he asked anyone else to work. The men who worked with him liked his pushing.

"Don't go to work there, they'll work you to death," a youngster was advised back in Clinton, Massachusetts, when he told some of the villagers he was going to work in G. F. Swift's meat market there in the early '70s. But the boy took the job regardless. He came to Chicago in the slaughterhouse gang which killed and dressed the first Swift beef at the stockyards. He grew up in the harness, became an important man in the company.

"G. F. worked me hard, but he never worked me to death," chuckles the veteran, today retired on his farm from which he frequently comes to visit in the office.

No man ever quit whom father wanted to keep. Probably the chief reason was that if he believed in a man, he would back up that man to the limit. Loyal support from the head of a business makes loyal men beneath the head. And if G. F. Swift did not believe in a man enough to back him up, then he wanted nothing to do with the man.

Certainly in the early days he did not hold his men by paying excessive wages and salaries. He paid small salaries for a good many years. The business was operating on so small a capital and clamoring so insistently for funds that he had to hold down the outgo. He would have been much more liberal if the needs of the business had permitted it. He was more liberal, by far, after the years of greatest expansion were past. But he held his men and kept them working for him loyally and intelligently by the force of his character and the high standards he set them. No one ever attained greater results from his men than he did, principally by the simple expedient of expecting them to deliver more than did other managers.

"No dead lines," was a saying he strongly favored —a dead line was what kept anyone from taking an interest in some activity with which his daily work did not bring him into contact. Everything was considered the concern of everybody. He would not accept the excuse "It wasn't in my department" or "I have nothing to do with the sales department." He wanted no tattling. But he wanted every one of his men to think of himself as a Swift man rather than as a lard department man or a hide cellar foreman or whatever his job.

Because father was the most important individual in the company, every Swift man must recognize a duty to him. That was why a Swift man who found G. F.'s buggy deserted beside a railroad crossing in the Yards was supposed to drive it to the barn.

"I VOTE NO!"

It was important that the buggy be in the barn ready for the chief's call—and it was the lookout of any employee that it get there.

How deeply this idea was ingrained in father's mind was brought out several times by incidents which in the light of today's attitude toward employees are downright startling. One was a time when his horse, left unhitched before the old Live Stock Exchange Building, took it into his head to run away just as his owner was coming out the door.

Down the crowded street ran the horse, the buggy swaying dangerously through the crowded traffic. Then out from the sidewalk dashed a workman, seized the horse's head, and, after being dragged a few feet, brought the rig to a stop.

Father had been only a few feet behind, on the dead run. He came panting up and addressed the man who had done the risky job:

"What's your name?"

"John Brown, sir."

"Who do you work for?"

With a world of pride in his voice and the realization that he had done a job for which he would doubtless he praised, the man answered: "I work for you, Mr. Swift."

"All right," declared his employer, by now in complete command of the situation. "Be about your business."

Chop-fallen, the workman went back to his job—doubtless believing that he worked for a curmudgeon with not an idea of gratitude in his head. Meanwhile that employer returned to the office, had the man given an increase in pay, called in the superintendent under whom Brown worked, and said, "Here's a man worth keeping an eye on. He just did so-and-so. He thinks quickly and acts quickly. Chances are he'd make a good foreman, first time there's an opening."

As for praising the man for bravery, it never entered his mind. The buggy careening down the street belonged to him, and hence was the particular lookout of any employee. Why shouldn't any man have tried to stop it? The point was that, by stopping it, Brown had shown himself a better man than the mass and hence deserved his advancement. The raise and the recommendation were not, be it noted, any tokens of gratitude for stopping the horse. They were for having the qualities which he showed when he stopped the runaway.

Another man, a clerk in father's own office, was blocked in a street-car tangle on Clark Street one evening. So he got out to walk. As he reached the sidewalk he saw his chief striding along in a great rush perhaps two blocks behind him.

He recognized immediately that his boss had been delayed by the car blockade in getting to his Kansas City train. The clerk knew he had an important appointment in Kansas City early next morning and that he must catch the train. So the youngster ran at top speed for the cab stand of the old Grand Pacific Hotel, several blocks up Clark Street. Then

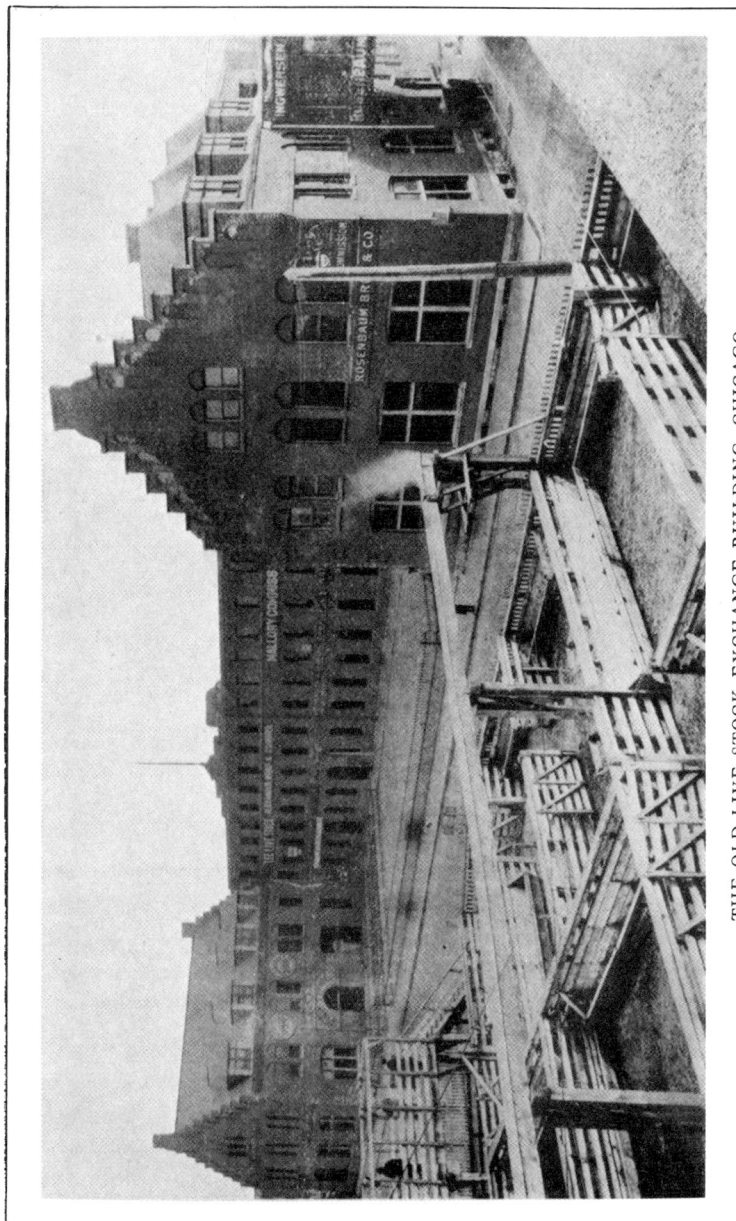

THE OLD LIVE STOCK EXCHANGE BUILDING, CHICAGO.

"I VOTE NO!"

jumping in the cab he ordered the driver to make fast time south.

Sure enough, he soon saw the tall figure of his chief striding along, at every step looking eagerly for a cab—and with very little chance of catching one in that latitude. The clerk pulled the cab up to the curb with a flourish. "Jump in, Mr. Swift," he directed. "Get to the Union Station in three minutes," he ordered the driver.

"Mr. Swift never said anything to me about that," says this man, who today occupies a place of large importance with us. "I knew it was regarded as a good piece of work, and I suspect it was behind a promotion which came to me soon after. But as far as G. F.'s attitude toward me was shown, he expected that sort of service from his people. Of course he knew he didn't get it from all of them, so when he got it he marked the man responsible as worth watching in future. But as for thanking the employees— that would have placed the whole transaction on a false basis."

He was, in his relations with the people under him, as in all his relationships, absolutely and meticulously fair. But he was never guilty of letting anyone believe that he expected from an employee anything less than the utmost. That would not have been good management.

Just as he did not believe in praising a man, so he did not believe in bestowing large titles on employees. He was so much and so thoroughly concerned with the realities of earning profits that the surface froth did not enter into his calculations. One of the surest ways to arouse his irritability was by going to him with such a question as, "What shall we call Mr. So-and-So's new assistant?"

"I've got no use for them titles," he would exclaim in some wrath, waving the interrupter out of the office with gestures of impatience.

Very few indeed were the titles bestowed.

Father harbored another deep conviction. "Swift & Company can get along without any man, myself included," he remarked a few times in my hearing. "This business will be bigger after I'm gone—that's what I'm building for."

It *is* bigger since he is gone.

But I know that it could not have become so big and so successful without the impetus it received from his management. Nor could its growth have been so steady and healthy, lacking the heritage of sound management methods and management policies which he built and gathered for it.

CHAPTER VII

HE HAD TO SPREAD OUT

WHETHER right or wrong, father *would* expand his business at every opportunity. He was a born expansionist.

But he was not a plunger. He knew his business, knew it intimately and in great detail. Because he could see where others could only grope, his vision was steadily ahead of his time.

"That crazy man Swift," the wiseacres called him when he came to the Yards from the East and set his whole energy and twenty years' saving to accomplishing something at which everyone else had failed. No one had succeeded in shipping dressed meat east and disposing of it at a profit. It was one of those things which everyone knew couldn't be done.

His partner Hathaway, of the Boston firm of Hathaway & Swift, could see no chance for success —and Hathaway had been in the live-stock business a good many years longer than had his younger partner.

Hathaway knew, as did everyone else, a thousand reasons why nobody could sell Chicago-dressed beef in the East, and why the East would continue to eat meat from cattle shipped alive for slaughter at the point of consumption. So vehemently did each feel himself right that the partnership had to be dissolved, though with no break in the friendship.

So the younger Yankee was left to build himself a business, to build it on his dream and his accumulated capital of thirty thousand dollars—which was not enough even in 1875 to operate the smallest conceivable packing plant for thirty days. He started under the handicap of inadequate capital. He was not willing as so many men are willing to give his capital a chance to catch up with the size of his business. He could have done this in the first very few years after he succeeded in accomplishing "the impossible." But he *would* keep spreading out.

Always his vision ran ahead of his fellows, of his competition, and of his capital. Always he had under way some enterprise which strained almost to the breaking point the supply of working funds he could command. And despite this ability of his somehow to keep ahead of financial difficulties, his mind ran ahead of his financing ability—he felt himself held back because he had not enough money to do this or that. It was always so.

Even if he had lacked his insistent urge to expand, he would unquestionably have become a successful packer. His other abilities were too great for him to have made anything short of a success. It was his creed of "Expand, and then some more," which kept him from using his $30,000 to build one of the smaller packing establishments, one of the scores doing a profitable business in tens of millions of dollars.

HE HAD TO SPREAD OUT

This creed it was which built him one of the very few transacting a volume in the hundred millions.

He always had an eye for business beyond the ken of others similarly situated. He was only nine years old, as a relative tells the story, when he walked into his grandfather's house and said, "Grandpa, I'll give you forty cents for the old white hen."

"All right," agreed his grandfather—and with no more ado the boy paid his money and went to catch his hen.

"Isn't that new business for Stave, buying hens?" inquired an older cousin who had been completely ignored by the nine-year-old intent on his job.

"Why," the grandfather answered, "he is here almost every day after one. He finds a customer somewhere. Seems to get enough out of it to pay."

There had to be some way for the boy to make money, if he was to have any for himself. Certainly there was no surplus for distribution among the twelve children on his father's sandy, unfertile Cape Cod farm. The best paying crop on Cape Cod today—almost the only paying crop—is summer boarders. For a good many years after Gustavus F. Swift's birth in 1839 the summer boarders had not begun their annual migration.

The boy saw little that was promising in life as a butcher's helper in a Cape Cod village. He had gone to work for his older brother Noble at fourteen and by his sixteenth birthday was making—be sure that he was earning—three dollars a week.

Even in those days of 1855 the golden goal of ambitious Cape Cod lads was Boston. He began to lay his plans for a move to Boston and the West.

His father objected. He saw for his son no great future in the big city, equipped as he was with no fund of education, of business experience, or of demonstrated ability. He held that strong sixteen-year old country lads were a drug on the Boston market. To back up his ideas he was willing to do a fair share —more than a fair share, perhaps, when one considers the value of a cash dollar in his circumstances of life.

"You really want to be in the meat business, don't you?" he questioned his son. "All right, Stave, I'll give you twenty-five dollars to start up in the meat business around home. That way you can get your start right here, instead of going away to the city."

With this twenty-five dollars was started the business which is today Swift & Company. The lineage is straight as an arrow. For, twenty-five dollars in his pocket, the boy of sixteen set forth to enter the meat business.

He made a neighbor an offer for a good fat heifer he thought he might butcher to advantage. It is characteristic of his shrewdness as a trader—shrewdness as far above his age as was his shrewdness above other business men's thirty years later—that he did not, boylike, offer his whole twenty-five dollars. Whatever his original offer, he actually purchased the heifer for nineteen dollars, as he told the story in

SALLY SEARS CROWELL
SWIFT, MOTHER OF
G. F. SWIFT.

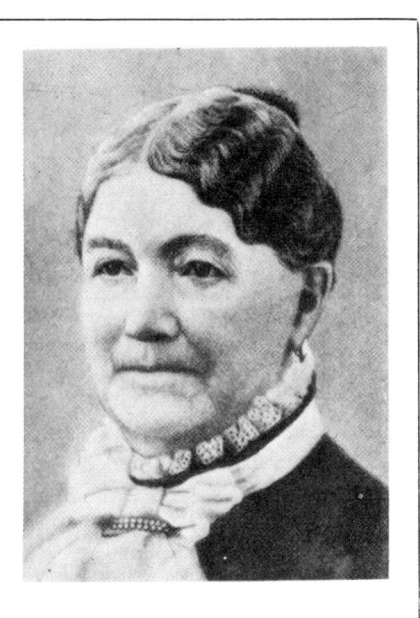

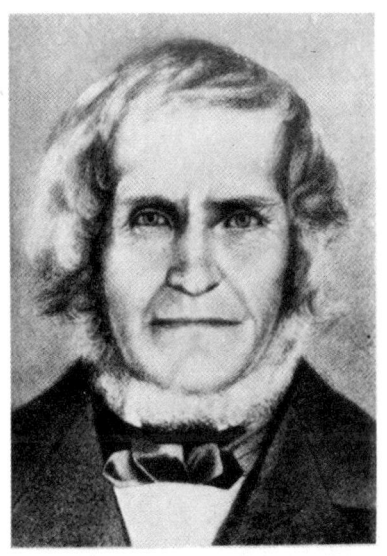

WILLIAM SWIFT, FATHER
OF G. F. SWIFT.

HE HAD TO SPREAD OUT

later life. He drove her home and slaughtered her in a shed. Now he was embarked in the retail meat business.

He cut up the beef, loaded the cuts into a wagon of his father's and set out to sell the meat in the neighborhood. Fortune favored the enterprise, another way of saying that he had used good judgment in buying the heifer, ample skill in cutting up the carcass, and sales ability in disposing of the cuts. He netted ten dollars out of the transaction for his time and trouble. Forthwith he went out to repeat the operation and the resultant profit.

For a few weeks or months he had ample capital— the only time in his business career when he had, except for the last two or three years of his life. But soon that active mind of his began to see larger opportunities which called for more working funds than he had been able to acquire by selling pot-roasts and steaks and ribs. He could always see the chance to make more money by doing on a larger scale.

The first occasion of this sort has been told by a cousin of my father's, E. W. Ellis, sixty-five years later. Thomas W. Goodspeed set it down[1] as follows:

"He called on Uncle Paul Crowell (son of Grandfather Crowell and village storekeeper). I obtained this information a few days after from Uncle Paul himself. Stave said, 'I want to borrow some money. Will you lend it to me?'

---
[1] *The University of Chicago Biographical Sketches*, Vol. I, p. 176.

" 'Oh,' said Uncle Paul, 'how much do you want?'
" 'Four hundred dollars,' said Stave.
" 'Whew,' said Uncle Paul, 'what you going to do with it?'
" 'I want to go to Brighton stockyards and buy some pigs.'
" 'Why, that will be quite an undertaking for a boy.'
" 'Yet,' said Uncle Paul to me, 'I could but admire his ambition.'
"Brighton yards, located northwest of Boston, sixty miles distant! Just imagine it! The worst kind of sandy, crooked roads. . . . . Well, in about ten days, he, with his drove, hove in sight at my father's home. He had sold some, but about thirty-five shoats were still with him. I looked over his outfit, which consisted of an old horse and a democrat wagon in which a few tired or lame pigs were enjoying a ride and a rest with their legs tied together. With him was another lad as helper, who was trying keep the shoats from straying. There was Stave, a tall, lank youth, with a rope and steelyards on his shoulder, also a short pole he carried in his hand that might do duty to suspend the squealers and steelyards between his shoulders and those of his customer. Father said: 'There is a good exhibition of ambition. Gustavus Swift will make a success in whatever business he undertakes. For he has the right make-up.' Gustavus made several such trips to Brighton for pigs, spring and fall, for two or three years."

The occupation of drover under these conditions was at best highly seasonal. Outside the spring and fall months, he might have lacked occupation. Instead, he worked out a procedure which gave him a business. He arranged for quarters at Brighton stockyards where he could slaughter his animals.

Each Friday he bought a steer on the market there and slaughtered it on Saturday. The quarters he hung over Sunday. Monday morning bright and early saw him in his democrat wagon with the meat, bound for Cape Cod. By Friday he had sold his beef and was back at Brighton once more, making his weekly purchase of one animal.

From his repeated Monday-to-Friday trips the young man accumulated a little money—a very little, no doubt, but enough to give him a foothold as a retail meat dealer instead of a wagon peddler. So he opened a market at Eastham, which shortly afterward he turned over to his brother Nathaniel. Then he opened a meat market at Barnstable and settled down as the meat dealer for this town of five hundred.

Father and mother, Annie Maria Higgins, had been married during the short career at Eastham. At Barnstable they and their growing family—there were four of us children by then—remained some eight years. But it was not the retail business which held G. F. Swift. Rather it was a broad business he had developed, leaving the market to be run by a clerk. Once more he was at his habit of expanding.

Beginning as he had at sixteen and continuing

without interruption as a cattle buyer, by the time he moved to Barnstable he had become an extremely good judge of cattle. There is no way to check up on the accuracy of a cattle buyer's judgment except to see how his purchases dress into beef. Even though his career had been active for only six or seven years, father had been seeing how each one of his cattle dressed—not only seeing it but also feeling with his own pocketbook the results of his judgment. In a man of his shrewdness the only possible result was that he became a remarkably good cattle buyer.

With his knack of seeing the opportunity for broadening out his activities, he had no sooner been set down in Barnstable than he began to wonder if he could not market Cape-Cod-raised cattle at a profit. The average farmer had only one or two head for sale in a season. The nearest market, besides the small local butchers like himself, was at Brighton beyond Boston. And it didn't pay to drive just one or two head to Brighton, even as low as the farmer valued his time.

So once more G. F. Swift ramified his business. To be sure, he kept the meat market, but this was now a side issue. He became a cattle dealer, buying on Cape Cod and selling at Brighton.

It is noticeable that, however he might expand or diversify his interests, he never deviated by a hair's thickness from the original direction of his work. Ever broader, ever making a little better living, ever building up his capital but spreading it just as thin as he safely could, he was on his way to founding the modern dressed meat industry!

By 1869, when he was thirty years old, he had accumulated enough to take his first step of any size. His capital was far from a fortune; it had taken him fourteen years to expand his original capital of twenty-five dollars into a sum sufficient for anything at all extensive. With this capital which he had sweated out by working sixteen hours a day father opened the meat market at Clinton, Massachusetts.

This enterprise has been described earlier in this book. It was a large store, for that time and place a pretentious, ambitious store. It developed quickly into a large and profitable retail business doing an annual volume of thirty-five or forty thousand dollars. It yielded him an income which in those days was unusually good for a small town.

But hardly had he attained for his store the momentum he had planned when his mind grasped other opportunities. Being a retail meat dealer involved pretty much killing his own meat animals and selling the cuts a few pounds at a time. But there were growing up, in some of the more thickly populated districts such as that around Boston, wholesale slaughterers and wholesale meat dealers who supplied neighboring retailers fresh dressed meats, thus saving the storekeeper the job of slaughtering.

Father was not unaware of this development, and of the related development which involved a shift of source of meat animals from local raisers to the grazing districts of the West. The ratio of cattle population to human population of the New England states had declined far below the point of domestic supply. The cattle to make up this deficiency were coming in from the West, which meant that someone was making a profit in handling them.

Never did a significant trend of any sort within the live-stock or meat industries escape G. F. Swift's alert mind. He saw a chance to become the slaughterer and wholesale supplier to his neighboring retail meat markets. Soon he was doing a considerable business in selling to the trade.

But even this development, with its improvement of a business already to be counted good, did not hold him for long. He had attracted the attention of two of the prominent figures in the New England live-stock and meat businesses. One was D. M. Anthony, a large wholesale slaughterer and meat dealer of Fall River. The other was J. A. Hathaway, a cattle dealer most of whose animals found their way aboard cattle ships bound for England from Boston.

Anthony wanted young Gustavus Swift in with him. So did Hathaway. The upshot was that the Clinton business was turned over to Edwin C. Swift to manage. And two new firms came into existence: Anthony, Swift & Company, of Fall River; Hathaway & Swift, of Brighton.

Shortly thereafter we went to Brighton to live. Father sold his retail market at Clinton to a man named Pope, while my uncle continued to manage the Clinton wholesale business. All of the Clinton butchers who were not needed for the wholesale business were now transferred to Anthony, Swift & Company's slaughterhouse at Assonet, just outside Fall River.

"Well enough" was never satisfactory to Gustavus Swift. He had been at Brighton only a year or two, buying cattle for Hathaway to ship and for Anthony to slaughter, when he decided that the advantageous way to buy cattle was near the source of supply. A big stockyards had been established at Albany. So he moved us to Albany, a peg nearer the source of supply.

However good Albany had looked to him as the primary market when he was doing business in eastern Massachusetts, it looked nowhere nearly so fine after he was on the ground. To be sure, cattle were there to be dealt in in great quantity. But to his analytical mind it was not right as a primary market.

He followed the railroad back to Buffalo, where another large stockyards was running. He kept taking short trips there to look over the market and to buy a few cattle. Buffalo was better than Albany, because it was nearer where the cattle came from. It left a good deal to be desired, though. Chicago was yet to be inspected.

The more father thought about Chicago, the more logical it sounded. The cattle on their way from the farms and the ranches and the plains made Chicago their first stop. Then why was not Chicago the place where, inevitably, cattle could be purchased to the best advantage? At Chicago must be the greatest selection, with the minimum of commissions and handling charges accrued against the animals.

So in 1875 he came to Chicago. Here he bought cattle for Hathaway to resell, for the Anthonys and Edwin C. Swift to slaughter and sell at wholesale. He also purchased cattle in Chicago on commission for Calvin Leavitt & Son, of Brighton, which sold these cattle to the Brighton butchers.

Wellington Leavitt, who is now and for a great many years has been Swift & Company's head cattle buyer, was the "Son" in the firm of Calvin Leavitt & Son. When Wellington Leavitt was still in business at Brighton with his father, he helped sell cattle sent down by my father from Chicago.

What cattle G. F. Swift purchased at Chicago that summer of 1876 all went east in cattle cars. But he conceived the idea of slaughtering the cattle at Chicago and shipping only the edible parts. Why pay freight on a thousand-pound steer? That steer would dress down to six hundred pounds of beef. Most of the remaining four hundred pounds were thrown away or were even an expense because someone had to be paid to cart them off.

Father tried it experimentally the next winter. He shipped box cars of dressed beef. Some of the cars were heated by stoves to prevent too hard freezing and accompanied by a man to tend the fires. Other cars were shipped with no stoves, completely

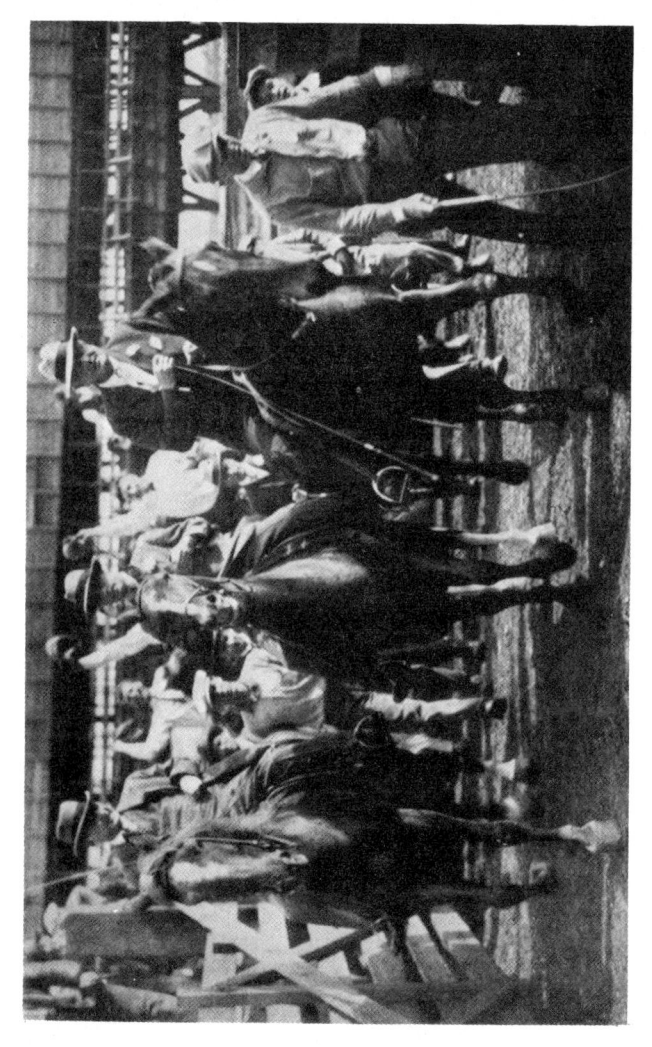

WELLINGTON LEAVITT, (LEFT) DEAN OF THE CATTLE BUYERS, WHO BECAME ASSOCIATED WITH G. F. SWIFT ABOUT 1875, THE PRINCE OF WALES, AND LOUIS F. SWIFT RIDING THROUGH "THE YARDS", OCTOBER 13, 1924.

dependent on the weather. All of the cars came through in good condition, with the beef all the better for hanging several days in transit.

From this the step to refrigerator cars was, in time, short. In difficulties it was long and wearying, too long for discussion at this point.

Every step of it, however, involved expanding, involved spending more money, involved a larger volume to make possible the savings or the profits or whatever the objective was for which at the moment he was striving. He had to lay all of the groundwork himself. No one else could obtain the funds he needed. No one else could improvise the thousand and one successful expedients which kept his business going upward.

For he kept the business climbing. Rather he raised it to ever higher points by projecting his creative imagination upward from one stage to the next, then taking the leap and carrying the business with him.

And he held absolutely to his own business. This is a basic reason why he succeeded in building up his business so fast. He went, everyone knows, at a rate considerably faster than a conservative man would have thought either possible or safe. He held absolutely to his own line. He knew what he was doing and why. His decisions were based on a meticulous knowledge of his own affairs and of the whole industry. He built in his own way and didn't wait until the time when he would have the money.

Each step of expansion was a definite progress along a charted road. Father had no idea at the outset that his business would or could become as large as eventually it did. But he was heading it always in its given direction.

He developed the idea of shipping beef instead of cattle. Right there he unquestionably selected his goal. He determined to head those who purveyed meat to the public.

He set his heart on being the leader, he set his mind to becoming the leader. This would have seemed a preposterous dream to anyone but himself, considering his lack of money and backing. No wonder they called him "that crazy man Swift." But if to others it seemed overreaching, to father it seemed so wholly reasonable that he attained leadership by a route straight as an arrow. He went that route, he reached his goal by strength of will and determination.

All circumstances were with him—particularly the times. If he had not exploited the refrigerator car, someone else no doubt would have succeeded with it in at least a few years. Others had already had some success with refrigerator cars without attaining leadership in the industry. With his early control of large-scale use of the refrigerator car and his remarkable combination of ability and energy, father had an advantage which he crowded to the limit. This limit was the leadership of his field.

How he pushed for sales outlets has already been described. His personal working methods by which

HE HAD TO SPREAD OUT

during the early days he concentrated sixteen or eighteen or occasionally twenty-four hours a day on overwhelming problems which harassed him—these have been told in a previous chapter. The summer of 1875 had seen the thirty-five-year-old Yankee come to Chicago's Yards as a late entrant in a race which seemed already settled. Fifteen years later he had sales branches or dealers in every strategic city of the United States. He was shipping great quantities of meat abroad in refrigerator ships. He had outlets all through the British Isles and in many Continental cities.

No longer was his enterprise confined to beef. He had put the company into mutton, into pork and provisions, into all of the by-product lines which had been an essential outgrowth. Swift refrigerator cars rolled by the thousands over every railroad in the country.

It was toward the close of the '80s that he raised the question of building branch plants still nearer the source of supply than Chicago. Beef cattle were coming principally from the West and Southwest. Why not slaughter them near their points of origin and thus effect savings comparable to the savings which had been attained when beef was dressed at Chicago instead of at Fall River?

At Kansas City, Kansas, was a stockyards of considerable size. Several concerns were operating packing plants there, one or two of them on a reasonably large scale. It was selected as the site of our first western branch. In 1888 the Kansas City plant went up.

It provided an excellent market for southwestern cattle. But Kansas City was not the most economical point for stock from the plains of western Nebraska and Colorado and the country farther north. So the Kansas City plant had been operated for only a few months when an identical plant was built at Omaha. The Omaha plant was completed in 1890. The plant at East St. Louis, Illinois, was finished in 1892.

The panic year 1893 gave the building program a set-back. But after a few months to recover his wind, father was once more aggressively at his plans for expansion. His next step was the St. Joseph, Missouri, plant, finished in 1896. Its start and its subsequent history well illustrate his way of tackling a problem when it presented itself to him.

St. Joseph is between Kansas City and Omaha. It is far less important as a railroad center than either of these larger cities.

An earlier effort had established the packing industry at St. Joseph, but while it had managed to struggle along it had not thrived. Kansas City with its large live-stock market offered stockmen a better chance to sell their animals. At Kansas City, buyers were actively competing and huge numbers of animals were dealt in daily.

At St. Joseph, only sixty-five miles away, there was little activity. Grass was literally growing in the yards there. The local business men earnestly

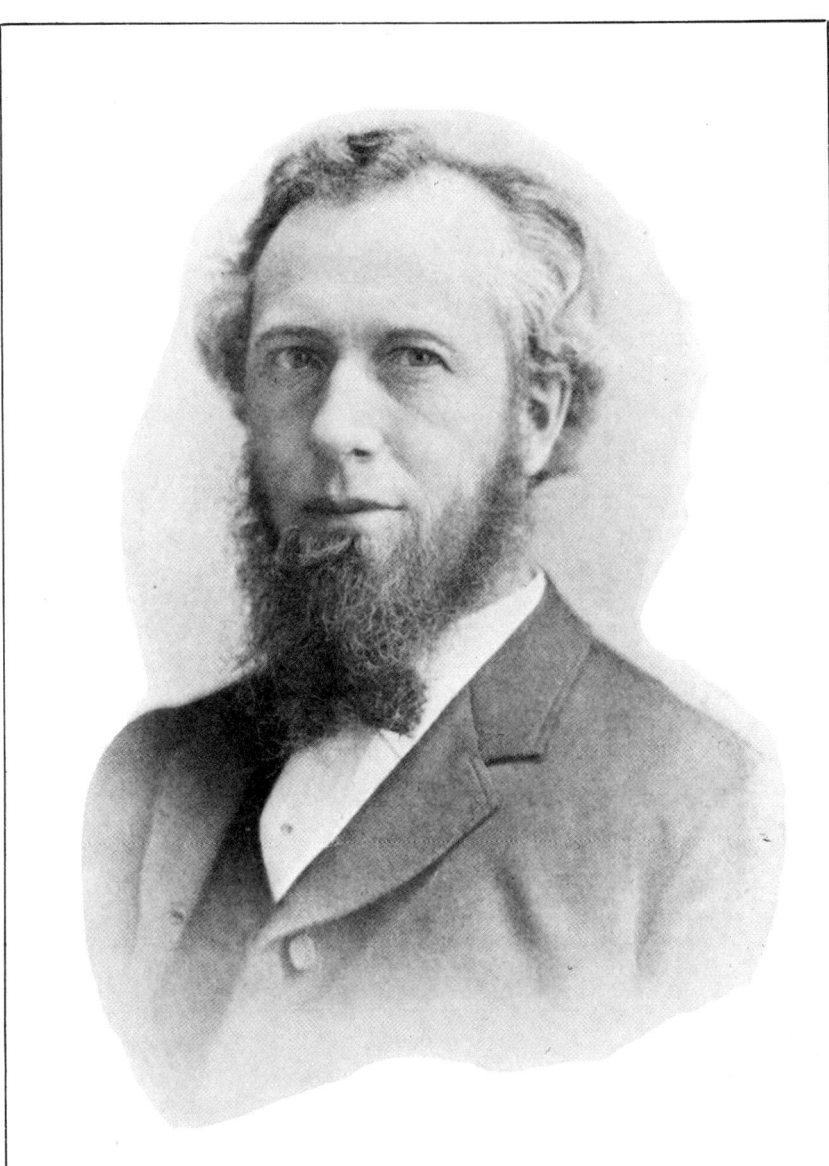

G. F. SWIFT, ABOUT 1885.

HE HAD TO SPREAD OUT 133

wished to bring in one of the larger packers with a large plant. And they approached the head of Swift & Company.

He did not want his information or opinions at second hand. He went to St. Joseph, taking with him a few of his lieutenants, and was feted and argued at. But all of that rolled off his mind like so much water.

It was at a banquet given him in St. Joseph that he made one remark from which has echoed many a chuckle. Frogs' legs were part of one course, but the guest of honor refused them.

"You'd better have some, Mr. Swift," urged one of the local hosts. "They're very tender."

"They ought to be," the partisan of beef came back at him with some heat. "All a frog does is sit on the bank and sing!"

Not the entertainments, but the personal investigations of himself and of his men, finally induced his decision. He studied the town, the people, the character of the country. For several days he drove around the surrounding country by himself or accompanied by that one of his own men who could contribute the most expert knowledge of whatever point he was studying.

The character of the soil. The local crops. The number of bushels to the acre. The kind of roads. The kind of farmers. The way the railroad layout would permit shipping stock to St. Joseph. All these points he studied until he probably knew a good deal more about them than did any local banker or other man around St. Joseph.

His investigations showed him that, even though it was within sixty-five miles of Kansas City, a good market at St. Joseph would divide the Kansas City and Omaha hog supply. He could buy the St. Joseph stockyards, which would give him an advantage here.

Everybody considered it a wild enterprise, even most of the men most closely associated with him. But the chief had made up his mind. "Folks think we're a little bit crazy," he told the meeting which had gathered to consider the purchase. "But there's lots of live stock down that way. They haven't got a real market there, so they don't get the animals.

"If we set out to make a market there, we'll make a market. We'll buy the stockyards and put up a plant."

It looked like a foolish move. The St. Joseph plant was built over the objections of a large share of his organization. But it paid—paid well. Like many of his most profitable expansions, in advance it seemed to almost everyone else absolutely wrong. He was simply ahead of the rest of us. He grasped all the facts and correlated them into a plan which brought dollars into his stockholders' pockets.

Immediately after the St. Joseph plant came the plant at South St. Paul. Here was a defunct packing plant which he bought because he saw something that others could not see.

People thought hogs could be raised only where

corn was grown—and the country around St. Paul was not then notable for corn. But father never did much loose thinking. He had a scientist's passion for indisputable facts. He checked up and learned that the farmers there had screenings and other small grains which did not grade up well. Consequently a farmer could more profitably turn this into pork than he could sell it as grain.

He was right. Almost invariably he was right in anything bearing on his affairs. Now South St. Paul kills more hogs than any other Swift plant except Chicago, which has of course remained the largest plant in every respect.

G. F. Swift could see further into the packing industry's future than any man I have ever known. He was very much the expansionist all of the time. He saw cheap live stock and he could not keep his hands off it. He had to expand to get facilities he felt he had to have—and he expanded so intelligently that he reached exactly the point he was aiming for.

Nothing was too big for him if it looked to show a profit. Sioux City stockyards offer an illustration. There had been a top-heavy boom at Sioux City, financed by eastern money. In every direction the plans had been laid along most ambitious lines—and eventually it blew up, of course.

Father wanted the stockyards. The creditors would not sell the stockyards separately. They would sell everything to one buyer or they would sell nothing. So he bought the whole thing, paying a large sum of money and taking along with his stockyards a number of enterprises he had no use for.

Here once more nobody would vote with him. Everyone knew he was wrong. But his vision showed him that the stockyards alone were a good buy at the price he had to pay for the whole—even if he had to throw away everything else about the property. As it was, the facilities which were not needed were gradually sold off, the last parcel years after his death. But as he had foreseen, this was an excellent buy. Today the stockyards are worth considerably more than he paid for the whole property. What he and subsequently his estate sold the rest for was clear profit on an already profitable deal.

Always he kept his affairs ahead of his finances and his plans ahead of his affairs. One reason, the principal reason he managed to carry the thing off, was that he knew his business and held to it exclusively. He had no interests outside live stock, packing, and closely related enterprises. A secondary reason why he succeeded where most men must have failed was that he knew the measure of everyone from whom he borrowed money in any considerable amount. The lender acted as the borrower counted on him to do every time.

When father started at Chicago in 1875, those in a position to size him up swore he would fail. When he began to expand, the dire prophecies were quite as confident. But he made every enterprise successful with which he was connected.

HE HAD TO SPREAD OUT

At the outset, he had about thirty thousand dollars from his share of the partnership of Hathaway & Swift. In 1885 his firm was incorporated as Swift & Company, with three hundred thousand dollars capitalization. Within two years he had to recapitalize for three millions, so rapid had been the young company's expansion.

By 1896 the capital stock was fifteen millions. By 1903, the year of his death, the capital was twenty-five millions. And every cent of the capital had come either from earnings or from subscriptions at par by existing stockholders whenever a new issue was made. The company's total sales in 1903 exceeded one hundred and sixty million dollars. Its president had seven thousand employees under him by that time.

For Gustavus Franklin Swift, while a dreamer and a visionary, based his dreams and his visions of expansion very much on the practical facts of life.

CHAPTER VIII

"I RAISE BETTER MEN"

"THERE'S an ice house down at Beardstown might be a good buy for us," G. F. Swift instructed one of his young men some thirty-five years ago. I want you to go down there and look it over carefully. Get the facts on its dimensions, ice capacity, construction, and everything else important."

So the youngster journeyed to Beardstown, spent the better part of a day there, and next day presented himself at his chief's desk. He reported a great assortment of facts.

Finally the boss interrupted him to inquire, "What kind of drainage is there off the roof?"

"Drainage?"

"Yes, drainage. What kind of spouts, gutters, and so on?"

The ice-house expert got red in the face. He did not answer.

"All right, now, you don't know, you don't know, do you? You get right on the next train and have another look at that ice house. When you come back, you be able to tell me all about that roof drainage and anything else you think maybe I ought to know that you don't know now."

So back to Beardstown the young man traveled.

He spent a day going over the ice house a second time. Half the day he spent on the roof. Next day he was back to report once more.

"You went up on the roof this time, didn't you?" inquired his chief after listening to a detailed description of every foot of tinsmithing about the premises.

"Yes, sir."

"I wanted to get you up on that roof," he declared with a dry chuckle. "I wanted to get you up somewhere near the top of this business. There's only one way a fellow like you can get to the top. If you don't do your job any better than you did first time I sent you, the only way you'll get to the top is by running the elevator."

Another time father was coming from the East to Chicago on a train arriving at night. At Cleveland the manager of one of our wholesale markets got on the car, going to some town near by. His chief joyously cornered him at once and began asking questions, as was his habit with any manager he ever succeeded in getting off by himself.

All went smoothly for a while. Then the boss asked, "How many windows on the west side of your cooler?"

"I don't know, Mr. Swift."

"Don't know! I never heard of a branch-house manager who didn't know how many windows he had in his cooler! You get off this train, go back to Cleveland and find out all about those windows. I'll expect you in my office at Chicago tomorrow morning to tell me how many windows there are and anything else I ask you. I guess we're slowing up now. See you in the morning." And he blandly waved the bewildered manager off at Sandusky.

Next day the man appeared at Chicago and underwent a rigid examination on all of the details of his cooler and its peculiarities. What's more, word of the episode spread through every Swift channel in the country. Managers who valued their peace of mind knew, thereafter, how many windows their coolers had. Moreover, they knew a whole lot more about their physical equipment than ever before.

At handling men, at selecting them, at training them to places of real responsibility—at all of these duties father's ability was superlative. His methods were in large measure unconventional. By their very lack of resemblance to the time-honored and time-worn they were the more effective.

When he sent a man back to have a second look at the roof drainage of an out-of-town ice house the employee learned for all time that on any assigned job he must do just as well as any man could. What is more, this lesson made him into a first-rate head of the ice department—a position into which the man developed and which he filled creditably for many years.

At one stroke G. F. Swift taught this lesson to a good many people besides the particular man who had to make the second trip. Because the punishment was so picturesque and at the same time was both laughable and appropriate, the story was passed along from employee to employee. It was something to chuckle about—and while he chuckled, every Swift man worth his salt applied to himself the standard of performance toward which the parable pointed.

The branch-house manager who returned home to count the cooler windows went for a parallel reason: a manager ought to know all about the equipment he is in charge of. The method the chief used here was almost exactly the same as that applying to the ice-house roof. Yet I dare say no thought of it came into his mind when he ordered the manager off at Sandusky. His mind worked so directly on a specific problem in handling men that he arrived forthwith at the proper answer. That the problem was similar accounts for the similar solution.

Father frequently asserted, "I can raise better men than I can hire." The proof of the assertion is in the present-day proportion of men trained under him who are in positions of high responsibility with Swift & Company more than twenty years after his death. He trained his men—"raised 'em," as he used to say—by methods which are as sound in principle now as they were then. Obviously some of the details would not fit this generation, which stubbornly believes that the boss is not invariably right.

A man who later had charge of one of our most important activities recently told of an experience with his chief forty-odd years ago. He had come to work just before Christmas of 1884, at a weekly wage of fifteen dollars. He had made a strong effort to get seventeen when he was hired, and failed. So after a year he asked for the two-dollar raise.

"G. F. took me out in the hall," he tells the story, "and walked me around a corner to a window. I can see him yet, as he put his cowhide boot up on the window sill and looked down his nose at me. 'You think you're worth more money'n you're gettin', do you?' he inquired rather savagely.

" 'Yes, sir,' I assured him.

" 'Well, you're not,' he told me. And then he started in to tell what he thought of me as an employee. It took him a long while. I had felt pretty sure of myself before I tackled him for the raise and I had a lot of good reasons why I deserved it. But I never got a chance to use them. He told me what was wrong with my attitude toward my work and he illustrated the general statements with specific examples out of my short career with him. He used the examples liberally, yet managed to give me the impression he had a lot more in mind which he wasn't citing because of the short time at his disposal for so insignificant a task.

"He literally took my hide off and nailed it to the door. When he got through with me, I felt real gratitude that he still tolerated my unwholesome presence in the office and was willing to let me continue drawing the same old fifteen dollars a week.

"I RAISE BETTER MEN"

When he had finished the job, after an hour and a half or perhaps two hours, I went back to my desk and went to work. I was full of the idea that I was next to useless. But G. F. had left a ray of hope in parting. He let me believe I might have a chance to become a productive member of the community if I really buckled down to the job of putting into use some of the advice I had just received!

"A year afterward, I got my two-dollar raise without asking for it. After that I steadily went along, taking on more responsibility and drawing bigger pay. It was some time after G. F. had raised me to ten thousand that he inquired very casually one day, 'Remember that time I took you out in the hall over in the old Exchange Building and told you what I thought of you?'

"I had supposed he had forgotten it years before. 'Yes,' I admitted—and I could feel myself getting red around the ears with the memory of it.

" 'Do you know why I did it?' he asked me.

" 'The only reason I know is that you were mad at me because I had been doing such a poor job,' I told him honestly.

" 'Why, no. That wasn't it at all,' he explained in some astonishment that I had not comprehended it long before. 'You were doing right well for a young fellow. Not bad at all. But I thought you had the makings of something better than an ordinary clerk and I wanted to see. I jumped on you that day just to put your feet on the ground. It made a man of you, that talk did. I could see it by next morning.' You know, I think he was right!"

Father did not believe in sparing overmuch the feelings of the man who needed correction or guidance or reproof. He felt that if a man needed talking to, the talk had better be strong and to the point. In these days employees were less sensitive, their sensibilities had not been so assiduously cultivated. Consequently his specific ways of going at such a job roughshod did the minimum harm and the maximum good.

But even though his methods would require some alteration to be usable today, the principle on which they were based is just as sound as ever it was. The man who hears promptly and forcefully about a mistake of procedure or of judgment has been caught at the right time and in the right way to make him remember the lesson. If he is the right kind of man he is better off for being corrected.

It is remarkable to look back now and see how large a proportion—how unbelievably large a proportion—of the men who came in for father's reformative measures have come up and up in the ranks. Some of the men he started in on could not stand the treatment and dropped out. Most of those who stuck it out became real assets to the company and have been rewarded accordingly.

Yet it was not always easy to reconcile a spirited man to treatment which he might feel was nagging. Those of us who were very close to G. F. Swift and had worked with him over a long term, knew that he never nagged. It was a mark of distinction to any man to have his chief return time after time to point out that individual's shortcomings and general uselessness.

One youngster was working as an assistant of mine when some failing or other brought him to father's attention. The boy was in a position where he was responsible for the work of a sizeable group of people, many of them a good deal older than himself and longer in the service. Consequently when he undertook to change their ways he had his troubles.

What caught the chief's eye was something that the youngster's subordinates were doing wrong. I happened to be out of town, else the first reproof would have come my way. As it was, he went after my helper.

It was his fashion, once some wrong method or weak spot claimed his attention, to check it up daily. The youngster did not make very fast progress in correcting his people's fault. So every evening, along about closing time, he was sent for. When he came to the front office he received a talk on his weaknesses as a manager. Finally the chief saw that some resentment was smoldering. So he inquired, "You think I've been after you pretty hard, don't you?"

"Yes I do, Mr. Swift."

"Well, I'll tell you. If you work for me long enough, some day you'll know something and you'll be some good to somebody." That was G. F. Swift's idea of a handsome way to make amends for all he had said before!

Finally, after ten days or so I returned from my trip. The youngster was just waiting for me to return so he could quit. But I had one argument that changed his mind. "Father doesn't go after a man day in and day out if he thinks he's wasting it," I told him. "You sit here every day, you hear the way he goes after me, so you know you aren't getting half as much scolding as I am. He's pretty careful about not going to a lot of trouble to correct a man if he doesn't think the man is worth correcting."

Before long the youngster was sent to England on a particularly important job—at the chief's suggestion. A little later he had to do some more foreign traveling. While he was still in his early twenties he was untangling hard knots for us all over the world. Today he is operating one of our largest plants. He is a fair sample of the results father got by his methods. They were effective even though they sometimes seemed harsh.

I doubt whether G. F. Swift consciously thought of himself as a teacher in his job of training executives. Certainly he was about the most effective teacher I have encountered. And while he was a terror to the man who was weak or wrong, he was extremely helpful to the man who tried hard.

One plant manager says of him: "When I first started to work in a place where Mr. Swift saw me, I was afraid of him and would go out of my way to

"I RAISE BETTER MEN" 147

avoid him. But after I really knew what I was doing, I especially wanted to see him when I came to Chicago. Before I planned a trip definitely I would generally try to find out if G. F. was planning to be there. Even when I didn't have any one thing to take up with him, I wanted to see him. For I knew that in the course of our talk he would give me some idea or other which would be valuable—more valuable than anything I was likely to get elsewhere."

When any of the leading men of the branch houses or even one of the more important beef salesmen came to Chicago, that man stayed at his chief's house. The custom had its start in the early days when transportation from the stockyards was slow and difficult, so that for convenience the men had to be kept at the house instead of being sent to downtown hotels. It was continued because father liked to keep right on with his business after the evening meal and he saw a really valuable way to employ this time in talking with his out-of-town men.

He would question the visitor by the hour until he had satisfied himself that the man was honest and knew his job. Then the more intensive questioning ceased. But in the earlier months of a man's tenure of his new job, every visit to Chicago meant so many evenings of cross-examination.

One new manager after his first experience of this sort went back home and prepared a good-sized pocket notebook in which he kept facts and figures of all sorts that his chief might require. A traveling auditor or someone of the sort brought back to Chicago word of this loose-leaf ready-reference compendium. It appealed to everyone, including father, as a huge joke. Thereafter he was extra careful to ask this man unusual questions. Tradition has it that for three years the notebook was maintained, that every time its owner came to Chicago he kept his hand on its reassuring bulk in his coat pocket—and that not once in that time was he asked a question for which he had the answer in his book!

After a new man in a new job had established himself as worth educating, his employer would proceed with the training. One of his methods was to go over a batch of random mail with the visitor, especially in the later years of his life when he used to have some of his letters sent over to the house. He would ask the guest what he would do about this request for charity, about that application for reinstatement. After a session like this the employee had a grasp on some of the basic rules of business which he had never before comprehended.

Once G. F. was convinced that a man should develop into someone of consequence, he kept trying and trying to do the job. It was seldom he failed. But occasionally he had, after a long struggle, to give it up.

There was one such man he sent to St. Joseph as assistant manager. The newcomer did not fit in and after a while was transferred to Kansas City. No matter how much time his sponsor would spend with this man, he could not bring him up to the mark. Also he kept trying to get both the St. Joseph manager and the Kansas City manager to say that the fellow was some good. Finally he gave it up. But he hated to do it.

"There isn't much use giving up a man too early if you think maybe he's going to be all right," he observed on this occasion and a good many times after. It became one of his precepts in developing men.

If he once sized a man up as having possibilities, he would not easily change his opinion. Occasionally this wasted a good deal of everyone's time in trying to develop a man who would not develop. Also it lost just so many months in getting the right man on that job. But more time is saved by patience in training men than by impatience. Few traits cost employers as much as the common failing of giving up a man for hopeless long before he has proved it. We try to inculcate in all our people this idea that there is no use giving up a man before he has proved himself worthless. As a result we develop the latent ability in a good many men and women who would not last two months if we were critical in the early stages.

In general father was not much on hiring men from the outside for jobs of any consequence. He preferred hiring his men young and bringing them up by hand. His inclination was to hire competent men on the outside only when they were especially equipped for some new enterprise with which we lacked experience.

Occasionally, though, he stepped right across the line and hired someone for a special reason. When our plant at St. Joseph was building, he made the acquaintance there of an eastern man, O. W. Waller, who was having an uphill fight to make his little packing plant break even. Father developed the habit of dropping in on Waller for a visit after his list of duties in St. Joseph had been completed and he was ready to leave by the first train.

One evening their visit continued until about half an hour before time for the Chicago train. It happened that Waller was also going to Chicago but had said nothing about it. Instead, once the caller was out of his office he hustled out the back way, jumped into his buggy, and drove home for dear life. At home he changed his suit, packed a bag, ate a hasty supper, and was driven up to the station platform at a gallop just as the train pulled in.

Quite a party of us were going in on that train, but father was fascinated by the performance of his rapid-moving acquaintance. It was so wholly like his own way of arriving with never a minute to spare. He deserted his own forces for the companionship of the St. Joseph packer after introducing us singly and recounting the speed with which this gentleman had traveled once he got started.

They sat together during all of the evening, in the

course of which father reminesced in great detail about his career from the age of nine down to date. This of itself was so unusual that we were all astonished. As they said good-night, father told him, "Any time you want to come to work for me, I've a good job for you."

Not long afterward Waller gave up the fight. He had not been able to overcome the handicaps of inadequate capital and inefficient plant. No sooner was he announced as going out of business than the head of Swift & Company was after him to take a job with us. Waller's ability to accomplish a great deal in a short time was so remarkably like his own that father recognized he would fit well into a place of responsibility.

So he was sent for to come to Chicago. And all around the offices the chief introduced him to everyone as "Mr. Waller from St. Joseph, who's come to work for Swift & Company."

"But I'm not working for Swift & Company," protested Waller.

"You mean to say you wouldn't work for us in the right kind of a job?"

"What kind of a job?"

"Manager of a packing house."

"It might be all right, if it was the right packing house," admitted Waller. "What one did you have in mind?"

"St. Louis."

"I wouldn't go there on a bet."

"Will you go for six or eight weeks?"

"Why, yes, if it's only for that long."

"I thought you'd go to St. Louis," exulted his new boss. "After that the new plant will be ready at St. Joe and you can take it."

So Waller went to St. Joseph as manager of our newest branch plant. He went on the chief's say-so and pretty much over the judgments of the other men well up in our councils, for he was a new man with us and it has never been our policy to put outsiders over old employees if the job could possibly be filled from within. But this once, G. F. Swift was convinced that he had hired a better man than any of the "raised" variety who were available. And he stuck to his conviction.

Because he did not want to take a single chance of being wrong after he had put an outsider in this place without consulting the judgment of his lieutenants, the boss proceeded to devote special attention to Waller. For the first year or so the St. Joseph manager was frequently summoned to Chicago and father went often to St. Joseph.

Since then Waller has occasionally told of his long sessions with his chief. From dinner time on, every evening in Chicago was devoted to talking over Waller's management problems, the affairs of the one plant and of the company. Father was always ready to counsel with him—though, in all justice it must be said there was no need for paying any extra attention to him. As usual, the head of the business had been absolutely right in his size-up of his man. Yet Waller declares today, no doubt correctly, that his lightning-like activity in catching the train at St. Joseph is alone what attracted the attention of G. F. Swift and brought about his offer of a good job.

In the early days the business kept calling for more and more men as it grew, and its head had to hire a good many men outside. His trade was shooting upward so fast that even his ability at training executives could not keep up with the demand. So he was always picking up likely looking men and putting them in training for jobs that needed filling.

For example, there was a grocer near where we lived. He had a good enough little business as neighborhood grocery stores went. But that discerning eye saw in him the material for a bigger place than ever his little store would afford. Father therefore advised him to sell his business and come to work for us.

First thing we knew the store had changed hands and the man was working in our wholesale market. He learned there how a wholesale market is run and the points which need watching. Presently he was going around our branch houses checking up on the managers, helping them to build up to the standard maintained in our Chicago packing-house market and picking up from all of them hints which he might pass on to the rest so that the wholesale organization would run more smoothly.

G. F. Swift's standing and reputation were such

that many a man gave up his own established business to come to us, with full confidence that he was bettering himself. That is how L. A. Carton came as treasurer in 1893 when the financial end of the organization loomed too big for its founder's continuing attention. It is how a good many of the best men came in the early days.

The man who could do better than most men some task which was part of our function was a man to catch his employer's attention. In the first years of the business this is how a good many of the men were found on the outside to take places of responsibility with us. All the way through it has been how men inside the organization have been chosen for larger positions.

There was one young man who came as a clerk in the president's office. At first his duties were chiefly filing. But he showed a real knack for keeping up with the work and for finding letters or contracts on the instant. Moreover he displayed an intelligent comprehension of the fact that he was there to save his chief's time and energy. Several times he used unusual gumption under circumstances where he might have been excused for letting things slide along.

So his boss noticed him. And one day when his secretary was away, with the youngster taking hold of the work as best he could, a cable announced that a ship which we were counting on to carry a load of beef to England had gone into dry-dock at

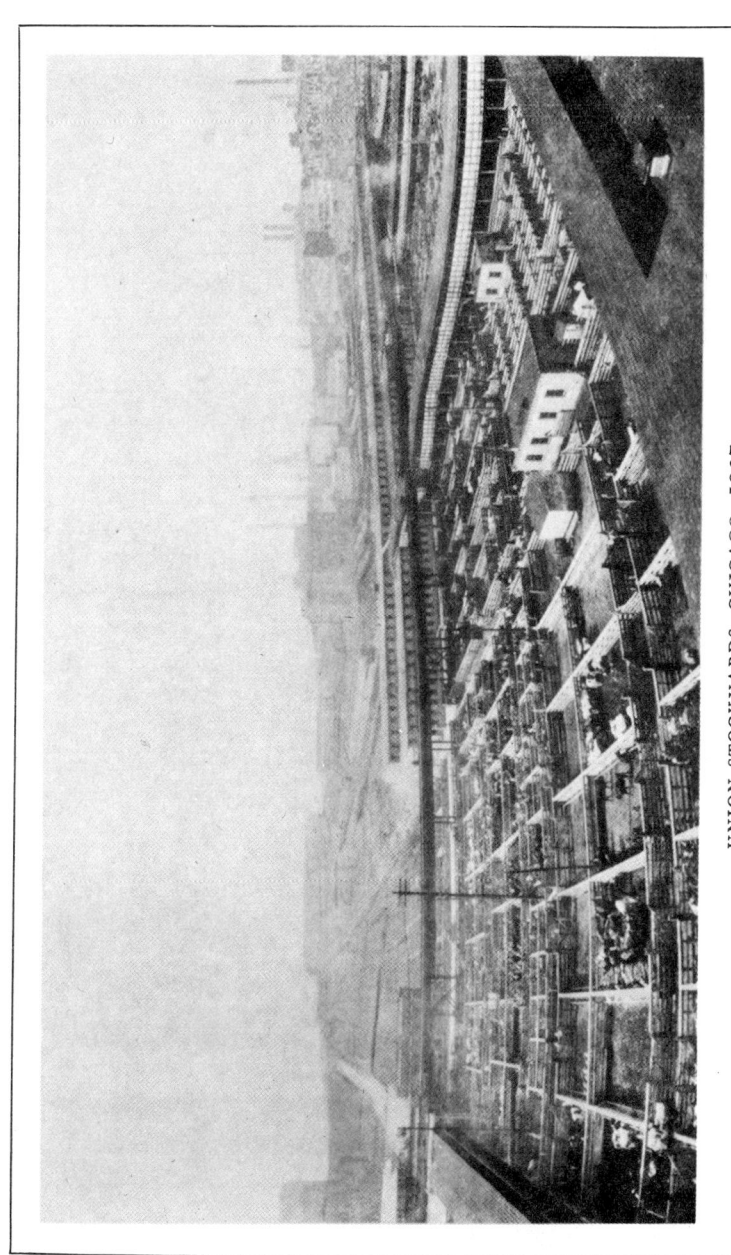

UNION STOCKYARDS, CHICAGO, 1927.

Liverpool and therefore could not meet its scheduled sailing date from Boston.

The schedule of sailings was handled in that office by another man under the secretary. The secretary always checked over this man's work and then submitted it to his chief. So the youngster turned over to the expert the job of rearranging the schedule of sailings.

But when it came to submitting this to the chief the expert would not. He was downright afraid, with that bone-quaking fear some clerks have of the big boss. So the report had to be taken in by the younger clerk, with the expert hovering in the background to handle any overtechnical questions.

Right away, of course, there came a question fairly bristling with technicalities. The spokesman said, "I don't know about that, Mr. Swift. Brown here can tell you."

"So you don't know, eh?" inquired the boss pleasantly. "Well, I don't know as I'd expect you to know all about that. But if you're going to come in here with reports you've got to know all about them. I don't want to have Brown explain it, as long as you're the one that's bringing it to me. You go along now and find out all about it. Probably Brown can make you understand it. After you do, come back and tell me. I expect to be in all morning. And if we come to something else you don't know, why I guess we can give you some more time to find that out."

One secret of his success in training men was the way he dealt with them. He knew all about practically every detail in the business, the standards to which every operation must be held. His microscopic eye for detail never overlooked any really significant points, even though he might not concern himself too immediately with them.

When he wrote instructions to a manager or a superintendent, he was explicit. Usually he closed such letters with the injunction: "Please answer and say if you will carry out these instructions." That phrase, winding up a letter, leaves no doubt in the recipient's mind as to what is expected of him.

At the same time, given a man in whom he had confidence, he would seldom overrule that individual's deliberate judgment. He preferred to let the man incur a loss, if necessary, to prove to his own satisfaction what would always have remained a doubt if it had had to be accepted on his chief's say-so. And he was seldom so cock-sure that he knew he must be right and his employee wrong.

The manager of a middle-western plant found a good market in San Francisco for dressed poultry. After a few experimental shipments he sent a man there to look after the dressed poultry business on the coast and one day mentioned to his chief that this had developed into a nice profitable venture.

It was the first father had heard of it. "You'll not make any money shipping poultry to San Francisco," he assured the manager.

"But we're making money at it now," was the rejoinder.

"You'll not make money on it in the long run."

"Do you want me to stop shipping and bring that man back here?"

"You'll not make any money at it."

"I think we can make money at it, Mr. Swift. Do you want me to stop it?"

"Oh, let's talk about something else," suggested the boss.

For a long while we made money at it. The manager was right, even though father had been so sure about it. His unwillingness to order a manager to go against his own judgment was one reason why he built up throughout the world a corps of representatives who handled his affairs superlatively well.

CHAPTER IX

THE FORBIDDEN YARDSTICK

ALL his life G. F. Swift was developing at a prodigious pace, developing in mind and skill and knowledge. Quite as naturally as a boy attaining manhood loses his awe toward many unremarkable adults who a few years before towered above him, so father found his standards always changing.

Men whose technical skill at one time represented his highest ideals of attainment became a few years later to his fast-marching mind a pack of fogeys. His own development had meanwhile gone to a point far beyond the ken of the mossbacked gentry.

First and last a good many of his men, most of them a deal younger than their employer, left him because they had failed to keep within hailing distance as he progressed. It took a nimble wit and a lust for hard work to hold that pace. Not that he expected every man to keep up with him. But the man in a key position—be he a department head or a superintendent or a clerk in the president's office—that man kept step or stepped out.

Only a good man could suit him for long. Father was sizing his people up all the time. He watched their performances in comparison with one another and in the light of what he knew about their abilities.

"The best a man ever did shouldn't be his yardstick for the rest of his life," was the maxim and the working rule by which he managed his men. The department head or superintendent who used that forbidden yardstick was not worth keeping.

Even more than in developing executives—and he excelled at it—G. F. Swift's knack of dealing with human beings appeared in his work with the rank and file of his employees. After all, it is easier to build up alert, ambitious individuals into competent executives and managers than it is to get a reasonable degree of work and intelligence out of the ninety-seven per cent of employees who never develop the capacity for authority and who never can. For the individual of managerial caliber is the exception and will do his best to help you push him ahead. The majority of inert people on the pay roll have an uncanny gift for using just enough gumption to hold their jobs and win little promotions, but they never show the traits which bring a man major responsibilities and major rewards.

The man of initiative and common sense quickly gains enough experience to appreciate the reasons behind his own promotions and reprimands. But the fellow down in the lower ranks of the business is usually more of an individualist. He lacks the training; and he has never tasted the rewards which come to one who subordinates personal preferences to the group's welfare.

Whether it was in the earlier days when father was

dealing direct with his workmen and clerks or whether it was in the later years when he could plan only the general policies, he displayed a genius for handling employees. To people in Swift & Company who did not know him well, or who had not worked with us long enough to understand what was at the bottom of his relationship with employees, the head of the business sometimes seemed an unpleasant, hot-tempered boss. He was unquestionably sarcastic. Sarcasm was his tool for keeping his subordinates alert and free from mistakes which should not be repeated.

But his irritability (as it seemed to some employees) arose out of disappointment. He was really disappointed, with a sense of personal error, when he found a weakness in an employee who he had not expected would have that particular failing.

One plan he followed constantly to minimize expensive errors was to get reports on all claims allowed our customers. These reports came to him on large sheets with brief particulars of each claim. Each summary described the error behind the claim and told who had made it.

Whenever he found a few unoccupied minutes in the day, he sent his office boy for a claim-sheet offender. Into his office would march some clerk he had never seen before. The culprit always knew, from the time the claim was allowed, that eventually he would be personally called to account by his chief.

Father would sit there for a moment sizing up

the man responsible for the loss. To the clerk it unquestionably looked as if his employer was racking his brain for a refinement of ingenious punishment. Actually the boss was looking him over to see whether he looked like a man who would habitually make mistakes and whether he was worth trying to save. His tendency was to err on the side of charity, to give the man a chance to make good.

After a moment he would speak. "So you're the young fellow who ordered out five hundred pounds of leaf lard and two hundred and fifty pounds of compound when a customer had bought two fifty of lard and five hundred of compound?"

"Yes, Mr. Swift."

"I suppose you know the customer claimed he used it up just the same way as if he'd got what he ordered and we had to bill it to him the way he ordered instead of the way we shipped?"

"Yes, sir."

"I suppose you think it doesn't make any difference if you make mistakes like that. Doesn't make any difference to a big rich company like Swift's if it has to allow a customer a claim of $13.47. We'd be in a fine fix if everybody made that kind of a mistake once a month, wouldn't we?"

The employee who emerged from the encounter with the least damage and still on the pay roll was the one who did not try to excuse the error, who acknowledged it and showed by his demeanor that he recognized it as a serious offense which he would carefully guard against in future. The man who tried to be flippant, or who took the attitude that anyone was likely to make mistakes and that a certain number of mistakes was allowable to any man—that fellow was likely to be through in a hurry.

Father did not consider any mistakes allowable in a well-managed business. That was his base on which he built the whole structure. He knew that errors would continue to be made. But none were allowable and no one would be retained who showed too strong a tendency to lose us money.

This is one of the really sound principles of business management. No mistakes are allowable and every mistake must be regarded as a serious lapse. If any other attitude is taken toward errors, then there is no controlling them.

It is always necessary to draw a definite line somewhere. It is impossible to draw a definite line on errors unless it is drawn right at the source. Allow it leeway in the slightest and it will move steadily away in the direction of more mistakes. And it is mistakes which lose money for a business.

If a concern is engaged in a sound line of business and if some fundamental change such as a new and monopolized invention which could not be prophesied does not render it suddenly unsound, then it may in general be said that it will always make money except when someone makes a mistake. The mistake may be one of judgment, of wastefulness, of carelessness, or whatnot. It may at the time seem important or unimportant. But the most basic mistake of all is to condone mistakes.

Twenty or thirty years ago it was no doubt easier to hold employees to a strict accountability. Discipline in the office and in the packing house was almost as strict as discipline in the family. And back in the '80s and the '90s the head of the family was obeyed or there was real trouble! Discipline was a part of the working code rather than a tradition of bygone days.

Father was a strict disciplinarian. Not always did his disciplinary measures bring about the results he had counted on. But he kept working along the same lines nevertheless.

He was walking through the cellars at one of our western plants one day with the superintendent when a negro trucker passed, whistling loudly. "Stop him whistling, stop him," the chief directed. So the superintendent called, "Hey, Sam, no whistling on the job"—which was the first ever heard of this on the plant in question. And the chief added, as explanation to the surprised negro, "If everyone whistles, we'll have no order."

A few minutes later they went to the hog-killing floor. The hog house was small for the plant and everything was done by hand.

The gang was composed of stalwarts every one—most of them southern negroes, with a few Irish at pivotal points. The day's schedule was six thousand hogs, a big day's work. Someone had started the negroes singing when the whistle blew that morning and the work had been turned out six hundred hogs an hour, ten a minute, right from the start.

"Here! Here! Stop it!" the astounded visitor had to shout to make himself heard over the ringing chorus of "Down in Mobile." So the superintendent called the foreman, who immediately silenced the singers.

"That will slow up the work, Mr. Swift," the superintendent told him. "We want to get out six thousand hogs today and we'll never do it without the singing. It helps those boys work."

"Never mind," directed his employer. "I think we can kill the hogs without any musical accompaniment. Yes sir, we turn out a lot of pork at Chicago without singing."

"You have conveyor chains, rolling tables, all the other facilities at Chicago for speeding up the work. If you need to turn out a little more than the usual production, you speed up the conveyors a little and the men speed up to keep pace."

"I think we don't need the singing. It's bad for discipline," was the final word on the subject.

But along later in the day as the visitor and the plant manager entered the superintendent's office, that practical soul took from his desk the production reports which had been accumulating during the day. They showed that from the moment the singing had stopped hogs had been killed at the rate of four hundred an hour instead of six hundred as before.

He handed the sheet to his chief without comment.

"Hm," came the decision after a considerable pause. "Hm. I guess maybe there's a little something in what you say. Maybe you might let those boys sing when they've got an extra lot of work to do. But—" regretfully—"it's mighty hard on discipline."

One of the cardinal principles which enabled him to raise better men than he could hire was his sparing use of compliments. He believed in seldom praising. His creed held that if a man does good work he deserves no praise for it, it is exactly what he is paid to do. If his work is exceptionally fine, still don't praise him. Give him a raise and a better job with more responsibility at the first chance. Thus you give the man the benefit he has earned by his ability. You have, as an employer, advantaged yourself of the employee's capacity. And you haven't spoiled him by telling him he is good.

The good man who came to us from another concern was likely to have been told that he was good and consequently to have had his head just a trifle inflated. The man who knows he is good is likely to be a bit sensitive about how he is treated. He requires an amount of dignity to support his best work. Father had his attention centered only on getting the work done and he had no time to think of useless frills. He did not build up non-essentials by compliments. That is one way he raised better men than he could hire.

He tried his best to hold his managers to the same point of view. He did not want them upsetting the apple-cart by giving out praise. Once at St. Joseph he was going over the plant with the manager when they encountered a negro janitor engaged in some job which, while it had to be done, yet was outside a janitor's regular duties. The manager praised him for his alertness in seeing the need and pitching into the job on his own hook. As they walked away he said to his chief, "There's one of the best men on this plant. He's always surprising me by doing better than I can expect anyone to do."

They walked on for a minute or two in silence. Then from the depths of his experience the older man offered his comment: "You're going to spoil a good boy—spoil a good boy, Mr. Donovan."

At another plant he was going through with a younger man, a foreman who has since become a plant superintendent. As they were standing by a long zinc table where they were doing the scraping by hand, he inquired, "Mr. Pratt, where do you think these hogs should be cleaned?"

"Right here where they are being cleaned," answered the foreman.

"We don't do it that way at Chicago," retorted his boss—this was the reply he used to squelch anyone at any of our other plants who stood up for an inferior way of doing. Chicago was at that time supposed to include all packing-house virtues developed to date. The other plants were the provinces.

"There are a lot of things you don't do at Chicago," replied Pratt. "We're scraping them while they're still hot from the scalding water. At Chicago they scrape the hogs on the rail. I think this is a great deal better than the Chicago way."

"Young man, you're right," his employer admitted. This was the highest praise he could bring himself to administer.

The veteran who went through this experience laughed about it many years later. And he commented: "I believe this is the only time Mr. Swift ever agreed with me about anything we discussed! Next time I was in Chicago, a few months later, I observed that he had them handling their hogs by our method."

It is noteworthy that the chief did not tell the man his idea had been adopted. He knew the originator would see it some time at Chicago. Meanwhile there was no use acting as if the man had done something to make a fuss over.

But if G. F. Swift was sparing of praise, he was lavish with advice about better ways to do things. He never overlooked an opportunity to instruct.

"How do you think these hogs are dressed?" he inquired of a plant man on another trip.

"I think the day's killing is well dressed," the employee told him.

"I beg to differ with you. That's all,"—and he waved the younger man back to his work.

Next day the plant man received a letter from the

plant superintendent, with the president's criticism attached. Busy as he was, father had gone into great detail about how the hogs should be opened straight through the center of the aitch-bone, split to show the loin and fin bones equally on each side of the hog, and the button of the neck split in the center. It was a constructive set of instructions on one operation of pork packing. Giving instructions took up a much larger part of his usual day than did praise.

One thing he insisted on was absolute honesty. Time and again he came to my desk or called me to his and pointed out some slip-up in shipping dates or a let-down in quality or something else which had the appearance of a sharp corner having been cut to get an advantage for Swift & Company. He would lecture me on the specific mistake. But always he would end up by talking about the need for being absolutely fair and honest all of the time. "We want character to go with our goods. And sixteen ounces is a Swift pound." I don't know how many times he said this to me; it must have run well up into the hundreds.

So it is not surprising that in the early days especially, before the spirit of fair dealing had been absorbed by all of our people, a good many men got through in a hurry. Usually it was for a lie or for misrepresenting to a customer. Father had no use for anyone who had any other standard than absolute honesty and sixteen ounces to the pound.

I recall one man who was fired for stealing. He

appealed to the front office. "I've worked for you for twenty years, Mr. Swift," he pleaded.

"You stole, didn't you?"

"Yes, sir."

"You worked for me twenty years too long then," was the decision.

There was another man, manager of a branch market, who got to drinking and committing a lot of the faults which so often accompany this overindulgence. He was sent for.

"Mr. So-and-So, how do you like working for Swift & Company?"

"Oh, very well, Mr. Swift." The employee went on to enlarge on the virtues of the house.

"You like your job, do you?"

"Oh, yes, I'm very well satisfied. I'm trying to do my very best. . . . . " and so forth. The chief waited for him to finish.

"Well, you've been doing a lot of things you hadn't ought to, a lot of things we don't stand for. I'm glad you liked your job, for you ain't got it now." And the man was through.

This kind of discipline was not inspired by any desire to be unkind. There was none of the cat-and-mouse idea in inviting the man to come from his eastern branch to be fired and in asking so solicitously after his liking for his job. Father knew the story would run through the whole organization and serve as a reminder that employees were not encouraged to behave themselves in ways which interfered with their usefulness. It was stern discipline, but effective.

Yet, rigid as were his ideas of discipline, he allowed them to relax for the worker who had earned special consideration or about whom there was some reason for not holding to too high a standard of expectation. There was a coachman who was discovered getting away with a little money.

Mother simply sent over to the cashier at the office when she needed money. This had long been the custom. The cashier handed over the money and charged it to "G. F. Swift Personal." Almost anyone was sent over from the house on occasion and the cash was always handed over—sometimes in rather larger amounts than the servant who got it was used to handling.

When the coachman was discovered knocking down money under this plan, he decamped. Father had him brought back by the police. And then he began thinking about how unbusinesslike the whole arrangement had been, how unfairly it placed temptation in the servants' ways. He couldn't keep the man in his employ. But he dismissed the charges against him and worked out a voucher system which made it unlikely that any such thing would happen again.

Another time the head of the ice department went to his chief to tell his suspicions that an old-time employee assigned to a minor but trusted place in his department had been dishonest. The old-timer was being used to pay off the ice-harvest gangs, always in cash. There was at the time no way to check up whether his payments and his amounts drawn for the purpose tallied.

"I think he's taking all of the ice-gang pay-roll money that's left after he pays off," the manager explained. "He isn't turning any in. Of course he may be carrying over the surplus from one gang and using it to pay the next, but I doubt it."

"The chances are he ain't," father admitted. "You know, he never had a very good education. Don't know the difference between his money and mine. But he's been a good faithful servant here and we can't expect maybe that he ought to be trusted with cash. He's always got a job here, though, as long as he lives. We may have to guard him from temptation, but he's always got a job here."

I think it is generally agreed by the men who worked with him that Gustavus F. Swift was one of the fairest, squarest bosses anyone ever had. He treated everyone alike, whether the employee was a member of his family or someone who had been placed on the pay roll only a week before. Some of us, in fact, suspected that he was more lenient to the ordinary run of employees than he was to his near relatives.

He was very much interested in the personal affairs of his people—a goodly amount more so than some employees thought was any of his business. He realized that a man's personal habits had a great deal to do with his ability and also that they shed light on what might be expected of the individual. When an employee got a share of Swift stock, the president of the company was likely to check up a year afterwards to see if he still had it. If it had been transferred, then he wanted to know why.

He wished his people to own stock. He was a pioneer in bringing this about in a big way. His was the first large concern to encourage its employees to become substantial stockholders.

A typical instance of the way he did it was when he called in one young man who had been with us for about a year. The youngster was doing well and gave every indication of becoming a valuable man. "Are you intending to stay with us?" was shot at the boy.

"Yes, Mr. Swift."

"Well, you seem a likely sort of young man. Maybe I'm mistaken, but it looks to me as if you might develop into someone who'd be of some use around here if you stay. Now, I want to have my young men partners, even if they can't do it in a big way. Like the idea?"

"Yes, sir."

"We're going to increase our capital stock. Got any money?"

"Only about two hundred dollars."

"All right. You can buy a thousand dollars worth of this stock if you want to. Pay down what you can and give me your note for the rest. I'll carry it for you and you can pay me off as fast as you're able."

So the employee got the stock. He still has it, I think, along with a good many more shares. That he was a likely young man was proved when he developed into a department head, then went abroad in charge of a substantial share of our business.

Father never overlooked an opportunity to place a few shares of stock with his people. When there was no other stock available, he would sell a little of his own to the employee, replacing it at the first good opportunity. But all of the time he kept in mind that the employee who is a partner is usually the keenest to make money for the firm.

Likewise he recognized that the concern which is owned by a very large number of shareholders is more stable than the company which is closely held. And its stock is more difficult of stock market manipulation.

Next in desirability as stockholders he rated customers. Swift stock was originally bought by eastern live-stock and meat men who constituted our first body of customers, the nucleus around which our dressed-beef business was developed. When new outlets were added, either as dealers or as agents, the newcomers were given the opportunity to buy a few shares. Thus the sales organization was built up with an undivided loyalty and a desire, founded on self-interest, that the company prosper.

I have said that sarcasm was my father's working

tool in handling employees. He might be and he generally was very personal in his remarks, but he meant them impersonally. No matter how hard he jumped us—I got just as large a share of this as anyone else—he left us with the feeling that it was all deserved. He left no sting but he left us convinced. No matter how hard he might jump, no matter how wholly unpleasant he might be in the tenor and tone of his remarks, next time he saw the employee the storm had blown over. The man who weathered one such talking-to generally got through any of its successors without having his feelings seriously abraded.

Another of his knacks in raising better men than he could hire was his ability at cross-examination. Whether the questioning took place in his office or at home or at the employee's desk or workbench, the procedure had its common characteristics. If the chief was seated, he looked as if he had been poured into his chair. He slumped down with his weight on the small of his back. But no matter how indolent his appearance, his lively blue eye kept roving.

His first questions would be so unrelated that the employee would wonder what on earth the boss was driving at. His succeeding questions would begin to shape up into a skeleton so that the man began to think he knew what it was all about. And then, when the conclusion seemed right ahead and the employee felt himself safely exonerated of all blame, father would with one or two well-placed queries turn an abrupt corner and skewer his victim neatly

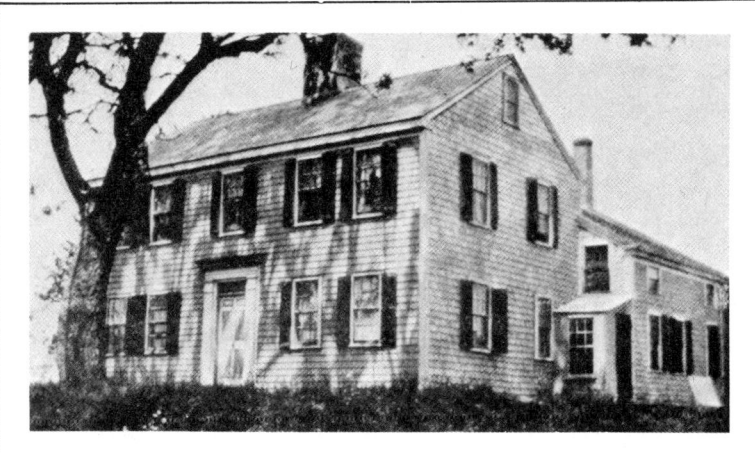

THE FARM HOUSE AT BARNSTABLE.

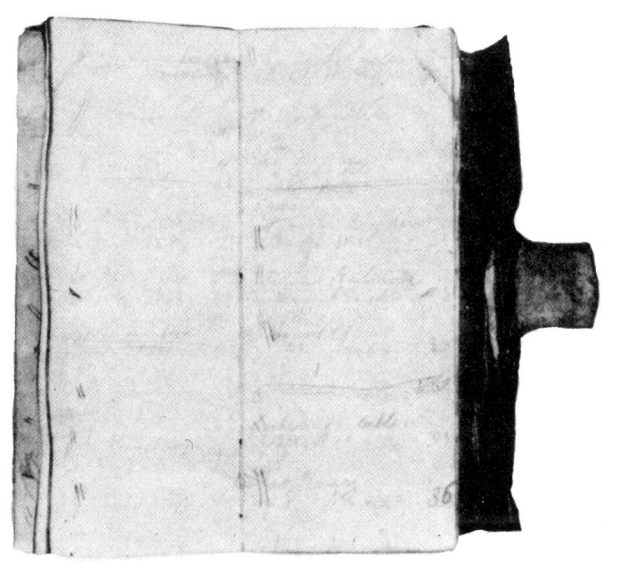

G. F. SWIFT'S ACCOUNTS, 1859-60, RECORDING
SALES OF MEAT FROM HIS BUTCHER CART.

on the sharp point of the cumulative admissions which conclusively convicted the man of something he had not even known he was suspected of. Never did G. F. Swift's questions indicate the direction in which he was working, until he had the answers so well in hand that there was no use denying his conclusions. His method might conscientiously be recommended to any earnest prosecuting attorney!

But if his questionings were devious, his instructions to employees were always direct. He said absolutely what he wanted done, in as clear-cut a way as anyone could devise. Then he left it to the employee to work out how he would get the results.

He was the driver, the dynamo of the business. He worked his men hard and treated them fairly. From time to time I have heard rumors of this or that employee who felt himself badly treated by father. But whenever I have been familiar with the facts, they have been all on the employer's side.

One instance was a man who came to us at a good-sized salary to improve our office routines. He was recommended as a first-class man and so represented himself. But like most men who set themselves up as experts, he soon showed that he knew considerably less than the good practical office men we had with us all of the time. So father had him fired.

Presently he appeared at the front office and was admitted. He was tremendously angry. He had, so he claimed, been hired for a year—and here he was fired within two months. "You're not getting the results you said you'd get, are you?" his employer inquired mildly.

"Not yet. But I was hired for a year, Mr. Swift."

"All right," the boss assented—not showing by his actions or manner what he thought of someone who failed to deliver what he had agreed to, but demanded his pay just the same. "You go over to Mr. So-and-So in the packing house. He'll have a job for you."

A telephone message got there ahead of the office man. When the one-year employee arrived, he was given a squeegee and instructions to keep the blood running into the blood-gutters. After a few hours there he had enough, even though he would have been drawing his stipulated pay as an office expert.

I have no doubt that this man felt terribly mistreated. There are instances of this sort which give rise to lurid tales of G. F. Swift's terrible temper and rank injustice. But I have never found a basis for it.

Over against this we can set the statement of a man who worked with him from the start at Chicago—who came out, in fact, from the slaughterhouse of Anthony, Swift & Company at Assonet to take charge of slaughtering at Chicago. He left us in 1897 to take a position with another concern which could temporarily afford to pay several times as much as we could for his specialized ability. Thereafter he had no connection with us, no reason for telling a good story about us.

It was almost thirty years after he left us and

fifteen years after he retired to live on his income that he told a man unconnected with our business:

"I worked for G. F. Swift for twenty-seven years. He was the squarest man I ever worked for. All that time I never asked him what he was going to pay me. I never had cause to complain. If you worked well for him, he saw that you got what you deserved in money and in every other way."

There, it seems to me, is the basic explanation of father's oft repeated assertion:

"I can raise better men than I can hire."

CHAPTER X

FIGHT WHEN YOU MUST

IF INDUSTRIES have birthdays, all record of them is usually lost in the snuffed-out memories of the dead. Seldom can you put your pencil on the yellowed page of an ancient calendar and say, "On this day began such-and-so an industry." These birthdays are difficult to mark.

But the birth record of the packing industry may be here written down with certainty and in no fear of contradiction. The modern dressed-meat business was born on the day after the Assonet butcher gang came to Chicago.

It was an autumn day of 1876. These Yankee butchers who had worked for Anthony, Swift & Company just outside Fall River came on a Grand Trunk pass, as was general in those times. Next day they fell to their task in the shed—by courtesy called a slaughterhouse—which G. F. Swift had purchased from one Billy Moore in preparation for their arrival. The lard refinery of the business he founded stands today on the site of Billy Moore's unprententious establishment.

The day can be marked as an industrial birthday because the beef those New Englanders slaughtered was placed in a box-car and shipped back to their home town. From this start came Swift & Company. I think we are not boastful in feeling that with it began the modern packing industry.

It marked a definite era in father's business career. It meant that he foreswore the live-stock business which during most of his life had been his livelihood. Instead of live stock as the merchandise he dealt in, he was substituting dressed beef. Because he envisioned an industry shipping beef from Chicago to feed the eastern states, he made dressed meat an industry.

His partner, D. M. Anthony, of Fall River, agreed with him—agreed, however, with a reservation of enthusiasm. Anthony was willing to risk a little money on his partner's idea, but he was not giving up his profitable going business to undertake a crusade for a new idea, even though that crusade might, as he hoped, turn out a moneymaker.

J. A. Hathaway, father's partner in his other firm of Hathaway & Swift, had no faith in the idea. It is not remarkable that he had not, for he was a cattle dealer. Anthony, a slaughterer and meat dealer, might have been expected to show more interest in a means of making money for handlers of meat. Hathaway could only look on it as an unsound plan. If this unsound plan should by any chance work out successfully, he knew it must ruin his line of business. It is human nature to take little stock in anything which might cost you your living.

Hathaway and his partner differed so radically on

this question that they dissolved their partnership. Their viewpoints could not be reconciled. Hathaway came to Chicago, paid cash for his partner's share of the joint interests, and returned to his cattle business at Brighton. He brought with him from the East a financial statement on which to base the settlement. "How do those meet your figures?" he inquired of his partner.

"I don't agree with you," the younger man told him. "I don't agree with you at all."

"Why, I'm surprised," declared Hathaway. "I thought I had my figures right. How far are we apart?"

"One cent. Your figures give me one cent more than I'm entitled to."

So they parted the best of friends. The older man brought along two gold watches. One of these he gave to father and the other to mother. They were fine watches and were treasured always as a memento of a friendly partnership which could not be continued.

Gustavus F. Swift was not a man who had many quarrels. "Use tact when you can—fight when you have to," was one of his working maxims. He always preferred going around a difficulty to going through it. He never threw a challenge into the other fellow's territory until he had made up his mind that arbitration or compromise would not settle the trouble.

One result of his tactful ways was that he had only

FIGHT WHEN YOU MUST

two serious labor troubles during his lifetime. The first of these was in the '80s, the other was the Pullman strike of the early '90s. With neither of these was he specifically concerned as an opponent of the strikers' demands. But when the strikes came and he saw that tact would no longer serve, he swung into the job of fighting with every resource he had.

If the disputes leading to these affairs had arisen out of conditions directly under his control, there would have been no strikes. When, however, the strikes threatened his prosperity through no fault of his own, then he proceeded to do everything he could to break them.

The first was a bitter strike. Particularly in those early days, father could not afford a shutdown and the consequent loss. He moved into the stockyards men who would work in spite of the strike. And he got his foremen to exert every influence to keep their men at work.

He was pretty well recognized as a leader in breaking that strike. Broken it was. After it was over, the foremen who held any considerable proportion of their men were noted for meritorious service. Not a few individuals who later rose to important responsibilities owed their promotions to the attention they attracted by holding their men at work.

The Pullman strike was altogether different. It was aimed not at us but at the Pullman Company. Its net result was to prevent the free movement of freight—which in the packing business means a shutdown in short order. The strikers were determined that cars should not move. G. F. Swift had a stubborn streak when anyone tried to tell him what he could not do. His determination matched the strikers'. He refused to be buffeted about in the rôle of innocent bystander.

The crisis as it affected us came one day when getting the cars rolling was especially important to us—it was July 3, or the day before Memorial Day, or some such occasion. The trainmen of the railroad which switched cars in the yards had been intimidated. Trunk railroads, however, were under United States military protection. If the cars were once placed on trunk line tracks we were reasonably sure they would reach their destinations.

So we organized an impromptu train crew, with guards, to move the cars from our loading docks and turn them over to the Michigan Central. Richard Fitzgerald, president of the Chicago Junction Railway, lent us a switch engine. An old employee who knew the workings of a locomotive served as engineer. The rest of the crew was made up of one or two high officials, such as the general superintendent, and the whole Swift family, including father.

To the accompaniment of jeers and, be it confessed, an occasional brickbat, we switched a train of refrigerator cars out of the stockyards onto the tracks of the Michigan Central. There a yard engine was waiting to take them. Then we all went back on the engine and tender and repeated the operation.

Feeling ran against us among those who sympathized with the Pullman strikers. A few of our empty refrigerator cars were burned up and a few cars of beef likewise.

But the meat kept moving out of the Yards—and when President Cleveland called out the United States troops from Fort Sheridan to protect lives and property, the strike was soon broken. It was a daring move for a man in political office. I can think of few who would have done it, however much right was on the side of law and order as against the strikers.

Difficulties with transportation had been father's daily portion almost from the time he came to Chicago. As soon as he began shipping dressed beef he ran into snags which were skillfully placed in his way. The railroads, in short, did not want his dressed-beef business. They wanted to continue hauling live stock, which gave them about double the tonnage. The basic idea of slaughtering at Chicago and shipping beef east was to avoid having to pay freight on the inedible portions of the cattle and to avoid the loss of weight to the cattle, due to the hardships of travel. But the railroads had not yet been educated to an appreciation that what is economically sound is in the long run most profitable to the carriers. It was this lack of understanding which eventually brought upon them the first governmental regulation.

Rate making in those days of the '70s and early

'80s was almost entirely a matter of bargaining between the individual shipper and the carrier. The Interstate Commerce Act had not yet appeared. And the carriers would not bargain on dressed-meat rates. They simply set a high rate and sat tight.

This was the group of old railroads, comprising the Trunk Line Association, which have the direct routes from Chicago to the East. They got the live-stock business, of course, for the shorter the haul the less shrinkage in weight of cattle on the hoof. The roads which reached the East by roundabout routes got none.

The Grand Trunk, running through Canada, had practically no live-stock business. So its officials were delighted to get a share of the traffic in meat since they could not have it alive. They were glad to set a fair rate on dressed beef. They welcomed the resulting revenue. One other railroad used occasionally to accept a little of our dressed beef for the East, but only in small quantities at the low rate.

Father used to meet in New York the chairman of the Trunk Line Association, a German named Albert Fink. He and Fink would argue the dressed-meat rate by the hour and never get anywhere. Fink had his orders from the railroads and could not budge an inch.

Because father saw that the only way he could possibly get anywhere was by tact, he used tact for ten years, or as close an approach to tact as was possible under the circumstances. Meanwhile his beef for points around New York City was turned over by the Grand Trunk to American roads at Buffalo and for New England points at other junctions nearer to this market. The American roads charged local rates on these hauls, which made them tremendously expensive as freight went in those days.

He kept this up until the Interstate Commerce Act was passed in 1887. Then the railroads had to take his commodities at a fair rate and had to desist from other practices which had stood in the way of freely shipping meat to the East. It closed a long argument between father and Fink!

His serious difficulties in shipping beef had started almost simultaneously with the first trouble on trunk line rates. G. F. Swift had shipped some dressed beef experimentally in box cars in the winter of '75-'76. He had not been at it long before the rate situation first blocked him, then turned him to the Grand Trunk.

Technical difficulties of carrying dressed meat a thousand miles in all weathers were, however, very real. The first car of beef he shipped was an ordinary box car with a temporary framing built inside to suspend the carcasses from. It was shipped in cool weather and the meat arrived sweet and edible.

Then followed experiments, directed at first to mastering the difficulties of winter shipping. A box car of beef might start out in zero weather and the meat be frozen stiff before it left the Chicago city limits. In Indiana it might encounter a warm wave and thaw out. Then it might freeze again and thaw again before arriving at Fall River or Clinton. After this it would be in a good deal worse condition than if it had gone all the way either frozen or chilled.

Cars were sent carrying small stoves with a man along to tend the stoves. Various wrappings and packings were tried. And finally the conclusion was plain that the beef lost in no way except appearance if it arrived frozen and was thawed out gradually.

This was in the winter before the butcher-gang came from Assonet to work in Billy Moore's slaughterhouse. The cattle that father sent dressed this winter were killed for him by G. H. Hammond for a slaughtering toll. When spring came in 1876 he gave up the experiment for a few months and went back to shipping cattle.

Hammond was, I think, the first man to ship beef commercially in refrigerator cars. He had at this time a handful of refrigerator cars which he used for shipping beef east. He was reasonably successful at it and had made a modest start toward attaining what father had in mind.

But G. F. Swift's energy and vision were destined to make a bigger thing of it than Hammond could make it. Hammond was using the idea as an auxiliary money-maker, something that yielded him a good steady little profit month in and month out. Father, once he had the device mastered, used it to build an industry such as had never been dreamed of before.

His first effort was to get the railroads to build

cars. The railroads as a class did not want dressed-beef traffic, much less were they going to encourage it. Finally it narrowed down to the Grand Trunk. But the Grand Trunk would not build the refrigerator cars, even if guaranteed a steady volume of traffic for them summer and winter. It was experimental.

Development of a satisfactory refrigerator car was being pushed from two sides at that time. On the one hand was the need to carry dressed beef from Middle West to East. But far more urgent was the demand for cars which would enable the farmers of the Pacific Coast to carry to eastern markets the fruits which they had in such abundance but could not sell. The coast had been growing in population and in fruit culture since the transcontinental railroads had been completed only a few years before. It was pressing hard for some means to market the perishable products of its fruit farms.

Outside the fruit belts of the United States, people seem to think of the refrigerator car as an appurtenance of the packing industry. Actually, by recent figures, there are several times as many refrigerator cars carrying fresh fruit, vegetables, and the like, as there are owned by packers and used principally for meat products. While G. F. Swift struggled to make progress to forward his ideas of shipping beef, a real effort was being made in many quarters to produce a satisfactory refrigerator car. Some had already been built which came pretty close to doing what they were supposed to.

Father rented such of these as he could get. In them he shipped beef east to his own wholesale market at Clinton, Massachusetts, and to Anthony, Swift & Company at Fall River. He even managed to get a couple of distributors and to keep them supplied with Chicago-dressed beef. The first two customers to push his product in the East—outside of the two firms which he owned or had an interest in—were Francis Jewett, of Lowell, and I. M. Lincoln, of Providence.

When the railroads refused to build refrigerator cars for him to ship in, he approached the Michigan Car Company, of Detroit. The McMillen family owned this concern. They were rich and had a leaning toward an undertaking which might make them a profitable future market if they took a little chance in the present.

Reduced to its barest terms, G. F. Swift's proposal to the owners was that they build him some refrigerator cars and let him pay for them out of their earnings. They took a chance with him, even though they did not know that the cars would earn. To be sure, they retained a hold on them—something on the order of a mortgage which was, I think, the forerunner of the modern equipment trust. But the cars would be worth little to anyone unless they could yield a profit. And if G. F. Swift could not make them pay, then the Michigan Car Company stood a slender chance of ever being paid for them.

He paid fifteen per cent down, as I recall the

FIGHT WHEN YOU MUST

transaction, with the remainder to be paid monthly out of earnings. It was a remarkable deal for those days. Car builders were used to getting cash for their products. The railroads had not yet been reduced to the intricate ways of financing which have become general as operating costs have risen.

Patents had offered a real obstacle, too. The patent situation on refrigerator cars was a maze. Hammond had certain patents which made his refrigerator cars satisfactory. There was a Tiffany patent, a Zimmerman patent. There was the Anderson car, the Wickes car. Not one of them was absolutely right for the purpose; all of them had some good features.

So father made what arrangements he could with the patentees and designed a car which seemed to incorporate the best features of them all. This was the design by which his first ten cars were being built in Detroit. Once he could have the cars rolling, he felt sure he would begin making money fast. The cars were completed and success seemed just around the corner.

But before they could be moved and put to work, Hammond brought injunction proceedings. He claimed an infringement and he tied up in the builder's yards all ten of those urgently needed cars.

Here they remained for several months. Legal procedure is always too slow to help much in a situation of this sort. No matter how father might fight it in the courts, at best it would take months or years before he could hope to have his cars released for his use.

Once more he resorted to tact. It was a blue time for him. But he managed to convince another wealthy man of the possibilities in those cars. This man lent him the money to put up as a bond with the court to guarantee Hammond against any damages the cars might do him. By hustling around, father soon had the ten cars hauling beef east for him. Eventually his claims were upheld. The courts ruled, "No infringement."

But even after it was working, almost nobody had much confidence in his plan of slaughtering cattle in Chicago and selling the meat in the East. "Stave's Wild West scheme" it came to be known among the Cape Cod relatives.

Within two years the Yankee had over a hundred cars running from the Yards to the East. They were all making money. Still no one took him seriously. Others before him had tried shipping beef east and had failed. Everyone prophesied that it would break him. He kept on, getting a tremendous head start while the others waited for him to fail. By 1880 the refrigerator car, and with it G. F. Swift's method of dressing beef in Chicago, was indisputably a success.

Once he got the refrigerator cars running, his difficulties were still on the increase. His technical troubles with the cars and with getting the meat chilled properly before hanging it in the cars very nearly broke him. Ruin was so close several times, in fact, that good active hustling was all that saved him.

Aside from these troubles, he had to develop all kinds of auxiliary equipment for his refrigerator cars and his beef coolers. He had to buy ice-harvesting rights in lakes all over northern Illinois and southern Wisconsin so that he might have the ice for cooling his beef and loading the ice boxes of his cars at Chicago. He had to develop icing stations all the way across the country to his markets in the East—the railroads would not build them. Then he had to get the ice-harvesting facilities to supply these stations. He had to build ice houses of huge capacity. His ice-consuming capacity was by the wave of a hand and the development of an idea greater than any other ice user's in the country.

These stations have, for the most part, long since gone out of our hands. The Interstate Commerce Commission ruled on complaint of other packers that we could no longer hold icing stations, since our icing stations gave us a small profit on all competitors' shipments. So the stations were sold to the railroads, which by then were glad to take them over. And refrigeration by mechanical means had displaced ice to such an extent that only a small percentage of all of our refrigeration requirements were supplied by natural ice.

But the means by which father built them, financed them, and maintained them—all of this is with us as vitally as it was then. For it comprised the principal essentials of building a business under great handicaps of inadequate capital. He built under those circumstances. What is more, he built both fast and sound.

CHAPTER XI

NEVER STAY BEATEN

"NEVER admit it even when somebody's beat you."

My father draped his angular person over my old-fashioned roll-top desk and gratuitously offered me this bit of friendly advice a hundred times, I suppose, during the '80s and '90s. To be sure, he vented a Jovian wrath more times than that when he had me beaten on some point and I would not admit it. But he seldom intended his generalizations of conduct to apply to his managers and his sons in their relations with him!

Had he been more the philosopher and less the man of action, father would have stated his advice a little differently. As he exemplified his maxim in daily life, in his idiom it should have been: "Never admit it even to yourself when somebody's beat you." He never admitted it, even to himself.

"Let's talk about something else," he would direct on those rare occasions when a manager or one of the boys cornered him and penned him in with heaped-up facts. Translated, this meant, "Go ahead, do it your way. But *I* won't admit you have me beaten!"

He was never small about it. He did not reserve this attitude for his subordinates or for the moments when, perhaps, a superintendent proved conclusively that his pet way of splitting a hog was far ahead of the plan his chief was sponsoring. What was true in the *minutiae* of his daily work was quite as noticeable in his moments of great crisis.

He would never admit a defeat, even to himself. He never knew when he was licked. If he had recognized a number of different occasions when he was genuinely worsted, his history must inevitably have been different.

Several times his business was in such shape that I cannot yet quite understand how he managed to pull it through. Certainly he would have lost it if ever he had recognized its hopeless state. In the early years at Chicago he was frequently so deeply involved that one marvels he came through at all.

A man who was associated with Gustavus Franklin Swift for many years, at first back in Brighton and later in Chicago, always declared that his friend and employer progressed as he did through two closely related reasons: "He had abiding faith in his ultimate success. He was afraid of nothing."

These are the only explanations I can offer for several extraordinary phenomena which acquaintanceship with his career brings to mind. How was he able to take hold of the refrigerator car—something which others had tried, which some in fact had used —and make it in his hands a tool a thousand times more potent than ever it had seemed? How did he manage, in a field where others were large and powerful, to grow from insignificance at a speed which even in this day of larger affairs seems dizzy, to overcome obstacles which from this perspective seem to have been insurmountable, and to become eventually the leader in his new industry?

His faith, his lack of fear, these made possible what he accomplished. He simply could not dignify discouraging circumstances by letting them discourage him. He went his way serenely ignoring what by all calculations should have disheartened him.

Had he recognized facts which were as plain as the nose on his face he would have quit and lost his business in '93. He would never have got past the discouraging times of the late '70s when daily he staked more than he could afford to lose. He staked it on the performance of faulty refrigerator cars which perversely failed to keep their perishable contents cold. He staked it on imperfect beef coolers which took the most inopportune occasions to obstinately refuse to chill the natural heat out of the fresh-killed carcasses in time for them to be shipped.

He was playing for big stakes, playing long shots to win. The odds against him were his faulty coolers and faulty cars. When he won, when a shipment got through in good shape, he made a good profit. When he lost, when a car of beef arrived good only for dumping into the bay at Fall River, then the loss should have staggered him.

But it did not. Such a loss failed to disturb him. "It will be all right," he would assure the rest of us as we discussed our bad luck in the depths of our discouragement. Then with all good cheer he would promptly entrust another half-dozen loads of the precious beef to his fallible cars. Probably this would get through in good shape and so would the next shipment. Then, just as he was getting in the clear with his profits on successful shipments, something would go wrong again.

It took only two or three cars of soured beef to wipe out his gains on a good many cars that arrived sweet and salable. Two successive losses of good size frequently put him in the red for an amount beyond the limits of any other man's credit. Somehow, though, he would keep his courage up, refuse to admit he was in a corner, get more money if the case was that desperate.

"The trouble is, we don't quite know how to do it right," he would admit with not a trace of discouragement. "We'll get it, though. We'll learn." Then he would set about experimenting some more, watching even more carefully than before to make sure that he overlooked no known precaution.

Many a hot July and August night he got on a horse and rode over to the packing house at midnight or later. He would go straight to the coolers and eye the thermometers. Then he would be after the foreman. "You've got to get those men to shoveling more ice and more salt," he would direct. "Let's see the temperature come down five degrees." And though it meant vigil to the moment of going to his

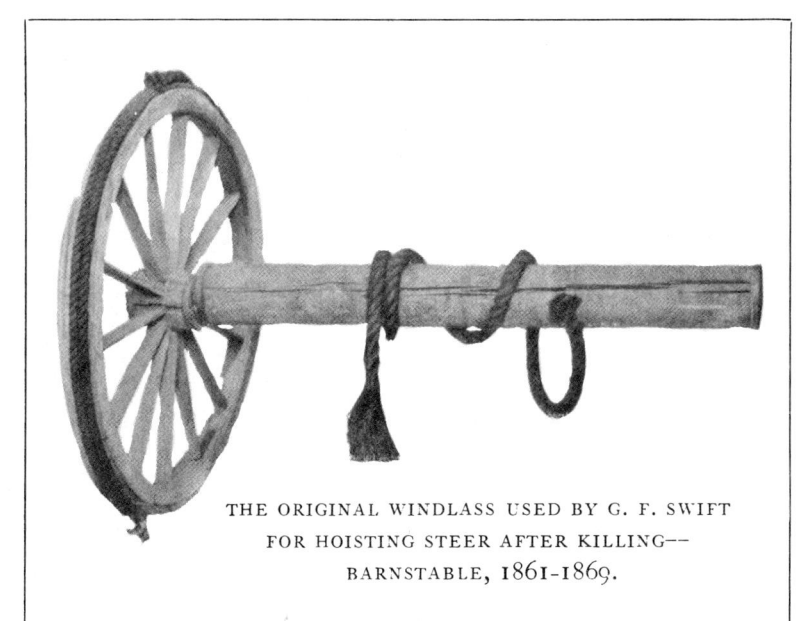

THE ORIGINAL WINDLASS USED BY G. F. SWIFT
FOR HOISTING STEER AFTER KILLING—
BARNSTABLE, 1861-1869.

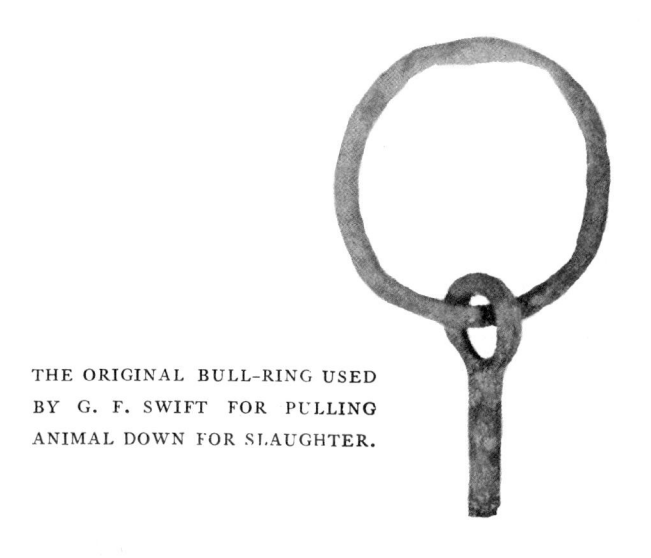

THE ORIGINAL BULL-RING USED
BY G. F. SWIFT FOR PULLING
ANIMAL DOWN FOR SLAUGHTER.

desk for the morning mail, father would walk among the men urging them to greater efforts until the telltale mercury column dropped to a reassuring depth.

Inventors busied themselves those days with coolers and refrigerator cars. Orchardmen beyond the Sierras clamored for something on wheels that would roll into Hoboken yards with its fragile freight all toothsome. Swift, the Yankee of the Yards, chafed for the chance to try any device which might serve surely to haul his Chicago beef sweet and edible to New England and New York. The world's mechanically minded worked to perfect the means.

But they seemed to crawl. Progress must be faster if this pioneer was to build an industry and control the large share of it his heart was set on. So besides having a look at any device brought to him, he likewise experimented on improvements to find what he must have.

Before he came to Chicago, he had at Fall River installed a refrigerator built by the Chase patent—then rebuilt it to make it work. At Chicago he built Chase refrigerators and Zimmerman refrigerators—and rebuilt them. He and his superintendent worked continually at improving these carcass chillers. They would build a model incorporating some hopeful idea for circulating air through every part of the compartment, the basic problem of refrigeration. Then they would send smoke through the chambers, so that their eyes might trace the currents.

Painfully, step by step they worked out the fundamental laws of refrigeration which are generally known today. They were not scientists looking for principles. They were practical packing-house men in search of ways to chill beef carcasses properly. Today we know that they discovered the principles and might well have written monographs and textbooks on refrigeration had they been so inclined.

All the while they were working with cars, too. Father tried out first, as I recall it, the Wickes car and the Anderson car. Anderson relied on the natural circulation of air through the ice chambers and the beef chamber—but the car was so built that this circulation took place only imperfectly. Wickes employed in his cars a contraption which hitched a fan to the car axle, thus blowing the cold air through the car.

It was an excellent device, barring a few flaws. When the car stopped moving, if it went on a siding or if the locomotive broke down or if a wreck stopped the train, then circulation stopped with it and consequently so did the refrigeration. Likewise if the belt broke or loosened. We lost a good deal of meat first and last in Wickes cars which were delayed. If the train kept moving, then the meat arrived in perfect condition—always assuming that the fan kept blowing!

Because the laws of refrigeration were not understood, we had difficulty in chilling carcass meats in quantity at the packing house. When we killed perhaps thirty or forty cattle a day, chilling was easy.

But as the day's slaughter mounted into the hundreds, the carcasses contained in the aggregate a great deal of heat when they came into the cold rooms. It was like bringing in so many loads of hot bricks. They raised the temperature effectively and frequently held it high through the night until the next day's fresh kill came in to reinforce them. If this kept up for two or three days, perhaps every carcass in the cooler was still warm to the touch.

When this happened and the warm meats went into the cars, they might be chilled in transit. But if a car happened to be one of the faulty ones, then its load was likely to sour long before it got to market.

In the late summer of '77 father got hold of the Zimmerman car, a great improvement over the others. But when he tried the same principle in a carcass chiller, it failed utterly.

Not until the summer of '79 did he get the proper design for his beef coolers. He had nothing but grief until then, when he got in an improved Chase patent refrigerator and added to it his own refinements for air circulation. Once this was working, he built on the same design several chillers of about one hundred-carcass capacity each. He insisted that beef must hang here between two and three days as a minimum.

Thus his Zimmerman car and his Chase cooler put him in what was by contrast with his previous experience extremely good shape. They left him free to work on other major problems. It was several years later that he discovered the Chase principle produced a better car, too.

But even when he had the Chase cooler and the Zimmerman car, the worst of his early troubles were over. He made money very fast. He could undersell the local slaughterers of the East and still make more profit per dollar of sales. He enjoyed a fixed differential in his favor, the saving he made by paying freight on only the edible portions of the beef animal.

The technical difficulty of getting chillers and cars to do what they were supposed to was only part of his troubles as a pioneer. Beef spoiled in transit or in the underchilled coolers. It cost him lots of money, too, when lots of money was exactly what he lacked—still this was only a beginning to his woes.

G. F. Swift's total wealth at the time he settled his partnership with J. A. Hathaway was around thirty thousand dollars. He had made little during the early years, for what he made on successful shipments he lost on the failures. And he poured good money after bad on experiments with coolers and cars—experiments which advanced his knowledge of refrigeration and so in the long run amply repaid their cost. But at the time they looked like dead loss. Dead loss was the one thing he could not afford.

Meanwhile he was having to put money and still more money in auxiliary equipment to further his refrigeration. Mechanical refrigeration was not in use then—at least not in packing houses. Our first mechanical refrigeration unit was built in our first pork-packing plant in 1887. It was our maiden step from our bondage to natural ice.

He had become by his adoption of the principle of slaughtering in one place and selling the meat a thousand miles away the country's largest user of ice. To supply ice in the quantities he needed and at the places he needed it, he provided the extensive facilities already mentioned.

Financing all this extension was a real burden. It came when money was most urgently needed in other divisions of the business—and before investors were eager to put in their money.

When father needed money in these days he usually went out and hustled for it. His presence inspired confidence. People usually believed in him from the first meeting. So, with his wide acquaintance in New England's beef and live-stock trades, he managed selling shares or borrowing money rather easily.

When everything else failed, he would go to D. M. Anthony and to John Sawyer in Boston. He always managed to get money from them. A good many times during those blue times of '77 and '78 their funds, wheedled from them by his persuasive enthusiasm, were all that saved him. But if he had ever let himself see there was doubt of his pulling through, he must many times have given in to the overwhelming odds.

His capital was habitually depleted. Frozen assets of one sort and another were almost the rule at first.

And while in a brisk market his business could have been sold on the auction block to yield enough for the creditors and leave a little something over for the owners, still he met the technical definition of insolvency. He could not have met his obligations at the time they fell due.

Somehow, though, he would fight through the troubles. He would not admit, even to himself, that he was beaten. So he was not beaten. He would go to a creditor for an extension, or to a banker with another note to replace the one which would soon fall due—and he would get what he went after.

These were growing pains, these financial troubles. The last of them and the most serious were the troubles of '93. He had got through one crisis after another by increasing the company's stock. The assets had grown considerably faster than the capital; book value was always considerably above par value. So he got more money into the business by issuing more stock when he needed it.

The business was coming to the place where it would need a lot more money to take care of its rapid expansion. Father saw this in '92. He also suspected the approach of the financial panic which appeared by May of '93. He did not, however, expect it so soon.

An unusually large cash dividend was declared at the end of 1892—something like twenty-four per cent, as I recall it. And, on the heels of this, the stockholders authorized a large increase of the capital stock. This issue was offered to the stockholders very soon after.

But it did not sell well at all. There had, of course, been in the directors' minds the idea that the big dividend would make the stock sell out in a hurry. But the stockholders were already feeling the pinch of the money tightness which was to clamp them three months later in the great panic. Thankfully they accepted the cash dividend and thankfully they used it to help themselves out of their other financial difficulties! As to the new stock issue, it would be a nice thing to buy, they figured. But when you haven't the money, you can't buy. So they didn't buy.

This is really why the panic of '93 hit Swift & Company hard. The treasury was bare of ready cash—and the proceeds of the stock issue which had been expected to yield plenty to carry through the slump failed to materialize. It was perhaps six months before the stock issue sold clean. By then the business was out of the woods. Father, aided by L. A. Carton, had managed to finance the business on its own assets. For half a year the business had been living, like the traditional desert camel, on its hump.

Details of that fight have been told in a preceding chapter. It was a magnificent struggle, the more remarkable that it was successful. If the head of the business had been willing to face the situation with a real recognition of how desperate it was, I do not believe he could have pulled it through. He would not admit even to himself that he was beaten. He laughed at the facts, though he relaxed meanwhile not an ounce of his effort to overcome them.

His attitude toward the whole affair came up one day in a conversation with his head butcher. The butcher was getting fifteen dollars a week—he wanted a raise. That a panic was raging meant nothing to him. The demand might have exasperated anyone at such a time. Strangely enough it did not annoy his chief.

"I'll tell you what I'll do," the boss countered to the astounded packing-house man. "I'll trade you my profits this week for your wages." On that jocular basis, the employee soon found himself good-naturedly agreeing that he didn't want a raise!

With the autumn of '93, Swift & Company was done with growing pains. Then it was that the business reached maturity. Within a year or two the continual shortage of ready money was over. Now its head could take his ease, with the business grown to a size greater than any other industrial concern in the country and with money plentiful.

It was the first time. From the very start, when he came to the Chicago Yards as a Yankee cattle buyer, G. F. Swift had been cramped for cash. When he started out in the dressed-beef business, then he was indeed of small financial importance beside Armour and Morris.

Armour & Company in 1875 handled no beef, no mutton. They were pork packers only. In cool weather they slaughtered, pickled, cured, and smoked pork products. These they shipped all over the world. When warm weather came once more they shut down their packing houses.

This, by the way, was true packing. The modern packer devotes only a part of his effort to packing. Packing involves preserving meats so that they will not spoil, at least not spoil easily. Hams, bacon, corned beef, smoked tongue, smoked sausage, salt pork, these are packed products. The dressed meat business is in no sense packing, though the word has come to include a great many nonpacking activities. G. F. Swift was in the dressed-meat business from 1876, but except in a very incidental way he was not a packer until 1887.

Morris & Company did no packing in 1875. It dealt only in fresh beef, as locally around Chicago as did Anthony, Swift & Company around Fall River. For beef could not be shipped dressed, a minor quantity always excepted which was salted and pickled principally for export.

P. D. Armour and Nelson Morris were rich men and older men than G. F. Swift. By the time they realized he was not going to fail, he had such a head start that they never overtook him.

From the time he had his refrigerator car lines going, he was the largest slaughterer of beef. He soon added mutton and was almost immediately at the top on this score. When pork was added, in 1887, he began dealing in huge quantities of fresh dressed pork—though it was a good many years before the pork products business, the hams and bacons, and the like, overtook that of his established competitors.

But even when the business was going well, he had his periodical troubles. One of these was the oleo oil patent suit. Father thought he had the rights to make oleo oil. A patent-holder thought that he had not. So the patent-holder brought suit for infringement.

The head of our company was put in the situation where he had to get that whole set of patents adjudged open to the world, else his business would have been liable for so much money that it could not have survived. This patent suit made little impression outside the packing industry. But every packer knew it was a fight to the death. By the time the decisions had been appealed and reappealed and a final unreversible decision handed down, anyone was at liberty to make oleo oil by any process he cared to use. Once more his refusal to admit he was beaten had won the day. For at the outset, if ever a lawsuit looked hopeless this one did.

Another set of troubles—minor perhaps but none the less obstinate—were those with the British distributors already referred to. They were willing to handle American beef. But because it was not native to the British Isles, their sound British instincts told them it must be inferior.

So they cut the meat differently from the standard way. This made it look inferior. Actually it was up to the standard of the best British beef ever produced anywhere. Ours was fine, clean meat. It did not take a cynic to have his reasonable doubts about the cleanliness of a good deal of the British beef.

Father was forever turning up at Smithfield market in the gray London dawn with his cheery insistence on having his beef cut properly. Although British conservatism seemed a hopeless obstacle, in time he wore it down—for he could not see the obstacle as hopeless.

He went at it cheerfully, won his point as he always did, and soon his beef was in demand as the finest obtainable. Before long he had to open branch houses all over Great Britain and Ireland to accommodate the trade.

He encountered a comparable task when he went at the job of feeding Chicago-dressed beef to the hidebound, rockbound conservatives of New England and New York. Eat meat dressed a thousand miles away? No Yankee had ever been served a steak which originated more than a few miles from the stove that cooked it, no sir, not if he knew it! To people accustomed to having a slaughterhouse just outside the limits of every town, the very idea of Chicago-dressed beef was repugnant. The meat was actually fresher in condition if not in time. It had been produced in cleanliness instead of in a filthy small-town shambles. The cattle were in better condition when slaughtered. But all this made little difference. Prejudice is founded on feelings, not on knowledge. When one puts his mind to work on a question, then prejudice cannot remain.

Father would not admit that a prejudice could stop him. He wore down that Yankee prejudice—mind you, he was doing this in the self-same weeks when he was watching his smoke currents eddy through embryonic chillers and refrigerator cars, on the day before or the day after he was buying an ice house with fifty thousand dollars which he confidently expected to get from selling stock to a friend. He was doing it between appointments at Brighton and Boston where he would somehow borrow the money to make up his losses on spoiled shipments. How any man could carry so many activities and perform them all so well has never been answered to my satisfaction. Yet I was with him several hours a day while he kept the equivalent of a fish-bowl, a cannon ball, and a live rabbit in mid air. It was uncanny.

His wide acquaintance in the live-stock and meat trade of the East served him in getting distribution, just as it served him in getting money. In fact, the two often went hand in hand. He would sign up a wholesale dealer to carry our dressed beef; then before he got through he would sell that dealer a small block of Swift stock. He got not only an outlet, but along with it the sincere loyalty of a partner. And he got the money he was needing so badly all the while. In the course of a few years he and his brother Edwin worked out several hundreds of these partnership arrangements, usually with a Swift interest in the distributing business as a double bond.

After the panic of 1893 had passed and money was easy in the business, an idea began to develop tending toward consolidation. The steel consolidations had just been completed. Consolidation was in the air.

So father, J. O. Armour, and Edward Morris formed the National Packing Company in 1902. It was capitalized at fifteen million dollars. Its components were a group of "small packers," the term which includes all but the handful of very large companies. The plan was to continue with the merger, taking in the smaller of the large packers. Then, when all of these were welded into one unit, the National Packing Company would absorb the "Big Three," Swift, Armour, and Morris. It was an ambitious plan.

But public opinion was too strong against it. Perhaps if father had lived, it might have gone through —though I doubt it. He died early in 1903. As public opinion rose against the enterprise, the terms on which the bankers would finance the merger rose at the same pace. Once the financing charges had begun their climb, the plan died of its own weight. Eventually by court order the National Packing Company was dissolved, and the smaller companies which composed it were returned to their previous owners.

So father's last great business dream fell through when he was no longer here to know it.

Of all the major plans he had ever made, this alone he failed to push through to successful, profitable completion.

Can there be a more forceful, compact way of summing up G. F. Swift's record?

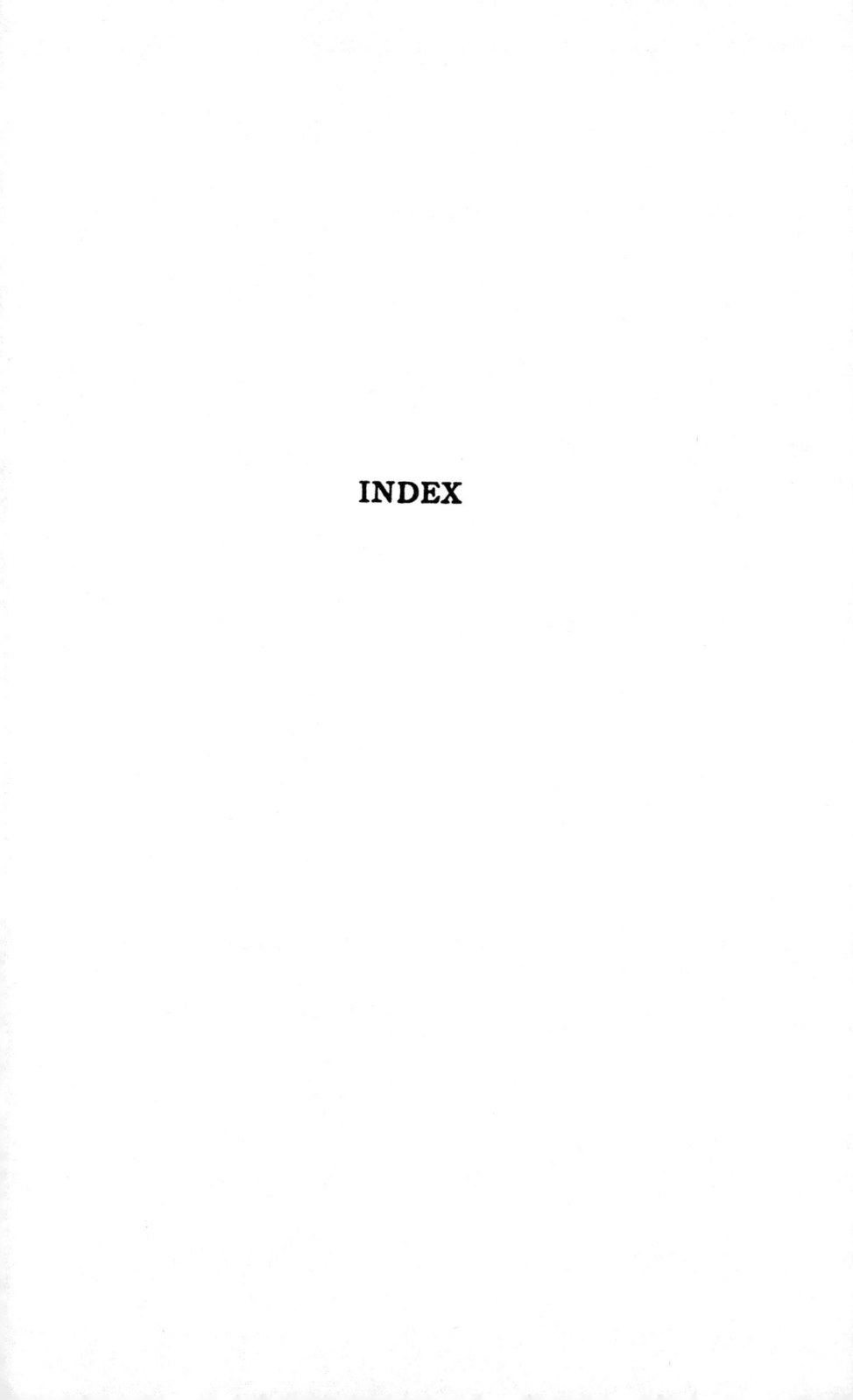

INDEX

INDEX

A

Albany, N. Y.   6, 8, 59, 127
Alterations avoided   13
Anderson refrigerator patents
    and cars   189, 198
Anthony, D. M.   10, 78, 126,
                              128, 179, 201
Anthony, Swift & Co.   10, 78,
                     126, 176,178, 188, 205
Armour & Co.   204-205, 209
Armour, J. Ogden   209
Armour, Philip D.   92, 204-205
Assonet, Mass.   107, 127, 176,
                                    178, 186
Auditor, Swift as   99

B

Back-of-Yards widows   101
Bankruptcy, rumors of   35-36
Barnstable, Mass.   74, 123-124
Bateman   16-17
Beacon Hill   47
Beardstown, Ill.   138-139
Beaten, never stay   193
Beef bags and tags   101
Beef coolers   9, 57, 72, 195-200
"Big Three"   209
Bigelow carpets   50
Blankets, horse   63
Blood   11, 176
Board of Trade   36, 37
Borrowing   29
    from employees   32
Bosses kept at work   15
Boston   6, 120, 122, 125, 155
Bran mash   62, 63

Brighton, Mass.   6, 59, 74, 90,
                 122-124, 126-128, 180, 194
British market   63, 91, 206
Bruise-trimming   47, 48
Bubbly Creek   3-5
Buffalo, N. Y.   6, 8, 127
Buggy, horse and   83
Bullock, splitting   59
Bureau of Animal Industry   7
By-products utilization 4, 10-12, 131

C

Cape Cod   iv, 5, 7, 8, 11, 49,
                      51-52, 74, 119-124, 190
Capital
    stock increased   27
    Swift's first   25
Carfare for boy   100
Cars, freight
    see Freight
Carton, L. A.   44, 154, 203
Casings   10, 98
Character, we want   168
Chase refrigerator patents and
    cars   197, 199-200
Cheating punished   97
Chicago
    in the 1870s   v, 6, 11, 127-128
    in the 1880s   3
    in the 1890s   3
    packers   11, 37-38
    stockyards   v, 5, 25-26, 29, 153, 204
    plant   17, 56, 59, 104, 145-146
    Swift comes to   6, 25, 127, 178
Chicago Board of Trade   36, 37
Chicago Junction Railway   182

Chicago Union Station	115	Duty first	112
Chicago World's Fair	39-40	**E**	
Chilling meat	191, 198	Eastham, Mass.	123
Chuck beef	57	East St. Louis plant	16-17, 47-48, 132, 151-152
Church, interest in	46, 62		
Claims examined	19, 160	Ellis Avenue	110
Clark Street	114	Ellis, E. W.	121
Cleanliness	47, 54	Emerald Avenue	110
Cleveland, President Grover	183		
Cleveland, Ohio	72-73, 139-140	**F**	
Clinton, Mass.	49-52, 78, 111, 125-127, 186, 188	Failure refuted	36
		Fall River, Mass.	10, 126-127, 131, 178-179, 186, 188, 195, 205
Coachman steals	170		
Compliments	165	Father starts Swift	120
Conference, use of	107	Faults, men's, corrected	144
Coolers kept attractive	57	Feet, beef	10
Cooling beef	191, 196	Filing	86-87
Covering wagons	18	Financing	27, 201
Credit maintained	28	Fink, Albert	184
Cross examination	147, 174	Fire in packing house	89
Crotch fat	56	Fitchburg, Mass.	70-71
Crowell, Grandfather	121	Fitzgerald, Richard	182
Crowell, Paul	121-122	Foremen visit Swift	97, 110, 147
Cure formula	104	Formula, pork cure	104
Customers		Fort Sheridan, Ill.	183
partnerships	80-81	Foster, A. C.	90
stock sold to	81, 173, 208	Freight	
Cutting beef	57	cars rented	188
Cut to sell	75	rates	9, 183
D		saving in	8, 24, 26, 128
		Frogs' legs	133
Decisions	129	Fruit cars	187
Defeat not admitted	157, 193		
Detroit	188-189	**G**	
Disciplinarian, Swift as	163	Glue	38
Dishonest employees	168, 170	Goodspeed, Thomas W.	121
Displaying meats	50, 51, 75	Grandfather sells hens	119
Donovan, John	166	Grand Pacific Hotel	114
Doud, Levi B.	42-43	Grand Trunk Railroad	178, 184-185, 187
"Down in Mobile"	164		
Drainage, roof	138	Great Britain	63-64, 91, 206-207
"Dummy-train"	84-85	Great Plains	6

INDEX

H

Halloway	77
Hammond, G. H.	186
patent suit brought by	189-190
Handling men	140
Hathaway & Swift	25, 78, 117-118, 126, 137, 179
Hathaway, James A.	25, 117-118, 126, 128, 179-180, 200
Heads, beef	10
Hearts, beef	10
Hides	7, 10, 38
Higgins, Annie Maria (Mrs. G. F. Swift)	123
Hoboken	197
Hogs	5-7, 60-61, 98, 122, 163-164, 166
Honesty	168
Horse	
and buggy	83
blankets	63
Horses	
see Swift, C. F., horses	

I

Ice, ice-houses, and icing	33, 138-141, 170-171, 191, 196, 200-201
Incorporation	27, 80
Injunction, car patents	189
Instructions made clear	156
Interstate Commerce Act	9, 184-185
Interstate Commerce Commission	191
Inventory reduced	38
Ireland	207

J

Jewett, Francis	188
Judge of men, Swift as	158

K

Kansas City plant	47-48, 54-55, 99, 103-104, 114, 131-132, 148-149

L

Lancaster ginghams	50-51
Lard	161
compound	161
refinery	178
Lawrence, Mass.	67
Leadership secured	130
Leavitt, Calvin, & Son	128
Leavitt, Wellington	90, 128
Lincoln, I. M.	188
Liverpool	154
Livers, beef	10-11
Live Stock Exchange Building	113, 143
Location studied	133
London	64, 91, 207
Longhorns, Texas	6, 72, 131
Lowe & Sons	70-71
Lowell, Mass.	67-68, 188

M

Managers	
must sell	65
trained	21
visit Swift	97, 110, 147
McKinley, President William B.	86
McMillen family	188
Meat carts	51-52, 121, 174
Meats	
fresh	7-9, 18, 49-52, 65-81
shipment of	8-9, 24, 130-131, 183-192, 195, 205-208
pickled and smoked	38, 103-106
Mechanics a luxury	13
Men	
handling	140
training	140, 146, 159
Michigan Avenue	36
Michigan Car Co.	188
Michigan Central Railroad	182
Midway	40

Milwaukee 92
Mistakes not allowed 162
Moore, Billy 178, 186
Morris & Co. 38, 205, 209
Morris, Edward 209
Morris, Nelson 92, 204-205
Mutton 131, 205

N

Napoleon iv
National Livestock Bank 42-43
National Packing Co. 209-210
Neat's foot oil 10
Negroes, whistling stopped 163
"Never admit you're beat!" 193
New York City 66-67, 184
"No dead lines" 112
Notes widely held 43

O

Ogden, Utah 80
Oleomargarine 11
Oleo oil 19-20, 47-48, 206
Omaha 62, 99-100, 104, 132
Outside men, hiring 149
Overcoat, foreman wears 54

P

Packing, true 205
Paint 63
Panic of 1893 28-45, 87-88, 202-204
Partnership dissolved 179
Partnerships 80
Patents
    car 189
    litigation settled 190
    oleo 206
Personal habits of employees 171
Pig buying 122
Piper, A. S. 33-35
Plant
    Chicago 17, 56, 59, 104, 145-146

East St. Louis 16-17, 47-48, 132, 151-152
Kansas City 47-48, 54-55, 99, 103-104, 114, 132, 148-149
South Omaha 62-63, 99-100, 104, 132
South St. Paul 104, 134-135
St. Joseph 14-15, 60, 104, 132-134, 148-153, 166
Pocket note book incident 148
Pony, small 58
Pope 126
Poultry, dealing in 156
Pork 131, 204-206
    cures 103-106
Praise, sparing use of 115, 165
Pratt, T. L. 166, 167
Prejudice against western beef 69, 206
Premium brand 106
Providence, R. I. 50, 188
Pullman
    company 181
    strike 181-183

Q

Questions, Swift asks 97

R

Raise refused 142, 204
Rank and file 159
Rates, freight 183
Refrigeration in 1869 50
Refrigerator cars 9, 27, 62, 130-131, 185-192, 195-201, 205
Reports, use of 102
Ribs 57
Rotterdam 47
Runaway horse 113

S

Sal soda 54
Salaries, small 112

INDEX

Sandusky, O. 140
Sandwich, Mass. 72
San Francisco 78-79, 156-157
Sarcasm used 53, 160, 173
Sawyer, John 201
Scraping hogs 60, 166
Self-reliance 94
Sell hardest first 72
"Sets," beef 10-11
Sewer wastes 4, 20
Shin-bones 11
Shortages 65
Singing stopped 164
Sioux City, Ia. 135-136
Slaughterhouses, local 7
Smithfield Market 64, 91, 207
South Boston 47
Statement to banks 41
"Stave's Wild West scheme" 190
Stealing 168, 170
Steamship dispute 95
Stock
  capital 27-28
  first issue **28**
  issue of 1892 203
  sold 27, 81, 172-173, 203, 208
    to customers 81, 173, 208
    to employees 172
St. Joseph plant 14-15, 60, 104, 132-134, 148-153, 166
St. Paul plant 104, 134-135
Strike
  of 1884 110-111
  Pullman 181-183
Superintendents visit Swift 110
Swift & Co.
  Chicago plant 17, 56, 59, 104, 145-146
  Cleveland branch house 72-73, 139-140
  eastern financial connections 28-29, 43-44, 208

East St. Louis plant 16-17, 47-48, 132, 151-152
incorporation and capitalization 27-28, 45, 80, 137, 202-203
Kansas City plant 47-48, 54-55, 99, 103-104, 114, 132, 148-149
loan from Morris & Co. 38
Missouri River plants 28
rumors of bankruptcy 35-36
South Omaha plant 62-63, 99-100, 104, 132
South St. Paul plant 104, 134-135
St. Joseph plant 14-15, 60, 104, 132-134, 148-153, 166
Swift & Company, G. F. 80
Swift Brothers 80
Swift, Edwin C. 67, 78-81, 99, 126, 208
Swift, Gustavus Franklin
  at Chicago plant 17-18, 59-61, 141-147
  at Cleveland 72, 139-140
  at Fitchburg, Mass. 70-71
  at Kansas City 47-48, 54-55, 99
  at London 64, 91, 207
  at Omaha 62-63, 99-100
  at St. Joseph, Mo. 14-15
  at St. Louis, Mo. and East St. Louis, Ill. 16-17, 77
  buying live stock 58-59, 121-128
  by-products development 4, 10, 12, 131
  church 62
  correspondence 86-87
  early slaughtering at Chicago 8, 10, 26, 128-129
  early years on Cape Cod 25, 49, 72, 119-124
  encourages stock ownership
    by employees 172-173
    by customers 81, 173, 208

Swift, Gustavus Franklin
(*Continued*)
   financing   24-25, 87-88
   horses   58, 62-63, 83-85,
        94-95, 100, 112-114, 196
   insists on cleanliness   48-56
   insists on dressing animals
      carefully   54-55, 57, 59-61
   New England and Albany
      until 1875   25, 49-52,
          74-75, 125-127
   personal appearance   3, 29, 193
   photographs of   *Frontispiece*, 132
   refrigeration and refrigerator
      cars   9, 27, 50, 57, 62, 107,
      130-131, 185-192, 195-201, 205
   sarcasm   53-54, 173-174
   selling   9, 63-81, 91, 109-110
   starting at Chicago   26,
      128-129, 136-137, 142-143
   starts at 14   7
   steamship rate arbitration   95-96
   teacher   21, 58, 140, 146, 167
   tendency to business
      expansion 24-30, 44-45, 117-137
   warring on waste   3-13,
                    18-21, 56-57
Swift, Louis F.   90
Swift, Mrs. Gustavus
   Franklin   91, 123, 170
Swift, Nathaniel   53, 123
Swift, Noble   119
Swift, Sally Sears Crowell
   (mother of G. F. Swift)   120
Swift, William (brother of
   G. F. Swift)   70-71
Swift, William (father of
   G. F. Swift)   120
Swift's Market, Clinton, Mass.
        49-52, 74-75, 78, 111

T

Tallying beef   19
Tankage   11
Teacher, Swift as   21, 58,
               140, 146, 167
Tiffany refrigerator patents
   and cars   189
Time saving   182
Titles   116
Tongues, beef   10
Trade wars   12
Training
   managers   21-22
   men   140, 146, 182
Tripe   10
   keg   56
Trunk Line Association   184

U

United States Steel Corporation   5
University of Chicago   121

W

Waller, O. W.   150-153
Waste   4, 20
Watchman challenges Swift 16-17
Weight tickets, loans on   42
Widows, work for   101
Wickes refrigerator patents
   and cars   189, 198
Wool   38
Worcester, Mass.   50

Y

Yards
   see Chicago, stockyards
Yardstick, the forbidden   158

Z

Zimmerman refrigerator patents
   and cars   189, 197, 199-200

DISCARDED

JUN 26 2025